AF520198

THE MATERIA MEDICA OF THE NOSODES

THE MATERIA MEDICA
OF
THE NOSODES

WITH

PROVINGS OF THE X-RAY

BY

H. C. ALLEN

BHARATIYA KALA PRAKASHAN
DELHI (INDIA)

First Published : 1910
Revised Edition : 2009

© BKP

All rights reserved, no part of this publication may be reproduced in any form or by any means without permission of the Publisher.

Published by **C.P. Gautam**
BHARATIYA KALA PRAKASHAN
3421-A, IInd Floor, Narang Colony,
Tri Nagar, Delhi-110035.
Phone : 32967505, Telefax : 011-27393083
E-mail : bkp3421@yahoo.co.in
Website : www.bkpbooks.com

ISBN : 978-81-8090-214-7

Printed by
Laxmi Offset Process, Delhi.

CONTENTS

PREFACE

Dr. Henry C. Allen was born in the village of Nilestown, near London, Ontario, and was the son of Hugh and Martha Billings Allen. On his paternal side, he was a descendant of that distinguished family of Vermonters of the same name, Gen. Ira Allen and Ethan Allen, both famous in the revolution. On his maternal side, the Billings' were well known among the Colonial families of Massachusetts Bay, and one of them, the great-grand-father of Dr. Allen, owned the farm lands on which the present city of Salem is built. After selling this property, the family moved to Deerfield, in the Connecticut Valley and were there at the time the Indians pillaged and revaged that part of the country.

He received his early education in the common and grammar schools at London, where he later taught school for a time. His medical education was acquired at the Western Homeopathic College at Cleveland, Ohio (now the Cleveland Homeopathic College), where he graduated in 1861, and later from the College of Physicians and Surgeons of Canada. Shortly after graduation, he entered the Union Army, serving as a surgeon under General Grant.

Afte the war he was offered and accepted the professorship on Anatomy in his Alma Mater at Cleveland, and it was here that he first started practicing medicine. Later he resigned and accepted the same chair in the Hahnemann Medical College of Chicago. In 1868 he was offered the Chair of Surgery to succeed Dr. Beebe, but was unable to acccept. He then located in Brantford, Ontario, where in December 24th, 1867, he married Selina Louise Goold, who, with his two children, Franklin Lyman Allen and Helen Marian Allen Aird, survives him.

—H.C. Allen

ADRENALIN (Sarcode)

Extract of super-renal bodies. Its cemical formula is $C_3 H_3 A_2 O_3$ and it forms shining prismatic crystals, which melt at a temperature of 207 lc.; it is most soluble in warm water. It has a bitter taste, which leaves a sensation of numbness on the tip of the tongue. In dilute acids it possesses a marked affinity for oxygen, and when exposed to the air it changes into oxyadrenalin which is poisonous, though not possessing the properties of Adrenalin. It is to this chemical change that constantly occurs in the tissues that the evanescent effect of the drug is due.

A number of cases of Addison's disease have been cured, and others arrested in their course, by Adrenalin. The most of these cases have occurred in the practice of other schools, and with large doses of the crude drug. Very few have been reported in the homoeopathic school, in fact, Raue says he has been unable to find an authenticated case of this disease cured, in our literature. As yet we have but one proving, made in 1904 by students of the New York Homoeopathic College, under the direction of Dr. V. L. Getman and the following provers: M. W. Macduffie, W. G. LaField, G. H. Clapp, J. B. G. Custis, J., G. C. Birdsall, and R. C. Miller. The day-books of provers are omitted.

Mind—

Despondent and nervous; lack of interest in anything; no ambition; disinclination for mental work; absence of 'grit'.

Aversion to mental work, cannot concentrate thoughts.

Head—

Hot headache in left side, extending to right, < by reading and in morning, with a feeling as though the eyes were strained.

Frontal headache, supraorbital, with congested nose and eyes.

Burning heat in head, feeling as though he wanted to open eyes wide.

Headache extending all over head but < on left side and over eyes across forehead.

Awoke with headache over eyes and left side of head as though he wanted to open the eyes wide and press on them.

Dull pain all over head, sometimes right-sided, sometimes left-sided, but always extending to eyes, causing a feeling as though he wanted to open the eyes wide.

Severe pain> by pressure on the eyes.

Headache with nausea and heat in face, without redness, < in the evening, but reappears as soon as pressure is removed.

Headache extending to the ears. All headaches are < in the afternoon or evening; in the evening they appear about 7 p.m. and last until relieved by walk in the open air or sleep.

If headache appears in the afternoon the time is 3 P.M., always > by walk in the open air, and somewhat relieved by eating and sleeping, but not so completely as by walk in the open air.

When the headache is worse it is also > by pressure on the eyes and opening the eyes wide, and is < by mental labor and indoors.

Dull headache over eyes; fulness in head.

Neuralgic headache; pains start from base of brain, go forward over the head to front and sides; pains are first shooting and seem to be just under the scalp, appear at 11 A.M. and last until 3 or 4 P.M., and disappear by eating, in open air, < in close, warm room.

Brain feels swollen as though it were too large for skull.

Congestion of brain during the day.

Dull aching in the eyeballs with the headache, > by pressure and by rubbing the eyes.

Headache coming on at 11 A.M., lasting until 12:30 at night, > by eating.

Fulness of the head in the afternoon and evening.

Flushes of heat in the evening over face and head, but face was only slightly red.

Dull feeling in the head from 3 to 6 P.M.

Frontal headache.

Eyes—

Strained feeling; congested; feeling as though he wanted to open them wide or press upon them.

Pain in the right eye.

Pressure on the eyes and opening them wide > the headache.

Hyperemia of the conjunctiva dissipated almost immediately when used locally; thus rendering operations possible.

Aching in eyeballs, > by pressure and rubbing.

Ears—

Aching in the left ear accompanies the headache; sharp pain in both ears at times.

Itching and tickling in right ear, > by boring into ear with finger.

Nose—

Congested, full feeling in nose.

Gelatinous mucus drops from the posterior nares, difficult to detach.

On going out into the cold air had a copious, watery nasal discharge, < on right side; when indoors, the nose felt full and stopped up.

Slight stuffiness in the nose, with full feeling at the root of the nose.

Face—

Feels flushed but is not red.

Flushes of heat over face and head; flushed throughout evening.

Mouth—

Bad taste on waking.

Mouth filled with dark brown mucus, which has nasty taste.

Tongue coated white, red edge and tip.

Tongue clean anteriorly; mouth dry.

Tongue coated white at times posteriorly.

Throat—

Much hemming and hawking to clear throat.

Vocal cords inflamed; laryngeal catarrh, profuse secretion from the pharyngeal glands of whitish gelatinous mucus which was difficult to loosen.

Right side swollen and sore, red and inflamed, < by swallowing.

Stomach—

Belching after meals.

Appetite increased.

Sensation of nausea as though he would vomit.

Pain in stomach passing from right to left, coming and going suddenly.

Nausea before meals, though appetite is good when he once began to eat.

Appetite increased; ravenous hunger.

Less thirst than usual.

Thirst at times for large quantities, increased in the evening.

Abdomen—

Rumbling in the intestines; borborygmus.

Stool—

Passage of foul flatus.

Stool loose, brown, semi-solid, passed quickly, with fetid odoright

Sudden spluttering diarrhea; all over in a minute, followed with burning in anus.

Urine—

Strong odor, hot and scalding; frequent, profuse, pale.

Burning before and during micturition.

Sudden urgent desire to urinate.

Amount of urine decreased, solids increased.

Crystals of sodium oxalate increased while sodium urate appeared during the proving, and was very prominent, no casts.

Pus corpuscles which were present at the beginning disappeared; no epithelia.

Hematuria with severe pain in the renal region; cured.

Urine more frequent than usual.

Male—

Spermatozoa present (in the urine?) at the beginning and during the first part of the proving, totally disappeared.

Sexual desire increased, without erections.

Erections; lascivious dreams all night causing waking from sleep.

Emissions in early morning without any bad effects.

Respiratory—

Cough, from irritation in supra sternal fossa.

Expectoration of gelatinous mucus, which is hard to detach.

Increase of respiratory movements, soon followed by suffocation and death from paralysis of medulla and pneumogastric (crude drugs).

Back—

Pain especially on the left side; better by sitting up straight or lying straight.

Extremities—

Slight rheumatic pains coming and going down leg.

Left foot, leg and buttocks go to sleep easily and feel numb; this numbness extends to both lower extremities but is < in the left.

Arms and legs go to sleep easily; numbness and tingling from below upwards.

Corns on the toes.

Aching in limbs on waking in the morning; aching in the calves.

Rheumatic pains in left elbow and little finger on waking.

Severe cramp in right heel lasting ten minutes, then the same in left heel, followed by stomachache.

Legs tired and ache, especially in the calves and below the knees.

Ankles feel weak and tired.

Painful swelling on first finger of right hand, resulting in a felon.

Tired aching in arms and legs on waking.

Dull pain in arms and legs.

Tissues—

It possesses powerful local action over dilated blood-vessels.

When injected into the circulation arteries become contracted and blood pressure rises.

Prolonged contraction of the general muscular system. Repeated injections cause atheroma and heart lesions in animals.

The skin becomes bronzed; great loss of strength; rapid emaciation; exceedingly rapid pulse; irregular intermitting heart beats; general marked anemia.

Sleep—

Great sleepiness and drowsiness.
Sleepy in evening and after a good night's sleep.
Dulness and sleepiness from 3 to 6 P.M.

Fever—

Flushes of heat over face and head.

AMBRA GRISEA (Ambergris)

Of doubtful origin, for years on the borderland as to its true classification, but probably a nosode or morbid product found in the belly of the sperm-whale, the *Physeter Macrosephalous*. It is often found floating upon the sea or thrown upon the shore of the Baltic, or on the coast of Madagascar or Sumatra. But, perhaps the best specimens are those which whalers cut out and are to be found in Boston and other whaling ports. It has many characteristics of intestinal or biliary concretions and has been considered to be of hepatic origin, probably a fatty excretion from its gall bladder. It was introduced by Hahnemann in 1827; proved by him and his friend, Count de Gersdorf, who personally obtained nearly one-half of the symptoms.

The so-called Oil of Amber (used by Dright Holcombe in hiccough) is Oleum Succinum, and should not be confounded with Ambergris.

Characteristics—

For children, especially young girls who are excitable, nervous and weak; nervous affections old people, nerves 'worn out;' premature senility; general functional impairment. Ailments of both extremes of life.

Lean, thin, emaciated persons who take cold easily; 'dried up;' nervous; thin, scrawny women (Secale); nervous bilious temperament.

Great sadness, sits for days weeping.

Great bashfulness, very characteristic; embarrassed in company, in sick room.

The presence of others, even the nurse, is unbearable during stool; frequent, ineffectual desire, which makes her anxious.

After business embarrassments, unable to sleep, must get up (Act., Sep.).

Retires weary, .yet wakeful as soon as head touches pillow.

Weakness; lassitude; numbness of single parts; one-sided complaints.

Ranula with fetid breath (Thuja).

Sensation of coldness in abdomen (Cal.); of single parts.

Cannot urinate in presence of other persons (Nat. mur.).

Discharge of blood between periods, at very little accident— a long walk, after every hard stool, etc.; nymphomania; severe pruritus, especially in lying-in.

Leucorrhea; *thick, bluish-white mucus,* especially or only at night (Caust., Mer., Nit. ac.)

Cough violent; in spasmodic paroxysms, with eructations and hoarseness; < talking or reading aloud (Dros., Phos., Tub.); evening without, morning with expectoration (Bry., Carb. v., Hep., Hyos., Phos., Puls., Sep.); whooping-cough, but without lcrowing inspiration; < when many people are present.

Relations—

Antidoted by Camph., Cof., Nux, Puls., Staph., X-ray. Ambra antidotes Staph., especially the voluptuous itching of scrotum.

Nux antidotes the potentized Ambra.

Compare—

Calc., Nat. c., Tub. (coldness of abdomen); Cast., Asaf., Psor., X-ray, Val, defective reaction; Coca, Fer., bashfulness and blushing; Mosch., Val., fainting, hysteric asthma; Act., Ign., night cough; lod., Nux, Tub., thin, emaciated, nervous, irritable persons; Ars., Tub., asthmatic affections; Phos., asthma, nervous, excitable, weak, irritable patient, tall and slender; Bov., flow every few days midway between the periods: Lach., Rhus, Sepia, < from overlifting; Cof., Croc., China,

Ign., Puls., Sec., Staph., Sulph., nervous hysterical affections; Kali bi., Iod., itching behind sternum in violent, racking, paroxysmal cough.

Carbo veg. and Petright in lack of reaction in acute disease.

In cases of women who are excessively nervous and fail to react in acute sickness.

Aggravation—

Warm drinks, warm room; in the evening; lying, especially on the painless side (Arn., Bry,, Calc., Puls., Rhus); reading or talking aloud; music; the presence of many people; after waking (Lach., Sep.).

Amelioration—

After eating; in the cold open air; cold food and drinks; rising from bed, resting upon affected parts.

Pains: tearing, drawing, sticking; with sensation of pressure.

The infant is weak, peevish and mentally deficient; thin and emaciated, the image of a little dried-up old man.

The hair turns gray and falls; the memory grows unreliable; comprehension is dull; hearing, smell and sight begin to fail; nervousness, anxiety, melancholy; aversion to company or indifference to family and the affairs of life are gradual steps in the path to senility. From defective assimilation the tissues become impoverished; from weak circulation there is coldness of the extremities, numbness and vertigo. These signs of senile decrepitude may be found to a greater or less extent in any stage of life, and this is the sphere of Ambra.—*Farrington.*

Mind—

||Memory impaired.

Comprehension slow, has to read everything three or four times and then does not understand it.

Is not able to reflect upon anything properly, feels stupid.

Confusion of the head; of the occiput.

Difficult thinking in the morning.

Distorted images, grimaces; diabolical faces crowd upon his fancy.

She is excited, loquacious; erratic talking fatigues her; was unable to sleep at night, or averse to talking and laughing.

Great sadness; despondent, does not want to live.

Forced to dwell upon most disagreeable things; sleepless in consequence.

Melancholy, sits for days weeping; with great weakness, loss of muscular power and pain in the small of the back and constipation.

Fears of becoming insane.

Despair; loathing of life.

Anguish and sweat all over, at night.

Anxiety, oppression, nervous weakness with irritability and impatience.

After business embarrassment cannot sleep, must get up and walk about (Rhus right, Sep.).

Hurries too much while engaged in mental labor.

Embarrassed manner in company; blushing, bashful (Feright, X-ray, Tub.).

Cough worse when many persons are present.

The presence of other people aggravates the symptoms.

Sensorium—

| Vertigo with feeling of weight on the vertex; < after sleep, < after eating.

She had to lie down on account of vertigo and sensation of weakness in the stomach.

Music causes the blood to rush to the head. Great weakness in the head with vertigo.

Head—

Pressure in forehead and vertex with fear of becoming crazy.

Tearing: in forehead; in left temple up to vertex; in right frontal eminence and behind left ear.

Extremely painful tearing on top of head and apparently in whole upper half of brain, with paleness of face and coldness of left hand.

Pressive drawing, ascending from nape of neck, and extending through head towards forehead, considerable oppression remaining in lower part of occiput.

Dullness in occiput.

Tearing pains predominate in head.

|| Rush of blood to head caused by music.

Weakness in head with vertigo.

|| Falling off of hair, hair turns gray early.

On the right side of the head, a spot, where the hair when touched pains, as if sore.

The scalp feels sore in morning, when awaking; this is followed by a sensation of numbness, extending over the whole body.

Eyes and Sight—

Dullness of vision, as if from looking through a mist.

Pressure and smarting in eyes, as from dust; lachrymation.

Pressure on eyes, which are difficult to open, and pain in eyes as if they had been closed too firmly, particularly in the morning.

Itching on eyelid as if a stye were forming.

Ears and Hearing—

Roaring and whistling in ears, in afternoon.

| Deafness of one ear.

Crackling in left ear (like the sound made when winding a watch).

| Hearing decreases; with cold sensation in abdomen.

Violent tearing pain in and behind right auricle.

Tearing in right ear.

Crawling, itching and tickling in ears.

Music aggravates the cough.

Listening to music brings on congestion to head.

Nose—

Dried blood gathered in nose.

Bleeding of the nose early in the morning.

Nosebleed with the menses.

Copious nosebleed early in bed, several successive days.

Nose stopped up and paining as if sore internally.

Long continued dryness of the nose, frequent irritation as from sneezing.

Face—

Paleness of face with headache.

Flushes of heat in face.

Heat in face with chill of other parts.

Tearing in the upper part of the face, particularly near the right ala nasi.

Pimples, and itching in whiskers.

Painful swelling of the cheek on upper jaw, with throbbing in the gums.

Jaundiced colour of the face.

Spasmodic twitching of the facial muscles, lower part of face; in the evening, in bed.

Lips hot.

Lips numb and dry, in the morning on awaking.

Cramp of the lower lip.

Teeth and Gums—

Drawing pain now in one and again in another tooth; increased by warmth,, momentarily removed by cold; not aggravated by chewing and passes off after a meal; at the same time the inner portion of the gums was swollen.

| Bleeding of gums.

Mouth—

Bitter taste in mouth in morning on awaking.

Sour taste after drinking milk.

Pain as if sore, folds under the tongue, like small growths, Ranula.

Tongue, bluish, lead coloured (Ars.).

Fetor of mouth, worse mornings.

Blisters in mouth, pain as if burnt; under the tongue, lumps like small growths, which pain like excoriation; smarting and cracked painful condition of mouth; on account of pain she could not eat anything hard.

Accumulation of water in the mouth with cough.

Rasping, smarting pain in mouth when eating solid food (Phos. ac.).

In the morning on awaking, tongue, mouth and lips as if numb and dry (sensation of numbness in throat, Mag., Sulph.).

Tongue coated grayish-yellow.

Throat—

Sensation of rawness in region of velum pendulum palati.

Rawness in throat with cough.

Tearing pain in palate, extending into left ear.

Dryness of throat in morning.

Sore feeling in throat during deglutition, and from outward pressure, not when swallowing food, with tension of glands of throat as if swollen.

Sore throat after exposure to a draught of air; stitching from the throat into r.ear; pains particularly from motion of the tongue.

Tickling in throat which induces coughing.

Tickling in throat and thyroid body, during act of coughing.

Accumulation of grayish phlegm in throat, which is difficult to hawk up, accompanied by rawness.

Hawking the phlegm from fauces produces vomiting and choking.

Papular-like eruption in pharynx.

Smarting at the back of the fauces when not swallowing.

When hawking up mucus in the morning, almost unavoidable retching and vomiting.

Stomach—

Thirstlessness.

After breakfast, nausea.

After eating: cough and gaping or gagging; anxiety; pressure in pit of stomach, as if the food stuck and would not go down (food descends slowly and gets into the larynx, Kali carb.); food is felt until it enters the stomach (Alum., Bry., Phos.).

Aggravation from warm drinks, especially from warm milk.

Better after eating: toothache; oppression in chest; chill, etc.

After drinking milk: sour taste; heartburn.

Belching with and after cough.

Eructations either empty, sour or bitter.

When walking in the open air heart-burn with balked eructations.

Eructations with cough, so as almost to cause choking.

Belching removes pressure under scrobiculum.

Hiccough.

Sensation of coldness in the stomach.

After exposure to the cold in a sleigh-ride, had suffered continually, summer and winter, for 14 years, with sensation of coldness in the stomach; had used all kinds of pads and warmers without relief; cured in 24 hours.

Heartburn: with abortive eructations; when walking in the open air; from drinking milk, especially warm milk.

Every evening, sensation of disordered stomach and acrid risings up to larynx.

Nausea after breakfast.

Vomiting and choking when hawking phlegm from fauces.

Pressure and burning under scrobiculum; belching removes it.

Pressure in stomach and hypochondria.

Tension and pressure or stitches and pressure in the stomach.

Concussion in pit of stomach with the cough.

Weakness in stomach accompanying vertigo; must lie down on account of vertigo and a sensation of weakness in the stomach.

Abdomen—

Pressing pain in a small spot in the upper right side of the abdomen, though not felt to touch.

Tearing pain in the region of the spleen, as if something were torn away.

Pain in right hypochondriac region > while lying upon it.

Tension and distension in abdomen after every mouthful he eats, even after every mouthful of fluid.

Distended abdomen; accumulation of much flatus, which subsides without being passed.

Sensation of coldness in the abdomen.

Coldness of one side of the abdomen (left); also with the deafness.

Colic, sometimes followed by diarrhea.

Pressure deep in the hypogastrium after the evacuation.

Stool and Anus—

First copious, soft, light brown stools, after a few days' constipation.

Constipation: Frequent ineffectual urging as in Nux vomica, but attended by much anxiety at stool and a sense of marked coldness in the abdomen, the patients being put to a great distress by the presence of others in the room (near presence of others unbearable while urinating, Nat. m.); after stool, aching deep in hypogastrium; itching and smarting in anus relieved by rubbing.

Diarrhea preceded by colic.

Stool not hard, though large.

Frequent ineffectual desire for stool; this makes her very anxious, at this time the presence of other persons becomes unbearable.

Large flow of blood with the stool.

Itching in anus.

Stitches in anus.

After the evacuation pressure deep in the hypogastrium.

Urinary Organs—

Frequent micturition at night (Lyc.) and in the morning after rising. Pain in bladder and rectum simultaneously.

Urine sour smelling; urine turbid even when first passed. Urine when emitted is clouded, yellowish-brown and deposits a brownish sediment, after which the urine looks clear and yellow; coffee ground sediment.

Sour smelling urine.

Urinates three times as much as the drink taken, especially in the morning; followed by a dull pain in the region of the kidneys.

Sensations as if a few drops passed through the urethra.

During urination, burning, smarting, itching and titillation in the urethra and vulva.

Male Sexual Organs—

| A man, aet. 80, gets asthma when attempting coition.

Impotence.

Violent morning erections without desire, with numbness in the parts.

Internal, strong, voluptuous sensation in genital organs.

Itching pimples over male genitals. Sore rawness between the thighs. Voluptuous itching on scrotum.

Female Sexual Organs—

Nymphomania: often with discharge of bluish-white mucus, < at night; stitching in vagina preceeding discharge.

Burning in sexual parts, with discharge of a few drops of blood.

Stitches in ovarian region, when drawing in abdomen or pressing upon it.

Discharge of blood between the periods, at every little accident, as every hard stool or after a walk a little longer than usual.

Menses early, the left leg becomes quite blue from distended varices, with pressive pain in the leg.

Lying down aggravates the uterine symptoms.

Is said to cause uterine atony.

Suppressed catamenia.

Menses too early and too profuse,

Menses appear seven days before time.

Severe itching on the pudenda, must rub the parts.

Soreness and itching, with swelling of the labia.

During urination: itching, titillation, burning of vulva and urethra.

Thick, mucous leucorrhea, increased from day to day, or leucorrhea at night, of bluish-white mucus; preceding each discharge, a stitch in the vagina.

During pregnancy: nervous, restless; pruritus vulvae.

Impending abortion.

Puerperal eclampsia.

Lessens the severity of the labor-pains.

In childbed obstinate constipation and tenesmus; abdomen puffed, causing much anxiety; so nervous she cannot attempt a stool in the presence of other people, not even the nurse.

Revillout compares the general action of Ambra with that of Kali bromatum. The effect appears quicker after Ambra, but that of Kali bromatum continues longer. Ambra, therefore, is preferable for the removal of severe reflex actions, infantile spasms, puerperal eclampsia. Ambra quiets beautifully the nervous restlessness of pregnancy and thus prevents convulsions; it also retards uterine contractions.

Revillout recommends Ambra in pregnancy:

1. To prevent eclampsia.
2. To diminish too severe labor-pains.
3. In too early labor or threatening abortion.

But Ambra given too frequently and in too large a dose may also produce uterine atony. Ambra given in large doses may generally remove convulsions, from whatever cause, and by diminishing nervousness acts favourably on nervous persons, infants and young girls.

Here, then, is another case of involuntary Homeopathy. Ambra produces in the healthy burning in the sexual parts, with discharge of a few drops of blood; menses set in a few days too soon; it produces discharge of blood at other times than the catamenia, also fluor albus, and also perhaps ovaritis. It also produces twitchings in muscular parts, spasms, restlessness, infirmity, anxiety, oppression, nervous weakness with irritability and impatience, twitching and jerkings in the extremities, with coldness of the body and great debility, a state so often found in females and excitable, weakly children, combined with sleeplessness; many dreams, frightened awaking, restless sleep at night, general restlessness, irritability, anxiety and despair.

Respiration—

Titillation in larynx with spasmodic cough. Titillation in throat, larynx and trachea, causing violent cough.

Hoarseness and roughness of the voice, with accumulation of thick, tough mucus, easily thrown off by coughing.

Itching, scraping and soreness of the larynx and trachea.

Reading aloud or talking aggravates the cough.

Itching in thyroid gland; itching behind the sternum causing cough.

Tightness of the chest, cannot take a deep breath or yawn deeply.

Oppression felt in chest and between scapulas; it subsides for a short time after eating.

Feeling of pressure in chest worse during exhalation.

Asthma of old people and children.

Asthma comes on while he is attempting coition.

Whistling in chest during breathing.

Get out of breath with the cough, which is spasmodic; rush of blood to the head.

Cough—

Spasmodic cough, loses her breath; with rush of blood to the head; finally some phlegm comes up.

Cough in spasmodic paroxysms.

Hollow, spasmodic, barking cough; worse from talking or reading aloud; with gagging after eating.

Spasmodic cough of elderly or emaciated persons.

Paroxysms of cough coming from deep in chest, excited by violent tickling in throat, evening without, morning with expectoration, generally of grayish-white, seldom of yellow mucus, of salty or sour taste; tough grayish mucus; worse in the morning.

Violent spasmodic cough, with frequent eructations and hoarseness; with pain in region of spleen as if something were torn off.

Lifting a heavy weight aggravates the cough.

Cough only at night, produced by an excessive irritation in the throat.

Cough with eructations of gas so as almost to choke the patient (Lach.).

Cough every evening with pain under the left ribs, as if something was torn loose there.

Accumulation of grayish mucus, difficult to hawk up, accompanied by rawness and almost unavoidable retching and vomiting.

Cough worse when many persons are present.

Cough causes concussion in pit of stomach.

Cough with emaciation.

A kind of whooping-cough; paroxysmal but without crowing inspiration. < after lying down.

Deep dry cough, with accumulation of water in mouth, and subsequent rawness of the throat.

Choking and vomiting when hawking up phlegm from the fauces.

Sputa yellow-white, cream-like; a 'sputum coctum.'

Collection of phlegm in the throat difficult to cough up.

Old coughs.

Scraping and tickling in the throat, larynx, down along the windpipe causing violent cough with sensation of tightly adhering mucus in the windpipe: during breathing whistling in the chest; rough and hoarse voice; collection of mucus in the throat, difficult to cough up.

Cough mostly only at night from violent irritation, with concussion of the pit of the stomach; cough sometimes in spasmodic paroxysms, with oppression of the chest, getting out of breath, great restlessness, and afterward a great deal of belching, a kind of whooping cough.

In nervous persons it causes titillation in the larynx and spasmodic paroxysms of cough; whistling in the chest; spasmodic short breathing; cardiac anguish and spasmodic palpitation.

Chest and Lungs—

Pain in lower part of right chest relieved by lying on the back.

Lancination in chest extending to back.

Oppression of the chest extending to back between the scapulae. Relieved a short while by eating.

Sensation of pressure deep in right chest; also in left chest or in upper part of chest.

Wheezing in the chest.

Sensation of rawness in chest.

Tearing pressure in left side of the chest.

Itching in chest.

Tightness of the chest, can neither yawn nor breathe deeply.

Sensation of a lump in chest.

Aching in the chest over epigastrium, as if parts had been beaten; relieved by eructations.

Violent, dull stitching pain in right mammae, interrupting breathing.

Burning in the external parts of the chest.

Pressure in upper part of the chest, coming in regular paroxysms.

Heart and Pulse—

Anxiety at the heart, causing oppression of breathing, with flushes of heat; oppression beginning in the heart.

Palpitation when walking in the open air, with paleness of face.

Violent palpitation, with pressure in chest, as if a lump lay there, or as if the chest was stuffed up.

Pulse accelerated, with ebullitions.

He perceives the pulse in the body; it feels like the tick of a watch.

Outer Chest—

Burning on the chest.

Neck and Back—

Glands of the throat tense as if swollen.

Burning in left scapula.

Tearing in the left, or in both shoulders.

Rheumatic pains in the right side of the back.

Painful tension in the lumbar muscles.

Stitches in small of back, when sitting.

Stiffness in small of back after sitting.

Pain in small of back, with loss of muscular power and constipation.

Upper Limbs—

Tearing in left shoulder joint.

Drawing, as if sprained and lame in the shoulder.

The arms go to sleep when lying on them, when carrying

anything in the hands or at night; with numbness especially of the left arm in rest; tingling in the thumb.

Tearing pains in the shoulder, elbow, forearm and hand.

Weakness of the fingers at night.

Stinging in hands and fingers, as from insects.

Drawing in fingers and thumb.

Itching in palms of hands.

Cramps in hands, sometimes only when taking hold of anything.

Tips of fingers are shrivelled.

Tearing, lancinating or itching in tips of fingers and thumb.

Skin on the fingers feels tense.

Long lasting icy coldness of hands.

Coldness of left hand with headache.

Finger nails brittle, with a very old man; they got soft, elastic and pink.

Lower Limbs—

Tearing pain, first in left then in right hip joint.

Sensation of contraction in right thigh; the limb seems to be shortened.

Tearing in nates, hip, knee, leg, ankle and foot.

Heaviness of the legs.

Strumming sensation in legs.

Sensation as if 'gone to sleep' in both legs; has no firm step.

Cramps in legs and calves nearly every night.

Cold feet.

Gouty pain in ball of great toes.

Itching on inner border of sole of the right foot, not relieved by scratching.

Sore and raw between the thighs, and in the hollow of the knees.

Left leg becomes blue from distended varices during menses.

Tearing or rheumatic pains, in parts of all the limbs.

Uncommon twitching and coldness of the body, at night.

Uneasiness, like a crawling, with anxiety, only by day.

Weariness, with painful soreness of all the limbs.

Nerves—

Trismus neonatorum.

Restlessness.

Jerks and twitches.

Convulsions.

Epilepsy.

Infantile spasms.

Spasms and twitches in the muscular parts.

Spasmodic complaints.

Arms and limbs 'go to sleep' easily.

Great lassitude, especially mornings in bed.

Fainting.

Weakness of the whole body; of the knees, as if they would give way; of the feet, with loss of sensation; in the stomach, so that she must lie down.

Great prostration after lingering fevers.

Chlorosis.

Loss of muscular power.

Vertigo and nervous apoplexy.

Paralytic complaints.

Numbness of the whole body.

When walking in the open air, an uneasiness in the blood and more rapid circulation, with greater weakness of the body.

Conversation causes fatigue, heaviness of the head, sleepless, oppression of the chest, sweat, anxiety; tremor and quivering; nervousness and irritability.

B. W., aet. 58, stout, florid, right side paralyzed for five years; walks with difficulty, dragging right foot; vertigo, *with feeling of great weight on vertex* for five years; worse after sleeping; sleepless after 1 A.M.; loss of memory; loss of sense of smell; numbness of right side; cold sweat on extremities, right foot colder than left; nausea in abdomen; has had much grief. Ign., Con., Ver. b.; little relief. Ambra 200 (two doses dry) removed pain in vertex, vertigo and nausea.

Sleep—

Cannot sleep, must get up; worriment from business embarrassment; insomnia of business men.

Cannot sleep at night, yet knows not why.

Sleepy on retiring; but as soon as head touches the pillow is wide awake for hours, restless, tossing, or simply unable to close the eyes.

Restless sleep, with anxious dreams.

Vexatious, anxious dreams and talking in sleep; awaken frightened.

Sleepless after 1 A.M.

Worse from too little sleep.

Twitching of limbs preventing sleep, and coldness.

Uneasy sleep from coldness and twitching.

Nearly every night cramp in calves.

Worse after sleep; vertigo; weight on vertex; whooping cough; feels weak; mouth dry; weary, eyes feel as if they had been closed too tightly.

When awaking: soreness of scalp; lips numb and dry; bitter taste in mouth.

Early in bed: nosebleed; great lassitude.

Temperature and Weather—

< from warmth: toothache.

> from cold: toothache.

< in warm room: cough.

> from motion in open airight

< from warm drinks.

After exposure to draft of air: sore throat.

When walking in open air: heartburn; palpitation; uneasiness in the blood; < weakness.

Took cold and had perspiration checked, after a thunderstorm, by north wind in face; tormenting cough for several weeks.

Fever—

Chill in forenoon, with lassitude and sleepiness; relieved by eating; skin of whole body cold, except face and genitals. Chill of single parts of the body, with heat of the face. Anxious flushes of heat returning every quarter hour; most violent towards evening.

Profuse sweat at night, worse after midnight and most on the affected side.

Profuse sweat, particularly on the abdomen and thighs, during exercise.

Malignant fevers.

Skin—

Itching.

Jaundiced colour of face.

Burning in skin.

The tips of the fingers become shriveled.

Soreness of a wart on the finger.

Numbness of the skin.

Burning herpes.

Leprous complaints.

Itching pimples in whiskers.

Sore and raw between legs and in hollow of knees.

Distended varices on leg during menses.

Reproduces the itch-eruption.

Nervous itching over the whole body, especially the mucous outlets of the body.

ANTHRACINUM (Anthrax Poison)

The alcoholic extract of the anthrax poison prepared from the spleen of cattle ill with the disease. A nosode rejected by the old school, and by a majority of the new, in spite of its being a remedy which bears out our theory, and one which has proved of the utmost use in practice. It has not yet been proved, but the frequent use made of it and the verification of the toxic symptoms by some of our best practitioners justifies its reception. The first preparation was made according to Hering's propositions (laid down in Stapf's Archives, 1830), by Dr. G. A. Weber, and applied with the most astonishing success in the cattle plague. He cured every case with it, and also cured men poisoned by the contagium. His report, a small treatise of 114 pages, was published in 1836, by Reclam, Leipzig. No notice was taken of it. Only the talented Dr. P. Dufresne, the founder of the *Bibliotheque Homoeopathique,* of Geneva, used it and prevented the further murderous spread of the disease, in a flock of sheep (among which it is always more fatal than among other domestic animals), and cured the shepherds as well (*Biblioth. Homoeop. de Geneve,* January and February, 1837).

The discovery of the bacteria and their incredibly rapid propagation, seemed to be of much more importance than the cure of cattle, and the loss of millions of dollars by this disease. In 1842 France sustained a loss of over seven millions of francs, and every year a small district of Germany had a loss of sixty thousand thalers, from the cattle plague; in Siberia, in 1785, 100,000 horses died with it; in 1800, one small district lost 27,000 horses. Radiate heat, proposed scores of years ago, for other zymotic diseases, by Hering, was discovered, in a very ingenious way, by Pasteur, to prevent the increase of bacteria. Now the heat (as it has done in hydrophobia), and the nosode may suffice to cure every case.

Doctor Kasemann had moral courage enough to introduce anthracin in gangrene and sphacelus, in 1852, and Doctor Raue has given it in carbuncles, since 1858 (see his Pathology and Diagnosis) and in gangrenic whitlow (see *Journal of Clinics,* 4, 142).

All symptoms produced by the poison on men are inserted, because the symptoms from the snake-bite and from the bee-sting have been proved to be useful in numerous cases as well as the toxic symptoms of Arsenic, Opium and other drugs.

Dr. Hering says: "Homeopathic practitioners of the greatest integrity, and trustworthy beyond a doubt, long ago cured splenic fever in cattle, flocks of sheep and their shepherds by Anthracin, an alcoholic tincture made from the blood of a bacteric spleen. Of course the alcohol killed the infusoria, but what remained dissolved therein cured the disease in animals and men." This proves conclusively:

That the crude poison and its alcoholic solution must possess similar pathogenetic properties; hence to a proving of Anthracinum must be added all the symptoms of uncomplicated splenic fever; to those of Hydrophobinum, the symptoms of every case of pure hydrophobia; to those of Syphilinum all those of pure syphilis, etc., etc.

2. That bacteria are not the cause but the effect of the disease, a doctrine which we hold to be true with regard to all parasites connected with deranged health, and that therefore their destruction by local application is not equivalent to the cure of the disease itself.

Characteristics—

In carbuncle, malignant ulcer and complaints with *ulceration, sloughing and intolerable burning*. Painful glandular swellings; cellular tissue indurated; anthrax-quinsy.

When Arsenicum or the best selected remedy fails to relieve the burning pain of carbuncle or malignant ulceration, study Anthracinum.

Hemorrhages: blood oozes from mouth, nose, anus or sexual organs; black, thick, tar-like, rapidly decomposing (Crotalus).

Septic fever, rapid loss of strength, sinking pulse, delirium and fainting (Pyr.).

Gangrenous ulcers; felon, carbuncle; gangrenous erysipelas of a malignant type.

Felon; the worst cases, with sloughing and terrible burning pain (Ars., Carb. ac., Euphorb., Lach.).

Malignant pustule; *black or blue blisters;* often fatal in twenty-four or forty-eight hours (Ech., Lach., Pyr.).

Carbuncle: *with horrible burning pains;* discharge of ichorous offensive pus.

Furuncles and all forms of boils, large and small. Some forms of acne; successive crops of boils or carbuncles on any part of the body; to remove the tendency.

Dissecting wounds, especially if tendency is to become gangrenous; septic fever, marked prostration (Ars., Ech., Pyr.).

Suspicious insect stings. If the swelling changes colour and red streaks from the wound map out the course of lymphatics (Ech., Lach., Pyr.).

Septic inflammation from absorption of pus or other deleterious substances, with burning pain and great prostration (Ars., Ech., Euphorb,, Pyr.).

Epidemic spleen diseases of cattle, horses and sheep.

Bad effects from inhaling foul odors of putrid fever or dissecting-room; poisoning by foul breath (Ech., Pyr.).

Hering says: "To call a carbuncle a surgical disease is the greatest absurdity. An incision is always injurious and often fatal. A case has never been lost under the right kind of treatment, and it should always be treated by internal medicine only."

Relations—

Antidoted by Apis, Ars., Camph., Carbo v., Carb. ac., Lach., Kreos., Puls., Rhus, Sil., Sali. ac.; Pyr. in malignant septic conditions.

Compare—

Anth. bovum, Anth. suum, Ars., Carbo a., Carbo v., Ech., Euphr., Tar. em., in the terrible pains of cancer, carbuncle or erysipelas.

It follows well: Ars., Carb. ac., Phos., Phos. ac., Phyt., Sec., in burning pains of ulcers.

Is followed well by Auright mur., Nat., Fluor, ac., Hecla lava, in periosteal swelling of lower jaw; by Sil. in cellulitis and grandular affections post-surgical.

Mind—

Anxiety, particularly in praecordia.

Delirium.

Excitement.

Loss of consciousness.

Depression, with debility, and chill.

Thinks she feels death approaching.

Animals howl, bite, run about, become greatly excited; followed by paralytic symptoms.

Disinclined to work.

Head—

Dulness in head as from narcotics.

Confusion.

Dizziness.

Dizziness with pain in head.

Loss of consciousness.

Headache, as if a smoke with a heating pain was passing through the head (fumee de douleur chaude); two shepherds who caught it from their flock.

Head is affected in an indescribable manner.

Uncomfortable feeling in head, slight chills, mild fever.

If fully conscious they complain of great pain in head.

Pain in head, dizziness; inner anthrax.

Here and there in all parts of brain small and large hemorrhages of embolic origin; after death from anthrax.

Membranes of brain exhibit circumscribed or symmetrically extended bloody infiltrations.

Headache with chill. Cerebral symptoms with carbuncle.

Flying gangrene.

Small swellings on temples and cheeks, extending through the orbital sutures and foramina to the dura and pia mater.

Carbuncles mostly on head, near the ears or temples.

Flying gangrene, head swollen (in swine).

Swelling of the head (sheep).

Eyes and Sight—

Great dilatation of pupils; inner anthrax.

A pale yellowish or greenish swelling, if in the eyelids, of a half-translucent aspect.

A pale redness above the brows along the forehead.

Ears and Hearing—

Ringing in the ears; inner anthrax.

Parotitis gangrenosa, after scarlatina.

Swelling extending backward over the angle of the right lower jaw, which could not be felt and up to near the ear.

Nose and Smell—

Nose swollen and red, fetid smell from it.

Bloody suffusions on mucous membrane of nose. Intense redness of the right half of nose, extending to the cheek.

Face—

Erysipelatous, dark brown redness and swelling over the whole right side of face, the nose and part of left cheek; swelling very hard, redness does not disappear under the pressure of finger.

Extending to cheek, redness from nose.

Could not move the lower jaw as usual.

Could open the mouth only so far as to put the point of the tongue out.

Impossible to open the jaws in the least.

Tearing in the right lower jaw.

Beginning of swelling was in the region of the right submaxillary gland.

A stony swelling around the right lower maxilla, the inner space of the mandibula filling up to half, reaches to nearly half the cheek, and disfiguring the face, extending backwards over the angle of the lower jaw; very little pain, not red, but sharply defined edges.

Swelling extending from the inner edge of the left lower jaw across the whole throat, in front and over the edge of the right lower jaw, and *au niveau* with the upper surface of the right lower molars.

A large stony, hard, pale swelling around the right lower jaw, nearly painless, disfiguring the face.

Gland under the chin painfully swollen.

Teeth and Gums—

On making an incision near second molar a mass of stinking, brown ichor is discharged.

Taste, Tongue—

Flabby taste.

Tongue often furred, with a thick brown coat; dry.

Mouth—

Offensive odor from mouth.

Mouth could not be opened.

Saliva increased.

Continued bleeding from the mouth; the blood shows a lack of power to coagulate; with inner anthrax.

Dark red, bloody ecchymoses of mouth.

Bloody suffusions and hemorrhagic collections on the mucous membranes of canthi of mouth and nose; inner anthrax.

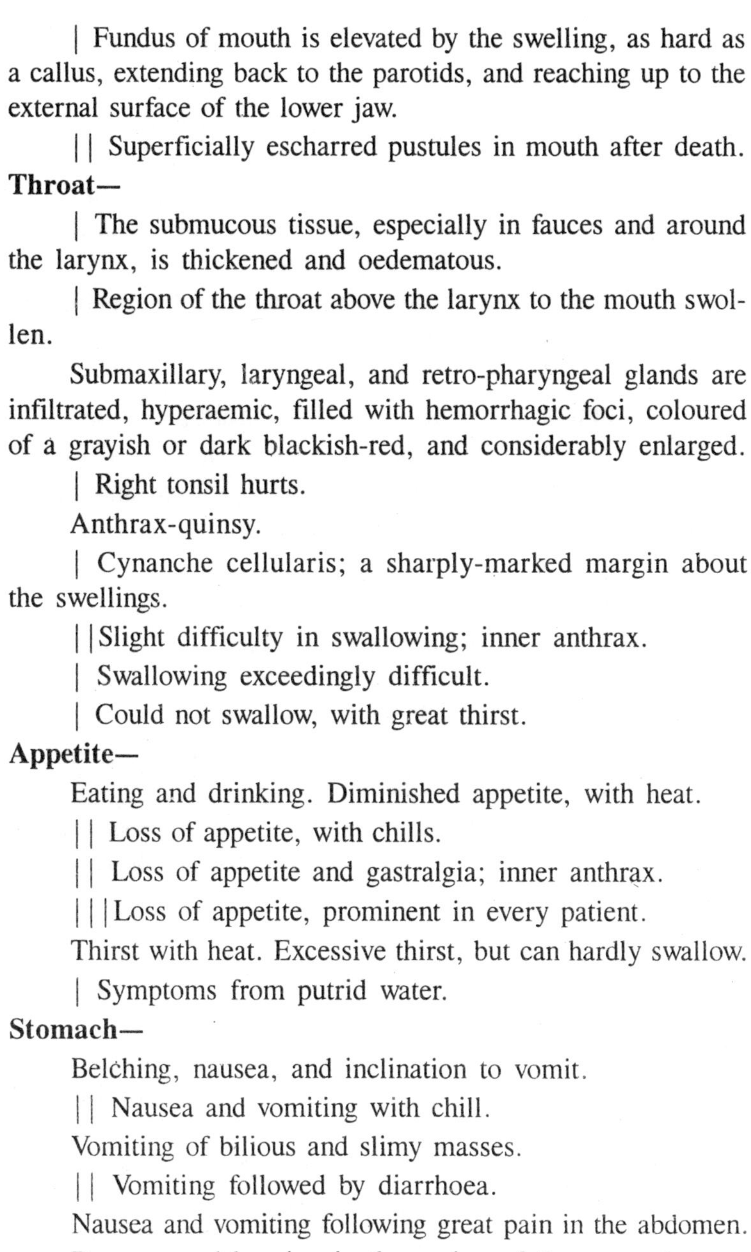

| Fundus of mouth is elevated by the swelling, as hard as a callus, extending back to the parotids, and reaching up to the external surface of the lower jaw.

| | Superficially escharred pustules in mouth after death.

Throat—

| The submucous tissue, especially in fauces and around the larynx, is thickened and oedematous.

| Region of the throat above the larynx to the mouth swollen.

Submaxillary, laryngeal, and retro-pharyngeal glands are infiltrated, hyperaemic, filled with hemorrhagic foci, coloured of a grayish or dark blackish-red, and considerably enlarged.

| Right tonsil hurts.

Anthrax-quinsy.

| Cynanche cellularis; a sharply-marked margin about the swellings.

| |Slight difficulty in swallowing; inner anthrax.

| Swallowing exceedingly difficult.

| Could not swallow, with great thirst.

Appetite—

Eating and drinking. Diminished appetite, with heat.

| | Loss of appetite, with chills.

| | Loss of appetite and gastralgia; inner anthrax.

| | |Loss of appetite, prominent in every patient.

Thirst with heat. Excessive thirst, but can hardly swallow.

| Symptoms from putrid water.

Stomach—

Belching, nausea, and inclination to vomit.

| | Nausea and vomiting with chill.

Vomiting of bilious and slimy masses.

| | Vomiting followed by diarrhoea.

Nausea and vomiting following great pain in the abdomen.

Pressure and burning in the region of the stomach.

| | Gastralgia.

| | Walls of stomach and intestine oedematous, discoloured, a cloudy red.

| | Mucous membrane of stomach and intestines reddish, swollen, with isolated or numerous oedematous, hemorrhagic prominent infiltrations, from size of a lentil to that of a coffee bean, showing a grayish or greenish-yellow discoloured surface, with a positively sloughing centre.

| | Numerous peculiar hemorrhagic and superficially eschared infiltrations of stomach and intestines; intestinal anthrax.

Abdomen—

Sensation as if the diaphragm was pushed forward.

Sensation of anxiety and constriction, most in the prascordia, liver engorged, slight hemorrhage here and there, spleen moderately enlarged, soft, full of blood, dark colour.

| | Enlargement of spleen.

| | Epidemic spleen disease of cattle or horses.

Preceded or followed with Arsenicum, Carbolic ac. or Euphorbium as called for by the symptoms.

| | The same disease in sheep. *Anthracinum suum* is better than *Anthracinum ovium* in the acute form, but in the chronic form *Anthracinum ovium* is better.

Sudden prostration with great abdominal soreness, mostly in the epigastrium with vomiting, cold limbs, dull head.

| | Bellyache with chill.

| | Colicky pains; inner anthrax.

| A horse fell down with colic, no motion except now and then bending the head towards the abdomen.

| | Mycosis intestinalis; intestinal anthrax.

| | In the intestines a thinly fluid material, slightly coloured with blood.

| | The retro-peritoneal and mesenteric connective tissue infiltrated, jelly-like, and of a yellowish-reddish colour.

| | Moderate serous or sero-hemorrhagic effusion and sub-peritoneal suggilations.

| | Simple hemorrhages, infarctions and foci on different parts of intestines.

| | Serous and sero-hemorrhagic infiltrations of the peritoneal and mesenteric connective tissue, walls of stomach and intestine, and of the mucous membranes.

| | Mesenteric and retro-peritoneal glands enlarged to the size of a walnut; form blackish-red masses, held together by a jelly-like congestive tissue, infiltrated with serum.

Dark red carbuncle in the omentum.

| | Peculiar pustular and carbuncular foci in the intestinal tract.

| | Swelling of the abdomen; inner anthrax.

Rectum and Stool—

Vomiting, followed by a painless, often bloody, diarrhoea.

Diarrhoea with bellyache.

| | Diarrhoea.

| | Vomiting followed by a painless, moderate, more or less intense, often bloody diarrhoea; inner anthrax.

| | With the diarrhoea sometimes a cholera-like collapse; inner anthrax.

Retarded stool.

Urinary Organs—

| Kidneys swollen, with oedema, sprinkled with small hemorrhages, engorged; suggilations in mucous membranes of the pelvis.

Respiration—

| Breathing frequent, laborious; quick, spasmodic; inner anthrax.

Lungs—

Pulmonary hyperaemia, ecchymoses.

| | Slight serous effusions into pleural cavities.

| | Sub-pleural ecchymoses with vascular engorgement, and a dark colouring of the parenchyma.

| | (oedema of the mediastinal lymphatic glands.

Heart, Pulse and Circulation—

Heart-beat frequent but weak.

| Her heart beats altogether different.

| | The beating of the heart stronger, more decided and more perceptible.

Pulse frequent, small, with violent action of the heart; soft; small and feverish.

| Soft, scarcely frequent pulse.

| | Discoloured lines over the veins, or red lines and stripes in the course of the lymphatics.

| | Cyanosis; inner anthrax.

| | Blood of a dark cherry red, generally fluid or with some loose clots.

| | Blood not coagulating.

Neck and Back—

Axillary glands swollen and painful.

| Swelling in the neck size of hazelnut, burning and fiery red; is pointed and hard.

| | | Carbuncle on the back, nine inches in length and five inches in its greatest width; with sloughing, abundant discharge of ichorous, terrible smelling pus, and blood-poisoning by absorption of pus.

Hydro-rachitis (Grubbe, Kreuzdrehe), a disease of sheep.

Upper Limbs—

Tetanic spasms of upper limbs; inner anthrax.

| Arms and hands covered with a crusty eruption, full of cracks, discharging pus and an acrid fluid, with painful, unbearable itching; checked for a while by the Old School, it had burst out again with terrible fury. After Anthracine, the crusts pealed off and were flying about like snow.

| The whole left hand (not the fingers) swollen, highly reddened, very painful; the redness extended over the whole hand and even the wrist, and a red streak ran up the forearm.

| On the middle of the palm of the hand a large blister, which, when opened, discharged a yellow watery fluid.

| | Felon, the worst cases, with sloughing; severe torturing pain and great prostration.

| Whitlow.

Lower Limbs—

Thighs livid to the nates, hard and painful; lower legs dark blue, feet oedematous; when the blisters break they discharge an offensive ichor.

| The whole thigh was swollen, most above the knee, and also the foot.

| Livid redness on lower part of the whole thigh, up to the buttocks, hard and painful.

| Above the knee, redness, swelling and pain, and later a large black blister on inside of thigh, extending four inches upward and inward; after being lanced bloody water ran out.

| On outside of knee a large fluctuating swelling, by pressure discharging a horribly smelling gangrenous ichor.

From the openings on lower leg, caused by the fracture, a copious stinking pus (like carious bones).

Bluish-brown spots which break open.

| The whole lower limb blackish-blue; the region of the blister (foolishly lanced) mortified, discharging much offensive ichor.

| Ulcers size of a hand on lower limbs; no antipsoric had relieved; Anthracinum helped very soon.

Carious ulcers. ,

| Foot oedematous.

Discoloured lines trace out the veins over the oedematous parts.

|| Severe pains in limbs and joints with the fever; intestinal anthrax.

Limbs as if beaten.

Limbs weak.

Nerves—

| Great restlessness.

Paroxysms of trembling.

Single muscles start or tremble.

||Epileptiform convulsions; inner anthrax.

Clonic spasms, trismus or opisthotonos; sometimes in serious cases.

Clonic spasms.

| | Tetanic spasms in upper limbs.

| | Opisthotonos; inner anthrax.

Debility and depression, with pain in the limbs.

| | Debility with chill.

| | Great weakness with the fever.

| | Debility and depression, with pains in limbs and general sense of malaise, followed by disturbance of intestinal canal; inner anthrax.

Debility and sweat all over.

| Completely exhausted, she thinks she feels death.

| | Cholera-like collapse after diarrhoea.

Collapse, with difficulty of breathing; loss of consciousness; death.

| | Sudden fatal issue, preceded by extreme collapse.

| | With cyanosis, asphyxia and the most extreme collapse, followed by death in all cases of bleeding.

| | Marked rigor mortis after death.

Sleep—

| Somnolence; inner anthrax.

Could not sleep for pain.

| Sleeplessness.

Restless sleep.

| Restless, irritated at night.

| | Restless sleep, with chill.

Delirium, sopor, then death.

Sleep short, not refreshing, more like a stupor.

Fever—

| | Chilly, with debility, headache, followed by a general malaise, loss of appetite, restless sleep, great debility and depression, and in eight or ten days carbuncles, most on the arm, forearm, head.

| | Decided chill, followed by bellyache, nausea, vomiting and in two or three days with the supervention of collapse and cyanosis; death.

| | Slight chills with fever and strange sensation in head.

With great prostration, chilliness, pains in the limbs, increase of fever and weakness, anxiety, restlessness, vertigo, delirium, dull head; stool retarded, urine scanty; skin dry, later covered with cold sweat.

| | Temperature very slightly elevated; inner anthrax.

| | Febrile movement, slight in the beginning, is often followed apace by high fever; great weakness, delirium, excitement, confusion.

| Moderate heat, little thirst, general sweat.

| Very much feveright

Heat, thirst, less appetite, suffering and fatigued.

| Fever with diarrhoea.

Fever attended by sweating.

| | Sweat all over with debility.

| Disposed to sweat; rather sticky.

| Copious sweat.

| | Cold sweats in serious cases.

Typhoid type, with rapidly sinking pulse, loss of strength, fainting, delirium.

Skin—

Dark-red spots (sheep).

Ecchymoses.

Cyanosis.

Skin of the affected part either hard or doughy.

| Skin dry, itching violently and burning.

Unbearable itching on arms and hands.

Itching with dry skin; violent as if mad (horses).

| Crusty oozing eruption, with the most violent itching.

| Crusty eruption discharging acrid fluid.

A small red spot, sometimes with a blackish point in the middle, gradually becoming more sensitive, has to scratch, it reddens more and more, swells and forms a small pustule or blotch.

|| A little red speck, like a flea-bite, with a central black point, swells gradually and changes into an itching papule, capped with a small, clear, reddish or bluish vesicle, gradually enlarging.

|| The excoriated spot dries up, becomes brown and livid and a local eschar forms.

By inflammatory swelling of the surrounding skin a red or violet raised border is formed, around it a bluish or pale yellow ring, upon which little vesicles, size of a hemp seed, appear surrounding the central eschar.

|| With an increase of the round thick eschar, one-fourth to three-fourths of an inch, the raised border also extends.

Excoriated surface dries and mummifies, but new blisters form all around.

|| Small and large epidermal vesicles filled with serum.

Blister on palm of hand.

|| The secondary vesicles contain a yellowish, reddish and blackish fluid.

|| Over the pustule a blister, size of a lentil, with a clear, bright yellowish, later a reddish or bluish fluid.

| Black or blue blisters.

|| Black blisters, fatal in twenty-four to forty-eight hours. Large black blister on inside of thigh.

|| In case of more than one detritus, the whole is swollen like erysipelas, and when cut it looks like the *Vespajas* of the Italian dermatologists.

| Erysipelatous inflammation about the carbuncle. |Erysipelas gangrenosa.

| Erysipelatous form of chronic anthrax. |

Small-pox of sheep.

Umbilicated pustules, yellow or bluish around, with the depression of a dark red hue, and hemorrhagic foundation.

If scraped off soon the excoriated spot dries, turns brown and livid and leaves a scar.

|| The dense or doughy soft papules or pustules, around and beneath the eschar, vary in size from a pea to a nut.

|| The papule promptly bursts and discloses a dark red base.

Sometimes blisters looking more like furuncles; a pus-like collection under the epidermis, which loosens and discloses decomposed matter.

|| Papules and pustules, with extensive oedematous and phlegmonous infiltration of the neighbouring skin and subcutaneous tissue.

|| The anthrax pustule penetrates deeply into the subcutaneous cellular tissue.

|| Anthrax pustules most on face, forearms, hands, fingers, neck, less often the ear, still less frequent the covered parts.

Anthrax carbuncles, with typhoid symptoms.

|| Little carbuncles; inner anthrax.

| Carbuncle.

|| Carbuncle darkish red, greasy, and is often more eroded than ulcerated.

Circumscribed carbuncle, hard large knots.

Diffuse, erysipelatous carbuncle.

|| Carbuncle on arm, forearm, head. See chill.

||| Carbuncle with horrible burning pains; or discharge of ichorous offensive pus.

||| Anthrax carbuncles cured by Anthracine, every day, also externally, in four days.

Anthrax contagiosus.

| Seventh day after the remedy several larger and smaller openings, discharging watery, sometimes bloody matter, very little pus; swelling less hard around the base.

| All openings run into one, discharge much pus.

| After having taken homoeopathic medicine for malignant ulcers, suddenly the greatest malaise, and a black blister formed below the knee with swelling all around, and feverish shaking chill through the whole body.

| Ulcus excedens (sheep).

Most malignant gangrenous ulcers (sheep).

| Chronic forms of anthrax with indurations like knots under the skin.

|| Large cutaneous eschars.

BACILLINUM

Mind—

Taciturn, sulky, snappish, fretty, irritable, morose, depressed and melancholic even to insanity.

Fretful ailing, whines and complains; mind given to be frightened, particularly by dogs.

Head—

Severe headache, deep in, recurring from time to time, compelling quiet fixedness; < shaking head.

Terrible pain in head as if he had a tight hoop of iron around it; trembling of hands; sensation of damp clothes on spine; absolute sleeplessness.

Meningitis.

Ringworm.

Alopecia areata.

Eyes—

Eczematous condition of eyelids.

Face.—Indolent, angry pimples on left cheek, breaking out from time to time and persisting for many weeks.

Teeth—

Aching in teeth, especially lower incisors (all sound), felt at the roots, especially on raising or projecting lower lip; very sensitive to air.

Grinds teeth in sleep.

Imperfectly developed teeth.

Throat—

Tickling in fauces, compelling cough.

Stomach—

Windy dyspepsia, with pinching pains under ribs of right side in mammary line.

Abdomen—

Fever, emaciation, abdominal pains and discomfort, restless at night, glands of both groins enlarged and indurated; cries out in sleep; strawberry tongue.

Tabes mesenterica; talks in sleep; grinds teeth; appetite poor; hands blue; indurated and palpable glands everywhere; drum belly; spleen region bulging out.

Inguinal glands indurated and visible; excessive sweats; chronic diarrhoea.

Stool and Anus—

Sudden diarrhoea before breakfast, with nausea.

Severe hemorrhages from bowels, cough.

Obstinate constipation.

Passes much ill-smelling flatus.

Stitchlike pain through piles.

Urinary Organs—

Increased quantity of urine, pale, with white sediment.

Has to rise several times in night to urinate.

Resipiratory Organs—

Slight, tedious, hacking cough.

Hard cough, shaking patient, more during sleep, but it did not waken him.

Pricking in larynx with sudden cough.

Single cough on rising from bed in morning.

Cough waking him in night; easy expectoration.

Expectoration of non-viscid easily detached, thick phlegm from air passages, followed after a day or two by a very clear ring of voice.

Sharp pain in precordial region arresting breathing.

Very sharp pain in left scapula, < lying down in bed at night, > by warmth.

Neck and Back—

Glands of neck enlarged and tender.

Lower Limbs—

Pain in left knee whilst walking; passed off after perseverance in walking for a short distance.

Tubercular inflammation of knee.

Generalities—

Great weakness, did not want to be disturbed.

Sleep—

Drowsy during day; restless at night; many dreams.

Fever—

Flush of heat (soon after the dose), some perspiration, severe headache deep in.

CHOLESTERINUM ($C_{26}H_{44}O$)

To the late Dright Wilhelm Ameke, of Berlin, we are indebted for the first mention of this remedy. From him Dr. Burnett obtained the suggestion and used the lower potencies with more or less success for several years, a description of which he gives us in his Diseases of the Liver. Unfortunately the remedy was either given in alternation or followed by other remedies in such a manner as to greatly mar the validity of its clinical work.

Swan appears to have taken his hint from Burnett's work and potentized the remedy, using a gall-stone for his preparations. Like many of the rest of the nosodes originally introduced by Swan, the work was necessarily empirical, yet he affirms after much experience that it is "almost a specific for gall-stone colic; relieves the distress at once." And this after failure with Nux, Cinchona, Carduus, Podophyllum and other apparently well-selected remedies.

Yingling reports some cures of gall-stone colic and other diseases of the liver in the *Medical Advance,* page 549, August, 1908, and arrives at the following conclusion:

> In gall-stone colic the patient suffers so severely that it is almost impossible to obtain symptoms. In such a case, when I cannot give a well-selected remedy, of late I rely on Cholesterinum, and thus far it has never failed. It should have a proving. Until then it can be used instead of Morphine in cases where the symptoms cannot be obtained for the proper selection of a remedy. Where a case of routine work is necessary, as it is sometimes, I believe

the homeopathic guess should be given the preference. It is very improbable that a person suffering from gall-stone colic will wait very long for the physician to study the case.

Clarke says, it is found in the blood, in the brain, the yolk of eggs, seeds and buds of plants, but is most abundant in the bile and biliary calculi. It occurs in the form of crystals with a mother-of-pearl lustre, and is fatty to the touch. It is soluble in both alcohol and ether.

Ameke claimed to have derived great advantage from its use in cases diagnosed as cancer of the liver, or in such obstinate engorgements that malignancy was suspected.

Burnett claims to have twice cured cancer of the liver with it, and "in hepatic engorgements that by reason of their intractable and slow yielding to well-selected remedies make one think interrogationally of cancer." In such conditions, where the diagnosis is in doubt, especially if the patient has been subjected to repeated attacks of biliary colic, Cholesterinum, he claims, is very satisfactory and at times its action even striking.

Yingling reports the following cases:

Woman, age 60. Frequent attacks of gall-stones, involving liver and region of stomach.

Attacks come suddenly and cease suddenly.

Pain is pushing in region of gall duct.

Vomits much odorless hot water.

Very pale, then became yellow.

Marked acidity of stomach since last attack.

Erratic rheumatism; pain < in damp, rainy weatheright

No appetite; food nauseates.

Region of liver sore, sensitive to touch or jar, < lying on the sides.

Before the attacks profuse urine; scanty and dark since.

Tongue coated dirty, yellowish white.

Heart becomes very weak, can hardly feel pulse.

Very weak, unable to breathe deeply.

This women was practically cured in a year, under various potencies of Cholesterinum, from the 2m. to the dmm.

Man, age 64, for three years has been passing gall-stones.

Vomits bile and becomes very yellow.

Has received Morphine which causes such disastrous after effects that he is away from business nearly a week. With one attack was in bed several weeks, and required a long time after to recover from bad effects.

Liver very sensitive and sore; pressure in front or behind very painful, worse in region of gall duct.

Bending or any sudden motion aggravates.

Had severe attacks of ague in Wabash bottoms when young. Is a large, portly man.

Cholesterinum 2m. not only promptly relieved acute attacks, but has effected a practical cure.

DIPHTHERINUM : AN INVOLUNTARY PROVING

BY J. E. FRASH, M. D., METAMORE, OHIO.

A girl nine years of age having been exposed, Nov. 13, to malignant diphtheria received Diphtherinum 1m. (Skinner) three times daily for eleven days, as a prophylactic, developing chilliness, high temperature, red face. She complained of being tired and cold, severe pain on swallowing and on the 12th day the tonsils and posterior walls of the pharynx were covered with dirty gray, yellowish membrane, corrugated vertically, like the surface of a wash-board turned up.

Thursday, Nov. 14, 1907, began powders, three each day for eight days, then two daily for two days.

Nov. 23, complained of being tired, sat down to rest three times.

Nov. 24, would lie down because tired, but after a while felt playful.

Nov. 25, temperature 103, pulse 148, full, with throbbing of carotids, eyes bright, face flushed, with center of cheeks almost purple.

Throat dark red, no membrane; but on posterior wall of throat, yellow, dirty cream colour with dry membrane in folds, up and down.

Monday night talks in sleep, with eyes wide open. Wanted imaginary objects taken from room, and to "make those people get away." Sat up and picked among bed-clothes for strap for her school books.

Nov. 26, temperature 101.2, pulse 116, membrane lighter and moist, thin in middle of throat.

Nov. 27, temperature 99.2, pulse 100. Throat clearing from middle. Jerking of single limb, or shoulder, or finger.

Nov. 28, temperature 101.2, pulse 116. Desired to have mother hold her hand. Tongue whitish, with exceedingly red tip (moist).

Nov. 29, temperature 10.2, pulse 116, breath offensive.

Nov. 30, temperature 99.4, pulse 100. Membrane white, and showing more to front. Clearing from center of posterior wall of throat. Tongue coated whitish, with red papille; very red tip, with a dark red spot in center of red tip. Slept well last night, until 4 A.M., then was restless and wakeful; moved and changed position, moved arms and legs often, snored and fan-like motion of ala nasi. Skin seemed dry, forehead moist along edge of hair, when first falling asleep.

Generalities—

Fluctuating temperature, very little pain, membrane in vertical folds on posterior wall of throat, when the membrane first appeared, spreading forward as far as border of the tonsils, and also began to fade and disappear first from center of posterior pharynx.

In center of the tip of tongue was a very dark red spot, also very dark red or purple spot in centre of very red cheeks.

The membrane from a case of malignant diphtheria, triturated with milk sugar to the 6th centesimal, then potentized by Swan. The diphtheritic virus, or diphtheria toxin, from which the serum anti-toxin is made. These potencies have been very effective, not only in malignant diphtheria but in many cases of post-diphtheritic paralysis and kindred nervous affections following the use of anti-toxin.

DIPHTHERINUM

Diphtherinum has made many brilliant cures of diphtheria and post-diphtheritic affections to its credit, yet to receive its place among the remedies of the homeopathic Materia Medica it must pass the crucial test that all others have encountered, viz., a careful and thorough proving of the dynamic potency on the healthy. Thus far, like its great congener Antitoxin, its use has been clinical and empirical, the distinctive difference being that its action has been dynamic, while that of antitoxin is Chemico-catalytic.

Yet the empirical use of Von Behring's Antitoxin is a great advance on the former empirical methods of the profession and has proved a blessing to humanity.

The indications here given are chiefly clinical and are tentatively held until verified or disproved by provings.

Characteristics—

Especially adapted to the strumous diathesis; scrofulous, psoric or tuberculous persons, prone to catarrhal affections of throat and respiratory mucous membranes.

Patients with weak or exhausted vitality hence are extremely susceptible to the diphtheritic virus; when the attack from the onset tends to malignancy (Lac c., Mer. cy.).

Painless diphtheria; symptoms almost or entirely objective; patient too weak, apathetic or too prostrated to complain; sopor or stupor, but easily aroused when spoken to (Bap., Sulph.).

Dark red swelling of tonsils and palatine arches; parotid and cervical glands greatly swollen; breath and discharges from throat, nose and mouth very offensive; tongue swollen, very red, little coating.

Diphtheritic membrane, thick, dark gray or brownish black; temperature low or subnormal, pulse weak and rapid, extremities cold and marked debility; patient lies in a semi-stupid condition; eyes dull, besotted (Apis, Bap.).

Epistaxis or profound prostration from very onset of attack (Ail., Apis, Carb. ac.); collapse almost at very beginning (Crot., Mer. cy.); pulse weak, rapid and vital reaction very low.

Swallows without pain, but fluids are vomited or returned by the nose; breath horribly offensive.

When the patient from the first seems doomed, and *the most carefully selected remedies fail to relieve or permanently improve.*

Laryngeal diphtheria, after Chlor., Kali bi. or Lac c.

Post diphtheritic paralysis—especially where Antitoxin has been used; many cases cured—after Caust., Gels., Nux, Secale and the best selected remedies have failed.

In post-diphtheritic paralysis and spinal affections following diphtheria many brilliant cures have been effected by the potencies. The same indications for its use in all forms of diphtheria that are used when Antitoxin is exhibited.

ELECTRICITAS
(Atmospheric and Static)

Caspari and his colleagues obtained the symptoms caused by Electricity, natural and artificial, and was first published in *Hom. Bibliot.* Later it appears in Jahr and has recently been republished, with additions by Clarke. Every medical man knows the extreme susceptibility of some persons to the electric fluid and the sufferings they experience on the approach of, and during, a thunderstorm, or the contact of an electric current.

The potencies are prepared from milk sugar which has been saturated with the current.

Characteristics—

Intense nervous anxiety; timid, fearful, sighing; screams through nervous fear; paroxysms of weeping.

Dreads the approach of a thunderstorm; suffers mental torture before and during an electric storm.

Heaviness and paralysis of limbs and entire body; feels as if she weighed a ton.

Electricity should not be used nor electro-thermal baths taken when suffering from a cold, especially if the chest be involved; fatal results have followed.

Relation—

Antidote: Morphia acetate, especially the potency. Clarke says: "I have found Phosphorus the best antidote to the effects of storms."

Compare—

The X-ray, Psor., Tub to remove the susceptibility.

ELECTRICITY.

Mind—

|| Weeping, timid, fearful; sighing, crying out through nervous fear. Paroxysms of oppressive anxiety.

Violent uneasiness; anxious, restless.

Dread at the approach of a thunder-storm; fear, internal anguish, especially of chest; nervous agitation.

|| Involuntary hysterical laughter. Rage. Ill-humor. Unable to comprehend time. Comprehension slow and difficult. Suffers mental torture before and during an electric storm.

|| Loss of memory.

Sensorium—

Loss of consciousness.

|| Loss of sensibility.

Looking around with haggard eyes.

Dulness of head.

|| Stupefaction. Giddiness, especially on stooping.

Head—

|| Headache; pressure in the forehead, from above downwards, as from a stone.

Darting from the vertex to the right side of the head.

| Tearing from the nape of the neck to the forehead.

Painful spasms in the head.

Sore pain in the occiput.

Disagreeable shocks, generally in the occiput.

Roaring in the whole sinciput.

Sensation of torpor in right side of head.

Outer Head—

Prickings in the scalp.

Undulating sensation under the scalp.

Feeling of coldness on the vertex.

Stinging itching of the head and thighs.

The growth of the hair is considerably promoted.

Eyes—

Gnawing in the left eye, or violent drawing, extending to the forehead.

Sensation as if the eyes were deep in the head.

Sensation as if something would come out of the eyeball.

|| Inflammation of the eyes; profuse lachrymation.

Wild rolling of the eyeballs.

Contraction of the morbidly-enlarged pupils.

Dim-sightedness.

|| Blindness.

Improved sight (curi. effect).

| Black point before the right eye.

|| Everything looks yellow.

A dark room looks as if brightly illumined.

Ears—

Darting in the right ear, from the throat.

Drawing from the jaws into the ears.

Redness and warmth of the ear.

Swelling of the inner ear.

Suppuration and small ulcers in the meatus auditorius.

|| Blisters behind the ears full of an acrid fluid.

Whizzing in the ears, or sensation as if obstructed by a plug.

Nose—

Tingling in the nose, or pressing from within outwards.

| Loss of smell.

Discharge of a milky fluid from the nose.

Face—

Expression of terror in the countenance.

Swelling of the face.

Scurf in the face, on the arms and body.

| Large blisters on the cheeks.

Chapped lips.

Eruption around the mouth and chin.

Teeth—

Tearing in the upper teeth, proceeding from the head.

Pain as from subcutaneous ulceration in old sockets of the molar teeth.

Rapid growth of teeth.

Mouth and Pharynx—

Soreness of the inner cheek.

|| Increased secretion of saliva.

|| Foam at the mouth.

|| The tongue is very sensitive, particularly at the tip.

||Swelling of the tongue.

Throat—

Loss of speech, inability to articulate.

Blisters on the palate, the epidermis becoming detached.

Constant titilation in the throat.

Inflammation of the pharynx.

Appetite—

Increased appetite.

Stomach, Nausea and Vomiting—

|| Heartburn.

Ptyalism.

Nausea, also after a meal.

Desire to vomit.

Vomiting with sore throat.

Hematemesis.

Stomach—

Sense of repletion in the stomach, after a slight meal.

Spasmodic contraction of the stomach.

Abdomen—

|| Cutting in the abdomen at the approach of a thunder-storm.

Stool—

Black-yellow, liquid stools, having a fetid smell.

Drawing up of the testes during stool.

Constriction of the anus, after stool.

Violent pressing in the anus (during menses).

Burning at the anus.

Flowing hemorrhoids.

Urinary Organs—

| Sensation as if the bladder would burst.

|| Frequent micturition.

Incontinence of urine.

Discharge of blood with the urine.

Female Sexual Organs—

Appearance of the menses (while in the electric bath).

| Black and thick menstrual blood.

Profuse menses, with pressing in rectum.

Leucorrhea, first thin, then thick, with coagula of the size of a hazel nut.

Larynx and Trachea—

Cough with violent titilation in the throat and pressing in the forehead from within outward.

Respiration—

Panting breathing.

Asthma all one's life, with palpitation of the heart and disposition to faint.

Chest—

Chilliness in the left side of the chest.

Palpitation of the heart, with fever, or with headache, or with oppressive anxiety and bright-red face.

Painful quick movement from the region of the heart through the chest.

Chest and arms become stiff, almost paralyzed; unable to walk.

Heaviness and stiffness of chest and shoulders, felt like marble.

Back—

Creeping in the spine.

|Boils in the back and nape of the neck.

Drawing through the scapula as with a thread.

Formication in a muscle which had become shortened by suppuration.

Stinging in a swollen cervical gland.

Upper Limbs—

Tearing in the right shoulder, going off in the warmth of the bed.

|| Frightful pains in the arms and lower limbs.

Jerking or tearing in the joints of the arms and hands.

|| Paralysis of the arms.

Swelling of one arm.

Crusty ulcers on the arms and lower limbs.

Violent jerking in the upper arm.

| Trembling of the hands.

| Swelling of the hand, also red, or sudden.

Red, smooth spot on the hand.

Whitish, itching spot in the palm of the right hand.

|| Feeling of numbness in the tips of the fingers.

Blister filled with a greenish, sanguineous fluid on the finger which discharges the bottle.

Lower Limbs—

Sensation in the thigh as if the flesh had become detached from the bone.

Tottering of the knees.

Tingling in the knees down to the foot.

Red, burning spot as if sore on the knee, or also itching elevation on the knee.

Tingling or languor in the tibiae.

Red spots on the skin.

|| Burning in the feet, up to the knees, particularly at night.

Coldness of the lower extremities up to the abdomen, in summer, during a cool wind.

Trembling and feeling of weariness in the feet.

Sense of numbness and distension in the feet, and as if they had gone to sleep.

Tingling in the soles of the feet. Sensation as of a broad ring around the malleoli.

Feet would patter rapidly on the floor during a thunder storm, could not be controlled even by husband sitting on knees.

Intense suffering of electric shocks through left foot and entire left side of body to head, repeated at every discharge during a thunder storm.

Sleep—

Yawning, with shuddering over the whole body.

Sleeplessness for two months.

Fever—

Shuddering over the body, every morning with yawning.

Chilliness, then dry, short heat.

Frequent alternation of chilliness and heat, with sore throat.

Chilliness with profuse sweat, with painful spasms in the head and along the back.

Warmth in the parts which were touched by the electric stroke.

Heat through the whole body, with chilliness on motion.

Heat in the parts which had been touched by the sparks.

Pulse intermittent.

Pulse quick and strong.

Accelerated circulation.

Excessive night sweat in an arthritic individual, without

relief; sweat with anxiety during a thunder storm.

Skin—

Itching or tingling over the whole body.

Violent pains and swelling of the foot which had been frozen twelve years ago.

Red pimples on the spot touched by the sparks.

White vesicles.

Itch-like eruption in the joints.

|| The skin becomes blackish.

|| Ecchymoses.

General Symptoms—

|| Pains in the limbs.

|| Drawing through all the limbs, extending to the tips of the fingers and toes.

Shock through the whole body, proceeding from the malar bone.

Tingling in the electrified parts.

Violent burning of the parts which are in contact with the chain.

|| General languor after a meal.

Relaxation of the nerves and muscles.

|| Fainting.

|| Stiffness of the limbs.

|| Paralysis of single limbs, particularly the lower.

|| Trembling of the limbs, particularly of those which have received the shock.

Subsultus tendinum.

Painful spasms along the back from below upward.

St. Vitus' dance.

Aggravation of the epileptic fits.

Intense suffering with paralysis of nervous and muscular system.

Heavy sensation as if she weighed a ton.

The following are reported by Seward (Trans. C. N. Y. S., *Medical Advance,* 1891, p. 150):

A lady had taken electricity for partial paralysis of left arm. During a thunder storm felt severe electric shocks through the left foot, the entire left side of the body to the head, repeated at every severe electric discharge, which left that side and limbs painful for days. The previous electrical treatment had rendered her more susceptible and its injurious effects will often last for years, or even during life, unless antidoted.

A young lady took an electro-thermal bath when she had a cold, and acute tuberculosis soon developed. She died in spite of the best homoeopathic treatment.

A lady who had passed the climacteric had taken electrical treatment, at first going to the office. Soon she became too weak to walk, her chest became weak and painful, and the arms stiffened and almost paralyzed; the entire body heavy and weak.

A young married woman had been under general and local electrical uterine treatment for several weeks, without benefit; complained of feeling so heavy, as though she "weighed a ton."

A woman received an atmospheric electric shock six or seven years before, and since had suffered in every electrical storm, even while it was miles away. It affected the whole body, but was worse in the lower extremities. During every storm her feet would 'patter' upon the floor, and her husband, sitting upon her knees, could not prevent it. She received three or four doses of Morphia acet. 200, and has never felt such effects from a storm since, now more than ten years.

My son, during the effects of a common cold, took an electro-thermal bath. Soon after felt a heaviness and stiffness of chest and shoulders he had never felt before; "his chest and shoulders felt like marble." An incurable tuberculosis developed and he died in two years. Did not know he had taken bath for over a year after.

A brother of Dright Hawley, while in New York in November 1890, took a severe cold, followed by rheumatic fever; was treated homoeopathically, without relief; advised to try electro-thermal baths, and became worse. Was removed to Syracuse and was under care of Drs. Hawley, Miller and Seward, with little or no benefit. His sufferings were intense, his voluntary muscular and nervous systems were paralyzed by electricity; could neither move nor feed himself. Was taken to his home in Illinois, and in May, six months later, could walk a little by dragging his feet. He fell, and had hemorrhage from the lungs. The doctor said there was no hope for a cure and gave him Morphine, as a palliation, in water. In a few minutes after the first dose he said: "I can use my hands better than at any time since the electrical treatment," and under the antidote recovered.

LAC CANINUM

Like Lachesis, and many other well known polychrests in the Materia Medica, this remedy met most violent opposition from ignorance and prejudice. It was for years looked upon as one of the novelties or delusions of those who believed in and used the dynamic remedy; yet its wonderful therapeutic powers have slowly but surely overcome every obstacle.

It was successfully used by Dioscorides, Rhasis and Pliny in ancient times, and Sextus recommended it for the removal of the fetus. Sammonicus and Sextus praise it in photophobia, otitis and other affections of the eye and ear. Pliny claimed that it cured ulceration of the internal os. It was then used as an antidote to many deadly poisons.

The use of the remedy was revived by Reisig, of New York, who, while traveling in Europe, heard it lauded as a remedy for throat diseases, and on his return used it successfully in an epidemic of malignant diphtheria. He called the attention of Bayard, Wells and Swan to the wonderful results he obtained during that epidemic, and induced them to give it a trial.

Reisig potentized it to the 17th cent. from which the potencies of Swan and Fincke were prepared. The profession is indebted to the indefatigable labor of Swan for its provings, which were made from the 30th, 200th and higher potencies, and published in a small volume by Swan and Berridge, from which it was published in the *Medical Advance.* The provings of this remedy have placed it among the polychrests of our school and verified and confirmed the clinical accuracies of the observers of ancient times.

Characteristics—

For nervous, restless, highly sensitive organisms.

Symptoms erratic, pains constantly flying from one part to another (Kali bi., Puls., Tub.); *changing from side to side every few hours or days.*

Very forgetful, *absent-minded;* makes purchases and walks away without them (Agnus, Anac., Caust., Nat.).

In writing, uses too many words or not the right ones; omits final letter or letters in a word; cannot concentrate the mind to read or study; very nervous (Bov., Graph., Lach., Nat. c., Sep.).

Despondent, hopeless; thinks her disease incurable; has not a friend living; nothing worth living for; could weep at any moment (Act., Auright, Cal., Lach.).

Cross, irritable; child cries and screams all the time, especially at night (Jal., Nux, Psor.).

Fears to be alone (Kali c.); of dying (Ars.); of becoming insane (Lil.); of falling down stairs (Bor.).

Chronic "blue" condition; everything seems so dark that it cannot grow any darker (Lye., Puls., Psor.).

Attacks of rage, cursing and swearing at slightest provocation (Lil., Nit. ac.); intense ugliness; hateful.

Coryza, with discharge of thick, white mucus.

One nostril stopped up, the other free and discharging; these conditions alternate; discharge acrid, nose and upper lip raw (Arum, Cepa).

Itching of roof of mouth (Puls., Wyeth.).

Diphtheria and tonsilitis; symptoms *change repeatedly from side to side.*

Sore throats and cough are apt *to begin and end with menstruation;* yellow or white patches; painful swelling of submaxillary glands.

Throat: sensitive to touch externally (Lach.); < by empty swallowing (Ign.); constant inclination to swallow, *painful,* almost impossible (Meright); *pains extend to ears* (Hep., Ign., Kali bi., Meright, Phyt.); begins on left side (Lach.).

Shining, glazed appearance of diphtheritic deposit, chancres and ulcers.

Very hungry, cannot eat enough to satisfy; as hungry after eating as before (Case., Cal., Cina, Lye., Stront.).

Sinking at epigastrium; *faintness in stomach.*

Menses: too early; too profuse; flow in gushes, bright red, viscid and stringy (dark, black, stringy, Croc.); breasts swollen, painful, sensitive before and during (Con.).

Stool: urging, but passes nothing but flatus or small black balls.

Discharge of flatus from vagina (Brom., Lye., Nux m.. Sang.).

Breasts: inflamed, heavy, painful; < by least jar and towards evening; *must hold them firmly when going up or down stairs* (Bry.).

Serviceable in almost all cases when it is required to dry up milk (Asaf.); to bring back or increase it (Lac d.).

Sensation as if breath would leave her when lying down; must get up and walk (Am. c., Grind., Lach.).

Loss of milk while nursing, without any known cause (Asaf.).

Palpitation violent when lying on left side, > turning on right (Lach., Tab.).

Sexual organs easily excited, from touch, pressure on sitting, or friction by walking (Cinn., Coff., Mur., Plat.).

When walking, seems to be walking on air; when lying, does not seem to touch the bed (Asar.); legs as if floating (Sticta).

Backache: intense, unbearable, across super-sacral region, extending to right natis and right sciatic nerve; < by rest and on first moving (Rhus); spine aches from base of brain to coccyx, *very sensitive to touch or pressure* (Chin, s., Phos., Zinc.).

RELATIONS—Similar: to Apis, Con., Murex, Lach., Kali bi., Puls., Sep., Sulph., Taren. and the X-ray.

Probably no remedy in the Materia Medica presents a

more valuable pathogenesis in symptoms of the throat, or one that will better repay a careful study.

"Acts best in single dose; if repeated, should be given at exact intervals."—*Nichols*. An observation frequently verified,

Lachesis and other serpent poisons are very analogous.

COMPARE: Amb., Lach., Nat. m., Staph., weak memory for what she has read, not for other things; Bov., Graph., Hepar, Lach., Lye., Nat. c., Nat. m., Nux, Sep., Tub., forgetful in writing, uses many words or not the right ones; Anac., Caust., Con., Dul., Lach., Nat. m., Sep., absent-minded; Cal., China, Graph., Hep., Lach., Lye., Med., Nat. c., Nat. m., Nux, Sep., Syph., cannot speak correctly half the time; Am. c., Cal., Sep., Sulph., Tub., substitutes name of objects seen for that which is thought; Nux, Sil., Sulph., very restless, cannot concentrate her thoughts or mind to read, wants to leave everything as soon as it is commenced; Cal., Pal., Sep., cried, fearing she was contracting consumption; Plat., Med., exalted sensation of sensorium.—*Lippe*.

Aur., Nux, Rhus, headache < in cold wind and > in warm room; Cal., headache < by noise, > by keeping quiet; confused feeling in head; Acon., Bell., Cal., Gels., Nat., Ruta, Stram., must have light, but intolerant of sunlight; Kali bi., Teuc., Thuja, soreness and crusting of nostrils; Nat. m., lips dry and bleeding; Apis, Lach., throat sensitive to touch externally; Ign., < by empty swallowing; Bell., Cal., Carbo an., Lye., Nit. ac., Phos., Phyt., Psor., breasts as if full of very hard lumps; very painful when going up and down stairs; Cal., Muright, sensitive to pressure; Mer., sensitive to deep pressure; Bell., Bry., Cal., Phyt., soreness and enlargement of; Mer. i. right, small round or irregular gray-white ulcers on tonsils and fauces; Apis, Diph., Mer. cy., diphtheritic membrane and deposits on vulva; Chel., Dig., Ign., Pet., Sep., empty, weak, all gone sensation in stomach; Bry., Kali bi., Nux, pain as from a stone or undigested food in stomach; Apis, Lil., Lye., Pal., pain in right ovarian region; Am. c., Grin., Carbo v., Opium, as soon as he falls asleep the breathing stops;

Asar., China, Cof., Nat. m., Nux, Opium, Rhus, Spig., Stram., Stic., Phos. ac., Thuja, when waking seems to be walking on air, when lying does not seem to touch the bed; Lach., Lac v. d., Sang., Sil., dream of going on a journey; Sec., spreads fingers wide apart in convulsions; Nic., Tab., Tub., retina retains impression of objects—ear retains impression of sound; Lye., Dubois., Hyos., red spot before vision; Bronx, Lye.. Nux m., Nux v., Sang., discharge of flatus from vagina; Bor., Sanic., < going down stairs.

Aggravation—

In the morning of one day and evening of next; alternate menstrual nisus; at night; cold winds and cold sharp air; motion; extension of limbs; after sleep; touch of external throat; of breasts, causing sexual excitement; descending.

Amelioration—

Cold applications; rest; lying down; warmth; bending of limbs; warm room.

THE WORK OF AN ARTIST.

Dr. Wm. P. Wesselhoeft says: No more appropriate tribute can be paid to the memory of Dr. Adolph Lippe than to show his great sagacity in the application of medicine in disease. It was not only his great knowledge of the finer and more subtle indications for remedies, as given in our Materia Medica, or his judicious examination of patients, which made him an acknowledged master of our art, but mainly that freer and wider application of our law which elevated him to the sphere of the true artist. His readiness and rapidity in getting at the gist of symptoms, even in the most complicated case, could never be called careless or hasty. It reminded me of the words of an eminent artist, who said: "The chief difficulty with most painters is that they see *too much,* and in seeing too much they get confused with endless detail, which leaves their work without character, and they have little to show for their pains."

He knew the value of our art so well that the common places of every disease were almost instinctively avoided by him, and he never lost time in noting worthless signs, always looking and finding with unusual rapidity the salient points in the case before him. He heeded and lived up to the greatest thought of the master: "The physician's business is only with patients, not with diseases."

The cure of the following case will demonstrate what I mean by a freer and wider application of our law of cure:

I had treated the patient more than eighteen months without improvment, except that his great liability to taking cold had become less.

I copy from my record, taken December, 1881.

G. R., aged forty-five, light brunette, married ten years, general appearance healthy.

For six years has had no discharge of semen during coitus.

Occasionally nocturnal emissions.

Erections usually weak, give out during coitus.

Burning in perineum, worse after going to bed, and when thinking of it.

Drawing pains in testicles, with sensation of weakness of genitals.

Occasionally itching, dry eruptions in crotch and inner upper surface of thighs and anus.

With the sensation of weakness of genitals his eyes feel weak.

Very sensitive to cold and changes of atmosphere.

Takes cold easily, usually affecting nose and throat first with dryness, then with watery catarrh and sneezing, or he has aching pains in different parts of the body and limbs, changing location frequently.

Twenty years ago had African fever.

Never had gonorrhea, syphilis, or other eruptions than those mentioned above.

All other functions normal.

While on a visit to Philadelphia he applied to Dr. Lippe, at my advice.

Dright Lippe wrote me the following letter:

"I find that your patient had diphtheria about ten years ago, and was treated with inappropriate mercurials and gargles by Dr. ——. The character of the attack was that it went from one side to the other and finally back again to the original side. Great weakness, almost paralytic, followed the attack, and he thinks he has never regained his full vigor and usual strength since this illness. His acute cold has always the character of shifting pains and change of location. I have given him a dose of Lac can. cm., which may be required to be followed by a dose of Pulsatilla."

Suffice it to say that my patient never needed the suggested dose of Pulsatilla.

In three months after his visit to Philadelphia his wife was pregnant. She has since borne two remarkably healthy children.

As far as we know Lac can has no sexual weakness. That fact disturbed Dr. Lippe very little in his selection. He looked deeper and found the cause and the remedy. *This is true homeopathic pathology.* All the knowledge in the world of the special pathology of this case could not have revealed the remedy to any one. To the homeopathic artist, however, it was revealed, and a man regained his manhood and became the father of two children, after ten years of impotence.

Mrs. J. E. B., aged 29, blonde. For a week has felt a sense of impending illness; weary, languid, depressed.

Sleepless, restless, frequent turning, because bed felt so hard.

Fever at 2 P.M. continued all night; chilly on movement; cheeks flushed and hot.

Soreness of entire body; "aches all over."

Throat dry, with thirst for cold drinks, which relieve.

Profuse saliva; slightly viscid and salty, wetting the pillow during sleep; frequent swallowing.

Throat: sharp pains on swallowing < right side; neck sensitive externally.

Pain and soreness begun on right side, extended to left.

Tonsils swollen, red, shining; membrane light yellow in colour, most on right side, in diffused- points size of pin head, but looking like lid of a pepper box; 25 or 30 points on right tonsil, about one-half as many on left. Points and larger irregular patches on posterior and pillars of pharynx.

Offensive breath, characteristic of the graver forms of diphtheria: Lac can. 45m., one dose.

The following symptoms, not in the pathogenesis, were cured: sensation as if bed were too hard; chill on movement; aching all over; great fatigue; desire for and relief from cold drinks. —*Stuart Close.*

Tommie H. ——: About three weeks succeeding the manifestation of diphtheritic disease in the case reported to the Society in which Lac caninum cm. proved curative I was consulted for a condition of paralysis of the muscles of the neck, which has become quite marked, so much as to cause a falling forwards of the head so that it rests on the upper portion of the sternum. There is return of fluid through the nose, and an evident weakness of the muscles of the upper part of the back. Phos. on general principles.

August 6th.—His father brings the boy back in a much worse condition.

Three weeks after recovery from diphtheria: Paralysis of muscles of the neck, quite marked, so as to cause falling forwards of the head until it rested upon the manubrium. Fluids return through the nose, and marked weakness of muscles of the upper part of the back. The paralysis becomes more pronounced, with staggering when walking; stiffness and soreness of the muscles of the neck. After Phos. and Rhus, though apparently well indicated, had failed, one dose of Lac caninum cured the diphtheria and > the paralysis.—*Baker.*

Mind—

Very forgetful; in writing, uses too many words or not the right ones; very nervous.

Omits final letter or letters of a word, when writing; in speaking substitutes name of objects seen, instead of object thought of.

Finds it very difficult to read understandingly anything requiring mental effort.

Very absentminded; makes purchases and walks off without them; goes to post a letter, brings it home in her hand.

Cannot remember what she reads, but can remember other things.

Cannot collect her thoughts; confused feeling.

Very restless; cannot concentrate her thoughts or mind to read; wants to leave everything as soon as it is commenced.

Is impressed with the idea that all she says is a lie; it seems to be very difficult to speak the truth, but continually distrusts things; when reading anything she rapidly changes the meaning, omitting or adding things.

Every time a symptom appears she feels very confident that it is not attributable to medicine, but that it is some settled disease.

| Sensation as if she were going deranged, when sitting still and thinking; sometimes she has most horrible sights presented by her mental vision (not always snakes), feels horribly afraid that they will take objective form and show themselves to her natural eye.

|| Thinks that she is looked down upon by every one, that she is of no importance in life, and feels insulted thereat.

|| Imagines that she wears some one else's nose.

|| Imagines to be dirty.

| Imagines she sees spiders.

Feels very short in morning; while walking; same in evening.

Woke at daylight feeling that she is a loathsome, horrible mass of disease (while the breasts were affected); could not bear to look at any portion of her body, not even hands, as it intensified feeling of disgust and horror; could not bear to have any one part of her body touch another, had to keep even fingers apart (cannot bear one foot to touch the other, Lac f.); felt that if she could not in some way get out of her body, she should soon become crazy; could not think of anything but her own condition; feels weak, and nerves thoroughly out of order.

|| After inhaling gas for extraction of teeth, very strange sensation in head (such as he felt when going off under gas); sometimes imagines heart or breathing is going to stop, or otherwise frightens himself, and this makes heart beat violently; occasionally very depressed, and fancies he is going out of his mind.

After menses, imagines all sorts of things about snakes.

Wakes at night with a sensation that she was lying on a large snake.

Sensation or delusion as if surrounded by myriads of snakes, some running like lightning up and down inside of skin; some that are inside seem long and thin; fears to put her feet on floor, lest she should tread on them and make them squirm and wind around her legs; is afraid to look behind her for fear that she will see snakes there, does not dream of them and is seldom troubled with them after dark; on going to bed she was afraid to shut her eyes for fear that a large snake, the size of her arm, would hit her in the face.

Worries herself lest pimples which appear during menses will prove to be little snakes, and twine and twist around each other.

Horrible visions, fears they will take objective form; when sitting still and thinking.

On lying down either by night or day begins to think how horrible it would be if a very sharp pain, like a knife, should go through her, and thought of it causes great mental distress.

|| Attacks of rage, cursing and swearing at slightest provocation.

|| Cannot bear to be left alone for an instant.

|| No desire to live.

Anxious.

Fear of disease; of consumption; of heart disease.

Sits and looks under chairs, table, sofa and everything in room, expecting yet dreading to see some terrible monster creep forth, and feeling all the time that if it does it will drive her raving mad; she is not afraid in dark, it is only in light where she can imagine that she can see them.

||| Fits of weeping two or three times a day.

|| Child cries and screams all the time, especially at night, and will not be pacified in any way.

|| When paroxysms of intense nervousness come on, feels like tearing off her clothes; takes off her rings; cannot bear anything to touch her, especially over left ovarian region, from which she frequently lifts bed clothes.

Depression of spirits, doubts her ability and success, thinks she will have heart disease and die of it.

|| Chronic 'blue' condition; everything seems so dark that it can grow no darker.

|| Gloomy feelings, < as headache gets worse.

|| Fears she will become unable to perform her duties.

|| Fear of death, with anxious expression of countenance.

|| Very nervous; constant dread; a feeling as if she was going to become unconscious.

|| Wakes distressed, and obliged to rise and occupy herself in some manner; fears she will be crazy.

Has great fear of falling down stairs at times.

Very cross and irritable only while headache lasts.

|| When awake, very irritable and cries constantly.

| Intense ugliness and hatefulness; writes to her best friends all sorts of mean and contemptible things.

|| Easily excited.

|| Too excited to allow examination of throat.

|| Feels weak, and nerves so thoroughly out of order that she cannot bear one finger to touch another.

|| Exceedingly nervous and irritable.

|| Very easily startled.

Maud R., aged 10, a light brunette, parents healthy, while playing one and a half years before, fell forward and hurt her chest. Nothing was thought of it at the time, but when brought to me she was pale, emaciated, capricious with no desire to play. Sleep disturbed by frightful dreams, during the day piteously begs her mother to take her, she is so afraid. She feels as though *snakes were on her back.* In response to advice, Lac can. 50m., one dose dry on her tongue, was given, and in 24 hours the child became more lively and cheerful, and very soon all abnormal sensations disappeared and never returned.—B. T. Balch, *Hom. Phys.*

Head—

Dizzy sensation with slight nausea.

|| After inhaling diphtheritic breath, light headed, with tingling on vertex and slight sore throat.

|| Constant noise in head, very confusing; < at night and at menses.

|| Wakes at night with sensation as if bed was in motion; noise in head bad beyond description; first thought on waking that headboard was swaying, and so occasioning distress, but found it arose from internal causes.

| Frontal headache.

Headache first on one side of the forehead, then on the other.

| On going into cold wind, terrible pain in forehead as if it would split open, > on going into warm room.

||| After midnight, very severe frontal headache, and a piercing pain on vertex.

||| Headache both frontal and occipital, < by turning eyeballs upward.

|| Headache over eyes, < when sewing.

Headache: in afternoon, principally over left eye; over left eye on first awaking.

Pain in forehead, afternoon, first on left side, then on right principally over left eye.

Throbbing pain just over right temple, then sharp pain in right socket of right eye and in right temple, disappearing quickly.

|| Pains and throbbing in temples.

|| Headaches mostly through temples, darting, stabbing; sometimes begin on right side and sometimes on left always going from one side to the other.

(Sick headaches beginning in nape; the pain settling gradually in right or left forehead), < on waking.

Pain in left occipital region running up when moving head.

Sharp pain like a stab in right temple, at 7 P.M.

| Pains in head during day, first on one side, then on other seem perfectly unbearable; > on first going into air, but soon grow <.

|| Headache from below eyes over whole head and top of shoulders.

|| Severe pressure on brain.

| Arose in morning with heavy, dull, frontal headache, and at 9 A.M., severe sharp pain on top of head, coming from nape of neck, then stretching across head forward; pain so severe that he presses top of head with hands; neck stiffened; bending head forward, or lying down, causes congestion, increasing pain; again pains subside for short time, and begin anew, either in front part of head, or in nape of neck, or all over head at once; when pain is frontal it causes lachrymation.

|| Darting pains from occiput to forehead; beating.

Darting pain across forehead and eyes.

|| Headaches seem unbearable, and are attended by pain in lumbar region; all pains cease as soon as throat gets <.

Headache < by noise or talking, > by keeping quiet; confused feeling in head.

Intense headache, entirely > by cold-water application, but soon returned, not, however, as severe.

Sharp lancinating pain, in a zigzag line from right side of forehead to an indefinite point in occiput; instantaneous, and sometimes repeated; as soon as it is felt, she lays aside whatever she is doing and lies down, from an indefinite dread that it will return; if at night, she goes to bed at once; has great dread of the pain, though not very severe; recurred for several days.

Sharp, throbbing pain in right side of forehead; then in left side of forehead, slightly.

Headache over left eye on first waking, and great pain in pelvis, most marked at right ovary.

Neuralgic pain in left side of head, followed by a film over left eye, wants to rub it off; not > by rubbing.

Headache in upper part of forehead, with sensation of a broad band pressed firmly across forehead from one temple to the other.

Headache over both eyes, extending back over left ear.

Slight pressure on vertex and over eyes, the day before menses ceased.

Dull pain in right temple and right eye, with pressure on vertex during menses.

Stiffness in occiput on turning head, with soreness on pressure.

Occipital headache, with shooting pains extending to forehead.

Headache commencing in occiput (3d day) and extending to vertex and forehead.

Sensation as if brain were alternately contracted and relaxed, several times rapidly; generally only when lying down; at various times all through proving.

Head very sore and itches almost all the time.

Sore pimples on scalp which discharge and form a scab, extremely painful when touched, or combing the hair < at night.

Excessive dandruff on head for past week.

Throbbing in forehead and temples, finally settling in eyes; eyes very sensitive to light during headache; eye-balls sore and painful, pains extending deep back into the brain with the headache.

Headache commencing all over head at once (second day) in the morning, a dull, heavy, confused feeling in head all day, becoming a severe ache towards evening, and settling in eyes and temples.

Headache worse from motion and stooping; better from cold applications.

|| Frequently wakes with sick headache, which seems to commence at nape.

|| Sick headaches, beginning in nape; pain settling gradually in right or left forehead.

Eyes—

Sharp pain in socket back of right eye, followed by tenderness in right temple; both transient.

Darting intense pain round left eye.

Heaviness of upper eyelid, with pain above left eye; burning in left eye; agglutination of left lids (rheumatism).

Eyes slightly swollen; profuse lachrymation; with catarrh.

Looking at different objects causes eyes to ache.

Pricking sensation in eyeballs; eyes sensitive to cold air.

Upper eyelids very heavy, can scarcely keep eyes open; very sleepy.

Pain in eyes when reading; followed by a film over them, apparently requiring to be wiped off before she can see.

| Tendency in retina to retain the impression of objects, especially of colours; or somewhat of the object last looked at is projected into the next.

| Sees faces before her eyes, < in the dark; the face that haunts her most is one that she has really seen.

Small floating discs before eyes occasionally, and showing primary colours at edge of discs.

| When reading the page does not look clear, but seems covered with various pale spots of red, yellow, green and other colours.

Occasionally when looking at an object sees red spots on it.

While looking at an object appears to see just beyond or out of the axis of vision an object passing across the field of sight; but on adjusting the eye to it, it is gone; it always appears as a small object, | | like a rat or bird, sometimes on the floor, at others in. the air.

Swelling and inflammation of upper and lower lids of both eyes, the left the worst.

Tired feeling in eyes, considerable lachrymation—both eyes—redness of conjunctiva, eye-ball sore, aching and painful; pains extending deep back into head, with headache; pains in eyes better from cold (wet) applications; eyes sensitive to artificial light.

| | Eyes sensitive to light.

| |Must have light, yet is intolerant of sunlight.

| | Sees big eyes and creeping things.

| | Difficulty in distinguishing objects; in reading, letters run together.

| | When looking in a mirror by gaslight, after exerting eyes, sees a green spot or a green band before her left eye, the band slanting downward from left eye to right cheek.

| |Square or round green spots or brown spots before left eye, when sun is bright; sometimes bright spots before left eye.

| | Frequent sensation of a film before eyes, with vertigo, and while thus suffering would see a small dark object, like a mouse or bird, coming up to her left.

| | Film over eyes when reading or looking closely.

|| Eyes blurred.

|| Heavy pain in the eye-balls with outward pressure.

|| Burning in left eye.

|| Eyes watery and discharging.

|| Eyes dull and lustreless.

|| Dark brown areolae under eyes.

Non-oedematous swelling of upper and lower lids; pink colour of lower lids; most noticeable on right.

|| Heaviness of left upper lid, with pain above left eye.

| Upper eyelids very heavy, could scarcely keep eyes open.

||Agglutination of left eyelids.

A dull aching pain in right eyeball, with sensation of dryness and tendency to lachrymation.

Ears—

Pain in right ear, sometimes intense.

Very sharp pain in right middle ear, while walking in wind; had to cover it with hand, which gave entire relief; sharp pain in right side also.

No pain during day, but is awakened several times during night by sore aching pains in middle and external ear of side on which she is lying; soon passes off when the pressure is removed.

||Green, odorless discharge.

Reverberation of voice as if speaking in a large, empty room; with pain in frontal region, first over one eye and then over the other.

|| Sounds seem very far off.

Ringing in right ear.

At night a buzzing in right ear.

Noises in ears; sensation as though ears were full; pains in both ears.

||More than any other remedy, relieved deafness from hereditary syphilis.

Earache the first time in her life on right side; aching

deep in ear, worse from cold air; had to keep ear covered all the time; pain in ear better by pressure with the point of the finger in the meatus; external ear sore and painful; soreness and swelling on right side from ear down side of face in region of parotid gland and angle of lower jaw, right side; soreness extending from right ear down side of neck to right shoulder, painful when turning the head.

Nose—

| Sore on right side of septum of nose; next day nose sore, constant inclination to pick at it and get the scab off; nose still sore on sixth day, and on seventh day was very painful to touch; but on eighth day scab came off nose, leaving it as well as ever.

Left nostril first dry, afterwards discharging a thin, ichorous fluid, excoriating nostrils.

Stuffed feeling in nose and throat.

Watery discharge, followed by dry sensation in nose. Fluent catarrh from both nostrils, with sensation of fulness in upper part of nose.

||| Profuse nocturnal nasal discharge, like gonorrhea, staining pillow greenish yellow.

||| One side of nose stuffed up, the other free and discharging thin mucus at times and thin blood; these conditions alternate, first one nostril stopped up and the other fluent, and *vice versa*.

Bad smell in nose.

Cannot bear smell of flowers; they seem to send a chill over heright

All drinks return by the nose, nothing being swallowed. || Fluids escape through nose while drinking.

Discharge of clear white mucus from nose and sneezing. || Nose cold.

||Epistaxis: when speaking or swallowing; at 4 P.M., returning at intervals.

| Considerable sneezing.

Head so stuffed she can hardly breathe.

Stuffed feeling in head, as of a severe cold in head. | Nasal discharge, excoriating nostrils and upper lip. Coryza, with discharge of thick white mucus.

Coryza; constant watery discharge from nose, excoriating nostrils and upper lip.

|| Nose became so bad that there was fear of destruction of bones; bloody pus discharged several times daily; nasal bones sore on pressure.

||Two very angry gatherings, one under left side of nose, and one on upper left nostril; both came to a head, and discharged matter and blood, and afterwards scabbed over; before discharge shooting pain.

Ozaena, mercurial or syphilitic, when the labial commissures and alae nasi are fissured, and when the angina is marked with the glazed appearance of mucous membranes.

Face—

Right cheek burns like fire, and is red after coming in from the cold.

Pain as from a knife-thrust from under left zygoma up to vertex.

Burning, flushing of face.

Marked pallor of face.

Lips dry and peeling off.

|| Jaw cracks while eating.

|| Face indicates great anxiety.

| Countenance pale and careworn.

| Face very red and then suddenly pale.

Face flushed; cheeks red.

Dark brown areolae under eyes.

|| Face flushed, swollen and hot; burns, feels dry.

|| In morning, left superior maxillary feels sore; most of time there is dull pain, < by exertion; sometimes throbbing pain, burning, throbbing, aching heat, sensation of fulness;

cannot wear her false teeth from soreness and swelling of maxillary; an exacerbation of pain leaves face very sore; pains > by warm applications, but only cold applications > soreness.

|| Red circular spot below right malar bone, burning to touch.

|| Flushes on left cheek.

| Lips dry and peeling off; dry and parched, but mouth constantly full of frothy saliva.

|| Seems to affect lower lip most, and blisters and fever sores on lip are amenable to its influence.

|| Submaxillary glands swollen.

|| Swelling of left parotid, with sore throat and loss of appetite.

|| Parotid gland first attacked, and disease extends to otherlands of neck; throat and sides of neck not tender to external touch.

|| Swelling of parotid passes from right to left, but more often from left to right.

Teeth—

Pain in left upper molars, coming through left temple through left ear.

Teeth sensitive to cold water.

|| Gums swollen, ulcerated, retracted, bleeding, teeth loose; caused by defective nutrition and exposure.

|| Paroxysmal gnawing pain in left upper canine, temporarily yields to any cold application.

Gums, upper and lower, very sore and red.

Toothache: severe pain came on suddenly about 10:30 every night. Would begin immediately on lying down, or getting warm in bed. Was obliged to arise and walk about the room for relief. Pain began in a much decayed right lower molar, soon extending to all the teeth on right side; > by application of cold water. Pain continued for a month, coming on each night; the teeth feel sensitive as if they were too long or too large. It was often daylight before I could get any sleep. Pain of a dull gnawing sensation like a worm gnawing at the teeth. It came on at same time, whether I had my evening meal early, late or went without it. If I retired earlier and fell asleep, pain would awaken me at 10:30.

Mouth.—Tongue coated brown.

Tongue dirty, deeply coated near back and centre, except on edges, which are bright red; at 9 P.M. tongue looks patched.

Taste: putrid; of lead, afternoon.

Swelling of left sublingual gland; ranula.

Mouth and throat covered with aphthous yellowish-white ulcerations, easily bleeding.

Itching of roof of mouth (Puls., Wyeth.).

Roof of mouth very sore, with blisters that break and leave loose skin; any seasoned food causes great pain.

Inside of lower lip feels tender and sore, and looks very red.

| Mouth very dry, without thirst.

Saliva: increased, slightly viscid; ran from mouth during sleep.

| Mouth constantly full of frothy mucus, but a constant inclination to swallow.

| Frothy mucus in mouth < by going into open air, and after eating.

Breath very offensive.

Talking is very difficult, and there is a disposition to talk through nose (nervous throat affection).

|| Nothing tastes natural, except salt food.

| Putrid taste in mouth.

|| Tongue generally red and moist.

| Tongue coated whitish, except edges, which are red.

| Tongue coated, dirty looking, centre to root.

| Tongue furred, whitish edges, centre and root darker.

|| Tongue: heavily coated, and dry to the tip; dirty coated,

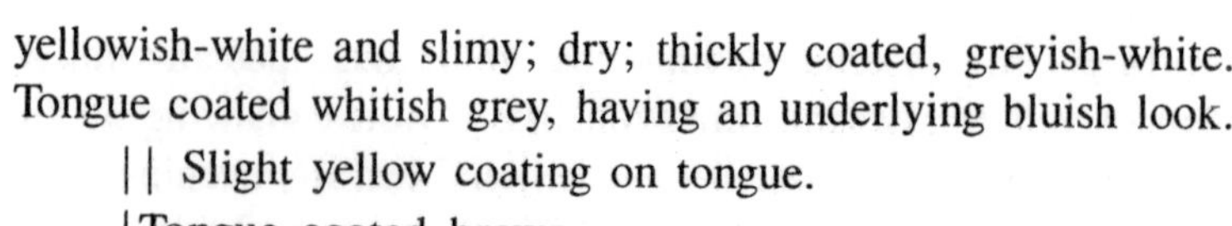

yellowish-white and slimy; dry; thickly coated, greyish-white. Tongue coated whitish grey, having an underlying bluish look.

|| Slight yellow coating on tongue.

| Tongue coated brown.

|| Difficulty in articulating, owing to a semi-paretic state of tongue, causing stuttering if she talks fast; has to speak very slowly.

|| Peculiar rattle in mouth, right along tongue; on attempting to hawk her mouth clear, mucus rattled along tongue quickly and continually; utterance was so indistinct as to be unintelligible, and every word she tried to speak was accompanied by this quick and continuous rattle along tongue.

|| Breath offensive, putrid.

|| Mouth dry and parched; drinks little and often. Increase in quantity of saliva which is slightly viscid.

|| Mouth constantly full of frothy saliva, lips dry, parched.

|| Constant spitting and drooling, very profuse, making chin and breast sore.

| During sleep saliva runs from mouth so as to wet pillow.

|| Stomatitis; stomacace; cancrum oris; nursing sore mouth.

Tongue coated white, breath offensive; sensation of a hair in back part of mouth on right side, which she tried ineffectually to wipe away; profuse expectoration of saliva.

Throat—

Quinsy: alternating sides; thick, tough pieces of diphtheritic membrane coming away, and new membrane constantly re-forming; swelling in throat so large and tense that mouth could not be closed.

| Throat sore; with severe headache; pain extending to chest; dry and sore; deep red colour on either side of throat opposite tonsils; on left side; painful to external pressure on both sides.

Sore throat, alternating sides, beginning and ending with menses.

Feeling of a lump in throat, which goes down when swallowing, but returns; throat < right side; < on swallowing saliva; afterwards, throat, which had been getting well, suddenly one evening grew rapidly <, but this time on left side.

Constant inclination to swallow, which causes pain extending to right ear.

Chill on movement; aching all over; great fatigue; desire for relief from cold drinks; bed too hard.

Shortly before going to bed, throat began to feel raw and sore; did not sleep well; next morning throat felt full and sore, somewhat < on right side; this condition continued two days, when it seemed to continue downward to chest.

|| Throat very sensitive to touch externally.

|| Sensation as if throat were closing and she would choke, sensation is between throat and nose; feels as if something in throat was either enlarged or relaxed; desires to keep mouth open lest she should choke; sometimes cannot swallow, because there seems to be a kind of muscular contraction in throat.

|| Paralytic symptoms strongly marked; as soon as he went to sleep would stop breathing, and was only kept alive by keeping him awake; apparently respiration was kept up by voluntary effort.

|| Talking is very difficult and there is a disposition to talk through nose.

||| Swallowing very difficult, painful, almost impossible; fluids return through the nose.

|| Uvula elongated and very much swollen, diphtheritic coating on it; tonsils swollen and coated; back of throat patched, extending up to hard palate; odor offensive and diphtheritic.

Constant inclination to swallow, causes pain extending to both ears.

Pricking sensation in throat, as if full of sticks.

Pricking and cutting pains through tonsils on swallowing, shooting up to ears.

| Pain in throat pushes toward left ear.

|| On swallowing acute pain at one time on right side of throat, and again on left side.

|| Throat > after drinking cold or warm; < by empty swallowing.

|| Throat sensitive.

| Tickling and sense of constriction in upper part of throat, causing constant dry hacking cough.

|| Sensation of ball or round body in left side of throat, and feeling that it could be removed with a knife.

Sensation of muscular contraction in the throat; sometimes inability to swallow.

Marked sensation of lump in throat on left side, when swallowing; pain extends to ear.

||Sensation of lump in right side of throat, with a feeling that she could take hold of it with her ringers and pull it out; accompanied by a very annoying pricking, stitching feeling; constant inclination to swallow saliva, which causes soreness of throat.

|| Lump on left side of pharynx below tonsil, causing an enlargement that filled each arch of palate, nearly to right side.

|| Most pain when swallowing solids, no aversion to cold drink; when swallowing solid food it seems to pass over a lump, with sore and aching pains extending to and into left ear.

| Soreness of throat commences with a tickling.

| Throat feels raw.

|| Sensation of rawness, commencing usually on left side of throat.

| Throat feels dry, husky, as if scalded by hot fluid.

|| Throat has a burnt and drawn feeling as from caustic.

| Pain in right side of throat in region of tonsil.

|| Wakes with throat and mouth painfully dry.

|| Throat very dry and sore, much inflamed, < right side; palate red, uvula elongated; very painful deglutition.

| | Throat sore, cedematous, puffed, tonsils badly swollen.

| Especially shining, glazed and red appearance of throat.

| | Sore throat, pains in whole body and limbs, severe headache.

| Sore throat on left side; painful to external pressure both sides.

| | Sore throat on right side, low down, and extending up to ear; pain when swallowing; sensitive to external pressure; slight coryza.

| | Throat sore, swollen, red and glistening.

| | Sore spot on left side of throat, only at night, removed by 1 A.M.; next night same on right side of throat; after 1 A.M. returned no more.

| Crusts on skin, with grayish yellow matter under them; mucous follicles of throat raised and swollen, and covered with whitish, cream coloured mucus; bloody pus discharged from nose several times a day; nasal bones sore to pressure.

| Partial suppression of urine; throat sore and of an oedema-tous, puffy appearance; next morning, pulse 130; temperature 102^0; tonsils badly swollen; great indisposition to take food or drink,

| | | Soreness of throat commences with a tickling sensation, which causes constant cough; then a sensation of a lump on one side, causing constant deglutition; this condition entirely ceases, only to commence on the opposite side, and often alternates, again returning to its first condition; these sore throats are very apt to begin and end with menses.

| | Sore throat just before menses for several years ever since diphtheria; small yellowish white patches of exudation on tonsil of affected side, with great difficulty of swallowing, and sharp pains moving up into ear; these patches are also present on back of throat and uvula; some are quite yellow and some are white; scraping them off makes them bleed.

| Shortly before going to bed, throat began to feel raw

and sore; did not sleep well; next morning, throat felt full and sore, somewhat < on right right side; this condition continued two days, when it seemed to continue downward to chest.

On waking in morning, throat felt as if there were lumps in it like two eggs, and sore all the time, especially when swallowing; cold water seemed to > momentarily; in evening, examination revealed both tonsils much swollen and very red, left most, and distinct patches on left tonsil.

Right tonsil red and swollen; pain in tonsil of gnawing character; < at night; dreams of snake in bed.

||| Tonsils inflamed and very sore, red and shining, almost closing throat; dryness of fauces and throat; swelling of sub-maxillary glands.

Quinsy just ready to discharge, disappeared without discharging, in an unusually short time; the trouble had been changing from one side to other and back again; has not returned.

| Sore throat, rapidly growing <; fever; difficult swallowing; right side <; right tonsil intensely inflamed, bright red and greatly enlarged, and a yellowish grey spot on inner surface; whole pharynx, uvula and velum much inflamed; spot became larger, and others formed in pharynx; left tonsil became nearly as large as right; fetid breath; subsequently a bright scarlet eruption on face, neck, hands and chest, like scarlatina; almost total inability to swallow, especially fluids; aversion to liquids, particularly water.

|| Quinsy: suppuration ran from left tonsil to right then from right to left then back again to right then both tonsils equally; and again one tonsil would > and the other grow <; whole posterior portion of throat was an osdematous swelling, rising-up like an insurmountable barrier; thick tough pieces of diphtheritic membrane were coming away, and new membranes constantly reforming; swelling in throat so large and tense that mouth could not be closed.

| | Mucous follicles raised or swollen, and covered with a whitish, cream coloured mucus.

| | Whole membrane of throat swollen, dark red, with grey patches and small, irregular shaped ulcers; membrane peeled off occasionally; articulation and deglutition intensely painful; < after sleep.

| | White ulcers on tonsils.

| Sore throat, beginning at left tonsil, swollen and ulcerated; throat feels swollen and raw, pricking and cutting pains shoot through tonsils when swallowing; submaxillary glands swollen, sore and aching pain in left ear; most pain when swallowing solids; food seems to pass over a lump; no aversion to cold drink; while drinking, fluid escaped through nose.

| | Sore throat commencing on left tonsil, which was swollen and ulcerated, and presented a depression covered by a white patch; the disease later extended to palate and right tonsil, the parts red and shining.

| | Throat highly inflamed, swollen, almost closed, grey diphtheritic spots on left side of throat.

| | Sore throat, ulcer on inner side of each tonsil, tonsils red and slightly enlarged, rest of the throat dry.

| | Ulcers increase in size and number, but neighbouring membrane looks clearer.

| | Small, round or irregular, grey white ulcers on tonsils and fauces, both sides.

| | Tonsils swollen as almost to close throat.

| | Right tonsil covered with ash grey membrane extending along free palatine border to uvula, which it had already involved; room loaded with diphtheritic odor; next day membrane had passed centre, involving whole arch of palate, and reaching far down on left tonsil.

| | Right tonsil raw, swollen; grey white membrane there and on fauces.

| | Whole of right tonsil covered with diphtheritic patch.

|| Both tonsils swollen and covered with spots of exudation, like the mould on preserves.

|| Tongue, fauces, tonsils, all swollen and covered with a dirty coating.

|| On each tonsil a very thick exudation, covering nearly entire surface; while examining a large piece of membrane was accidentally detached from one tonsil, followed by considerable hemorrhage.

|| Throat very sore, tonsils enlarged, especially left very large white patches; tonsils and pharynx deep purple red; putrid odor from throat; after patches were expectorated, they left throat very sore, raw and bloody.

|| Throat very sore, < left side; large greenish ulcers on both tonsils, surrounded by grey white exudation, parts not covered are a deep purple red; swelling externally on both sides; after exudation on tonsils disappeared, a raw, bloody surface was left.

|| White patches, like eggs of flies, on both tonsils, extending thence to back of throat; tonsils enlarged and deep red; felt she would suffocate at night from full feeling in throat, which prevented sleep; swallowing toast gave some pain, but seemed to clear throat; and she had to gulp it down.

|| Gargling with warm water brought up a stringy mucus.

|| Whole membrane of throat highly inflamed, swollen, and glands enlarged on both sides.

|| False membrane in throat, thick, grey, or slightly yellow, or dark and almost black, or white and glistening, almost like mother of pearl, or fish scales.

|| Dark red, angry streaks of capillaries in fauces, giving place to shining, glistening deposit, or tough membrane; half arch is filled with sticky, fetid saliva.

||| Diphtheritic membrane white like china; mucous membrane of throat glistening as if varnished; membranes leave

one side and go to the other repeatedly; desire for warm drinks, which may return through nose; post-diphtheritic paralysis.

Glossy, shining appearance; disposition on part of membrane to change its position in fauces.

|| Ulcers on throat shine like silver gloss, symptoms went from side to side; croupy symptoms not well marked; after exudation was cleared off, a deep excavation was left.

|| Diphtheritic deposits look as if varnished; exudations migratory, now here, now there.

|| Thick membranous mass lying on soft palate, left side; diphtheritic masses covering uvula and posterior wall of throat; next day, membrane on soft palate thicker, dirty brown on uvula and posterior walls and pillars of throat, much more extensive and offensive; very difficult deglutition; a large membranous mass, which threatened suffocation, having been removed by forceps; on following morning a second membrane had taken place of first, and walls of throat were covered with a dirty grey exudation; uvula almost black, and coarse shreds of membrane hanging from it.

| In morning throat very sore; right tonsil covered with ulcers and patches, which extended over palate and covered left tonsil; next day membrane extended across posterior wall of pharynx; uvula elongated, accompanied by chilliness, high fever, pains in head, back and limbs, great restlessness and extreme prostration. This was pronounced to be "severe diphtheria," but it soon got well.

|| Throat sore, but little swelling, tonsils very slightly enlarged; soreness of throat, first chiefly right then left; well marked diphtheritic membrane on both sides of the throat situated on an inflamed red base, 3/4 inch long, 1/4 inch wide, 1/2 inch thick, and the same length and width as at the base; anterior edge a dirty yellow; centre more organized, pearly, glistening, white like cartilage; membrane on right side seems more firm and dense, and disappeared later.

| Severe chills, headache, pain in back and limbs, restlessness and sore throat; three days later right tonsil covered with

ashy grey membrane, extending along free palatine border to uvula, which it had already involved; peculiar diphtheritic odor in room; pulse small; skin clammy; rapid vital exhaustion; next day membrane involved whole arch of palate and passed down to left tonsil.

| Roof of mouth and back wall of pharynx coated with a greyish yellow deposit, greater part of which soon disappeared, lasting only about an hour; throat very much > by noon, deposit had nearly disappeared, but < again by night.

| | Throat covered with diphtheritic membrane; uvula elongated, swollen and covered with black and white or grey diphtheritic deposit; back of throat extending to hard palate, all covered; breath very offensive; left side of neck swollen and almost even with jaw; great difficulty in swallowing-; after throat began to improve, disease seemed to work through whole alimentary canal, for uvula and parts were very much swollen, and every little while there would be involuntary discharges of diphtheritic matter from uvula and rectum.

| Patch of diphtheritic membrane appeared first on right tonsil, then on left and frequently alternated sides; swelling of neck (submaxillary and lymphatic glands) also alternated in like manner; < during and after a cold storm from northeast; tickling in throat when drinking; one side of nose stopped up, the other free and discharging thin mucus at times and thin blood; this condition of nose also alternated; non-oedematous swelling of eyelids, pink colour of under lid, particularly of right eye; breathing hoarse and croupy, at times entire stoppage of breath; often snoring, and only possible through mouth; obstinate constipation, frequent desire, with darting pains in rectum, no power to expel; stool large in size, whitish, rough, scaly, hard; could not bear to be left alone an instant; saw big eyes and creeping things; must have light, yet is intolerant to light of sun; urine scanty, infrequent, no desire, coffee coloured; 80 per cent, of albumen and much mucus; quantity less than a gill in twenty-four hours.

| Fever: bathed in warm perspiration, especially about

the face, neck and hands; anxious expression; eyes watery and discharging; wants to sit up in mother's arms; cries and desists at every attempt to nurse; reaches for water, yet refuses to take it; respiration hoarse; crying whispered and broken, often no sound at all; pulse 170; tongue, fauces and tonsils swollen and covered with dirty coating; drooling from mouth; throat tender to touch externally; thick, dirty, grey, diphtheritic membrane, covering free border of epiglottis, and extending off to each side; child refuses to swallow and sputters out the medicine, some returning through the nose.

Soreness of throat, accompanied by intense heat; pulse scarcely to be counted; prostration so complete that patient refused even to make an effort to take medicine; temperature 102.6°; great sensitiveness of throat externally; symptoms after sleep; very thick exudate, covering nearly entire surface of each tonsil, which, if forcibly removed, is followed by considerable hemorrhage.

| Throat highly inflamed, swollen, almost closed; grey, diphtheritic patches on left side of throat; difficult breathing, at times suffocative spells, pulse 140; face flushed, swollen and hot; tongue dry and thickly coated, greyish white.

On third day right tonsil swollen and on it a small diphtheritic patch, rest of throat inflamed; on fourth day both tonsils swollen and covered with diphtheritic patches, with difficult deglutition; high fever, restlessness, cried out and talked in sleep; complained of pains in head, back and limbs; bright scarlet redness on chest and around neck, which, on fifth day, extended all over body and legs; disease now at highest point; skin, in large patches, assumed a dark red colour bordering on purple; whole body swollen; membrane, swelling and soreness on right side; deglutition impossible; refusing to drink while complaining of intense thirst; characteristic fetor in room; soreness on right side decreased and commenced on left; left tonsil and posterior wall of pharynx covered with membrane; posterior nares invaded; marked sensation of lump in throat on left side, when swallowing, with pain extending to left earight; tongue coated dirty, yellow white and slimy; absence of prostration; improvement commenced on seventh day and remedy was discontinued. .

| Pains in limbs, small of back and head disappear, and throat becomes more painful, but looks better; often ulcers increase in size and number, but neighbouring membrane looks clearer; < by empty deglutition; throat feels stiff; > after drinking, warm or cold, no thirst, but dry mouth; pain pushes toward left ear; right tonsil raw, swollen, grey white membrane there and on fauces; epistaxis when speaking or swallowing, in one case; sweat all over; great exhaustion with poisoned feeling; frequent micturition, urine dark; restless, legs and whole body; face burns dry; constant spitting, drooling;, ulcers small, round or irregular, grey white; voice hoarse, interrupted by weakness and hoarseness.

|| Throat filled with substance that looked like "smear kase;" throat, tongue, roof of mouth, gums and cheeks completely lined with this substance; mouth and throat filled with loose particles; horrible odor.

| Heaviness, and stomach bloated and tender; enlargement of tonsils, left tonsil <; feels weak; cannot eat or drink anything without pain in pit of stomach; shortness of breath and general languor.

|| Membrane would leave throat, and a very severe interstitial hemorrhage of bright red blood would ensue; hemorrhage would slowly improve, and membrane appear again in throat; these had continued to alternate for several days.

|| False membrane, thick grey, yellow or dark, surrounding mucous membrane dark or bright, may be < on either side, or inflammation shift from side to side, generally < on left.

|| False membrane, thick, yellowish grey, often greenish.

||Pharyngeal inflammation, with wholesale destruction

of epithelium, viscidity of saliva, heat of palms; absolute necessity for constant change of position.

|| Thick, dirty grey diphtheritic membrane covering free border of epiglottis, and extending off to each side.

|| Uvula pretty free from membrane, but intensely sore and bleeds.

Uvula coated (in seven cases).

|| After membrane exfoliates, mucous membrane appears raw and bloody, with increased deglutition.

|| In most cases of diphtheria, the throat symptoms begin on right side.

|| Inflammation, ulcers and swelling shift from side to side, generally < on left.

||| Diphtheria and diphtheritic croup; membranous croup.

Awoke about four A.M. (second day) with a feeling that she was going to have sore throat; rawness and soreness in throat on right side.

Swollen feeling in throat.

Feeling as if she wanted to expectorate but could get nothing up.

Sensation of a sac (lump ?) in her throat on right side which seemed to descend when she swallowed, and scraped or rubbed against the mucous membrane as it went down; returning after deglutition.

Fauces and tonsils very sore and red.

Right tonsil appeared puckered and drawn up from circumference to centre.

In centre of right tonsil, a small black spot about the size of a pin-head

Two long shaped ulcers on right tonsil, toward inner edge.

On third day a ring of small yellow blisters around each ulcer, which later presented appearance of a false membrane.

False membrane on right tonsil but not on left.

Left tonsil became sore and inflamed on second day, when the right was not nearly so painful; by evening pain and soreness returned to right side when left side was relieved. This alternation from side to side continued one week when the painful symptoms wholly subsided.

All deglutition painful, but worse when swallowing solid food.

Pain extends to ear when swallowing.

Pains in throat worse in cold air.

Throat feels stiff as a board.

Feeling of lump in throat which goes down when swallowing, but returns; throat < on right side.

A lady, aged 50, a widow, mother of one child, is syphilitic, and has suffered very much with inflammation and ulceration of the tonsils and fauces—which are completely honeycombed by abscesses—and for the last month the pain and soreness has changed from one side to the other every day. For instance, the side that was sore yesterday is well to-day, and the side that was well yesterday is the sore one to-day. She has been treated a long time for this disease without benefit, by a professed homeopath.

Four doses, 200th, of this remedy were given, two each day, when improvement set in, and in ten days she was well, and has so remained without further medication.

"Right to left, and from left to right"—daily. — *Wakeman.*

One of my cases was little Moody, son of Moody, of "Moody and Sankey," sick with scarlatina "for the third time" (so reported). His throat was full of large, foul, grey-yellow patches, deglutition extremely painful after sleep and from swallowing acid fruits, lumpy sensation in throat, unrest, delirium with undefined fears, considerable bright-red, fine eruption on face and chest, itching with dry skin. (I do not remember to have seen a case of diphtheria, so-called, fairly well defined, but some eruption appeared at some time during the disease). Lac can. cm., one dose dry, and in forty-eight hours after a dry powder of cmm. potency, cured promptly without any other remedy.

In the use of Lac can. in diphtheria I have observed an interesting point: "It was twenty-four hours from the appearance to the entire disappearance of the patch in the throat" in the original proving. In prescribing I was just twenty-four hours before repeating the dose or reconsidering the case. If no better at end of twenty-four hours, with symptoms still pointing to Lac can., I give another powder of a different potency. I have thus obtained much more prompt and satisfactory results than when the remedy was given in water and repeated every three or four hours.—*Nichols.*

Appetite—

Appetite improved; increased.

Cannot satisfy her hunger.

| Desire for highly-seasoned dishes, which is very unusual; has used pepper, mustard, and salt freely.

No appetite.

Considerable thirst.

Great hunger for large quantities, often.

|| Craves milk and drinks much of it.

Aversion to anything sweet.

No appetite or thirst.

|| Thirst for a little at a time, but often, as throat is so dry and hot.

|| Thirst.

|| Great thirst for large quantities, often.

|| Desire for warmish water with a pinch of salt in it.

|| Aversion to liquids, especially water.

|| Appetite and strength failing; dislike to food, especially fat or greasy.

Stomach—

| Nausea, with headache, on waking; continuing all morning.

Nausea > by eructations of wind.

At 5 P.M. while smoking a cigar, great nausea with severe pain in stomach-pit; vomiting seemed imminent, but the sensation ceased in four or five minutes.

At 10:15 A.M., empty, weak feeling in stomach-pit; next day, same at 6 P.M.

| Weak, sinking feeling at stomach-pit, on waking in morning.

Burning in epigastric region, feeling of a weight and pressure of a stone in stomach.

||| Great faintness of stomach and nausea.

|| Nausea at beginning of diphtheria.

The almost constant diphtheritic discharges from mouth and nose nearly ceased, and she almost immediately had spells of sickness of stomach, and would occasionally vomit pieces of membrane.

|| Frequent attacks of severe vomiting, and when not so, always feeling of nausea, and fear to eat.

|| Gnawing, hungry feeling, not > by eating; everything she eats, except fish, makes her worse; the thought of milk makes her sick.

Dyspeptic pain, as from a stone, or undigested food, in stomach-pit at 9:45 P.M.; followed by a stabbing pain in right lung, just below nipple.

| Burning in epigastric region; feeling of weight and pressure of stone in stomach; very thirsty; abdomen swollen and burning, with bearing down pains therein; mucous, yellow, liquid stools; pulse 100; pains and throbbing in temples; flushes on left cheek; red, circular spot below right malar bone, burning to touch; no appetite, cannot bear food; jaw cracks while eating.

|| Stomach tender and bloated; cannot eat or drink anything without pain in stomach-pit.

|| Beating in stomach and bowels.

|| Severe throbbing in region of solar plexus; when it

becomes very severe, which it did daily for hours at a time, it would seem to extend or continue upwards to head, when dizziness and lightness of head would supervene, requiring her to lie down at once, otherwise she would fall violently to the floor.

| | Gastralgia or cardialgia, < at menses, so she would drop to the floor, comes and goes suddenly.

Abdomen.—Pain in right side of pelvis; while it lasted there was no pain in left side.

Pain and burning in left side of abdomen and pelvis, with weight and dragging on that side; clothes feel very heavy.

| |Feeling of tension in left groin; does not want to walk or stand, as it < the sensation; > by flexing leg on abdomen.

Very acute pain in left groin, extending up left side to crest of ilium; > by stool; sometimes the pain is in track of colon.

Abdomen swollen, and sensitive to deep pressure, which also = nausea, the nausea passes off when pressure is removed.

Felt as though abdomen and chest were firmly compressed all over, as if the skin were contracted.

Abdomen very sensitive to pressure and weight of clothes, entirely > by removing them, during very profuse menses.

Pains in abdomen intermittent.

Pain in pelvis, principally over right ovarian region.

Headache (left) on first waking, and great pain in pelvis, most marked at right ovary.

Pressure from within outwards, as if contents of abdomen would be forced out literally, just above pelvis.

Sensation while walking as if abdomen would burst.

Severe burning pain right hypochondriac and iliac region and corresponding part of back, extending across back to left side of abdomen; < when on feet or when fatigued, > lying down.

| Abdomen very hard and swollen, in evening.

|| Abdomen swollen and burning, with bearing down pains therein.

|| Extreme heat in abdomen.

| Severe shooting pain in abdomen, passing in all directions.

|| Intense sharp pain in left side of abdomen, with nausea while leaning forward.

|| Pain and burning in left side of abdomen and pelvis, with weight and dragging on that side; clothes feel heavy.

Pain in pelvis, principally in right ovarian region.

| Headache over left eye on first waking, and great pain in pelvis, most marked at right ovary.

| Pains in abdomen intermittent.

|| Pain in abdomen, < leaning forward; > leaning back.

|| Smarting in right groin; pains seem to be in pelvic bones, uterus and limbs.

| Very acute pain in left groin, extending up left side to crest of ilium, > by stool; sometimes pain in track of colon.

Stool and Rectum—

Frequent desire for stool all through provings.

When having a soft passage great tenesmus; rectum does not act as if it had lost power, but as if it could not expel faeces because they are soft, and adhere to the parts like clay.

Constipation; occasionally natural passage; urgent desire for stool, but passes nothing but wind, or possibly one or two small pieces like sheep-dung; considerable wind in abdomen, with rumbling, but never any pain.

Profuse diarrhea, with colic pain; diarrhea watery, profuse, coming out with great force.

Great constipation before and after menses; bowels very loose (not diarrhea) during menses.

|| Mucous, liquid, yellow stools.

| Constipation.

|| Obstinate constipation; frequent desire with darting

pain in rectum, no power to expel; stool large, whitish, rough, scaly, hard.

Frequent urging, passing only flatus or small black balls.

Urinary Organs—

Urination causes intense pain in urethra, soon passing off.

Sensation after urinating, as if bladder were still full; continued desire to urinate.

Frequent desire to urinate, which if not immediately attended to causes pain in bladder; a numb, dull sensation; if not > by urination it spreads over abdomen and left side to ends of fingers; never in head; would frequently wake at night dreaming of the pain, and would have to urinate to > it.

Constant desire to urinate, passing large quantities frequently; at night she dreams of urinating, and wakes to find an immediate necessity; a less strong and healthy person would probably have wet the bed.

(Nocturnal enuresis, a specific.)

| | Constant desire to urinate, with intense pain.

| Constant inclination to urinate which was restrained, as urination caused intense pain when coming in contact with vulva.

| Urine unusually frequent and dark.

| Urine frequent; especially at night; scanty, high coloured; red sediment.

| | Urine very scanty and dark.

| Urine dark, heavily loaded with thick reddish sediment that adhered in different coloured circles to bottom and sides of vessel.

| | Great difficulty in urinating.

| | Urinating only once in twenty-four hours, and then copiously, but with some difficulty and slight irritation.

| | Urine scanty, infrequent, coffee coloured, no desire to urinate, quantity less than a gill in twenty-four hours, eighty per cent, albumen, with much mucus.

| | No urine for 47 3/4 hours, bladder pretty full, parts fearfully swollen, and irritation on urination very great.

| | Urine partially suppressed.

| Constant desire to urinate, urine scanty.

Males Sexual Organs—

Sexual desire quite marked.

Right spermatic cord, low down, sore to touch.

| Chancre on prepuce, left side of frenum; penis greatly swollen; chancre like a cauliflower excrescence, red, smooth, and glistening, granulating rapidly from centre to circumference.

(Small sore at entrance of urethra; parts of glans around urethra an open ulcer, exhaling most fetid smell, and with most excruciating pain; red, glistening appearance.)

| | Gonorrheal pains, intermittent, in front, middle, or posterior part of urethra; when the gonorrhea is >, catarrh sets in.

| | Large chancre on dorsum of penis, with a fungoid bacteric mass covering whole of corona glandis, which was at first of a glossy, shining white appearance, and later covered with a fungus, looking like fully developed aphthte, edges of swollen prepuce covered with nodosities and itching.

| Penis enormously swollen, and a chancre on glans like a cauliflower excrescence, over half an inch in diameter; it was red, smooth and glistening; no pain; in a week there appeared two small chancres, deep, sharp edges, clean, and with same shining appearance.

| | Small sore at entrance of urethra; kept getting <; prepuce involved for about half an inch, and parts of glans around urethra an open ulcer, exhaling most fetid smell, and with most excruciating pain; hemorrhage at 10 P.M. every evening, and during day when removing dressings; constant desire to urinate, with intense pain; no sleep for a fortnight, red, glistening appearance.

Prepuce involved for about an eighth of an inch, and parts

of glans penis around urethra an open ulcer exhaling most fetid smell; pain excruciating; hemorrhages at ten every evening and during day when removing dressing; desire to urinate constant, and accompanied by intense pain; had not slept for a fortnight; red, glistening appearance of ulcer.

|| Buboes and chancres.

Females Sexual Organs—

Menses scanty; terribly cross and impatient first day, severe paroxysmal pains in uterine region, causing nausea; occasional pain in left ovarian region, passing about half-way down thigh, on upper part of it; all these pains > by bending backward; pain and aching in right lumbar region when leaning forwards (as in sewing) even for a short time; entire > when bending back.

Menses scanty at first; with pain in left ovary.

Menses very profuse; abdomen very sensitive to pressure and weight of clothes, entire > by removing them.

Several cases of membranous dysmenorrhea.

Dysmenorrhea, pain in left groin, with bearing down and nervousness.

Leucorrhea all day, but none at night, even after taking a long walk.

Slight leucorrhea during the day, < when standing or walking.

Severe pain in right ovarian region, completely > by a flow of bright-red blood, which lasted an hour, and did not return.

In afternoon, intermittent, sharp pains in right ovarian region.

Constant pain in right ovary.

Sharp pains beginning in left ovary, and darting like lightning either towards right ovarian region, or else up left side and down arm, or sometimes down both thighs; but generally down left leg to foot, which is numb; pains like labor-pains;

accompanied by great restlessness of legs and arms, and great aching in lumbar region; (5th d. after premature labor).

|| Sharp, lancinating pains like knives cutting upward from os uteri, and as these were being relieved, sensation as of needles darting upwards in uterus.

| Escape of flatus from vagina.

Pressure on anterior part of vulva, entire > by sitting; sensation as if everything were coming out at vulva; with frequent desire to urinate and smarting in urethra.

| Itching in left side of labia, with rough eruptive condition on left side of vagina, with acrid leucorrhea; excoriating severely.

Great swelling of left labia, and terrible pain while urinating (from gonorrhea).

| Intense painful soreness of vulva, extending to arms, coming on very suddenly about noon, and lasting for about two hours; came on again during evening; could not walk, stand or sit; > by lying on back and separating the knees as far as possible.

| Raw and bad-smelling sores between labia and thighs, in folds of skin; < when walking, would rather keep still all the time; these sores are covered with a disgusting white exudation.

Sexual organs extremely excited; very much < from the slightest touch, as putting the hand on the breast, or from the pressure of vulva when sitting, or the slight friction caused by walking.

After-pains very distressing, extending to thighs, rather < on right side.

Menses very stringy and sticky, cannot get rid of them.

Urination caused intense pain in vulva, when even the least drop of urine came in contact with it.

Breasts very sore and sensitive to pressure for a day or two during menses.

| Breasts very sore and painful, with sharp, darting pain

in right ovarian region extending to knee, very painful and must keep leg flexed (1st d. after miscarriage at 6th month).

Constant pain in breasts, they feel very sore when going up or down stairs.

Constant pain in nipples.

Breasts sensitive to deep pressure.

Breasts painful; feel as if full of very hard lumps < going up or down stairs.

Loss of milk while nursing, without known cause.

Calactorrhea (many causes).

Dries up the milk when nursing.

Given for an ulcerated throat to a nursing woman, it cured the throat and nearly dried up the milk.

After two doses of c. m. rapid decrease in size of breasts and quantity of milk in a lady who wanted to wean her child.

Heat in ovarian and uterine region (with menses); inflammatory and congestive condition of ovaries before menses; especially of right ovary, with extreme soreness and sensitiveness, which makes every motion and position, even breath, painful.

|| Pain in abdomen principally in right ovarian region.

|| Sharp pain in right ovary.

| In afternoon, sharp pains in right ovarian region, not constant but intermittent.

| Severe pain in right ovarian region, > by flow of bright red blood.

| Pain in left ovarian region; across lower part of abdomen.

|| Constant burning pain in left ovarian region, extending from left leg even to foot.

| Inflammatory and congested condition of uterus, with extreme soreness and tenderness, that made every motion, position, and even breath painful.

|| Parenchymatous metritis (two cases), in one, uterus

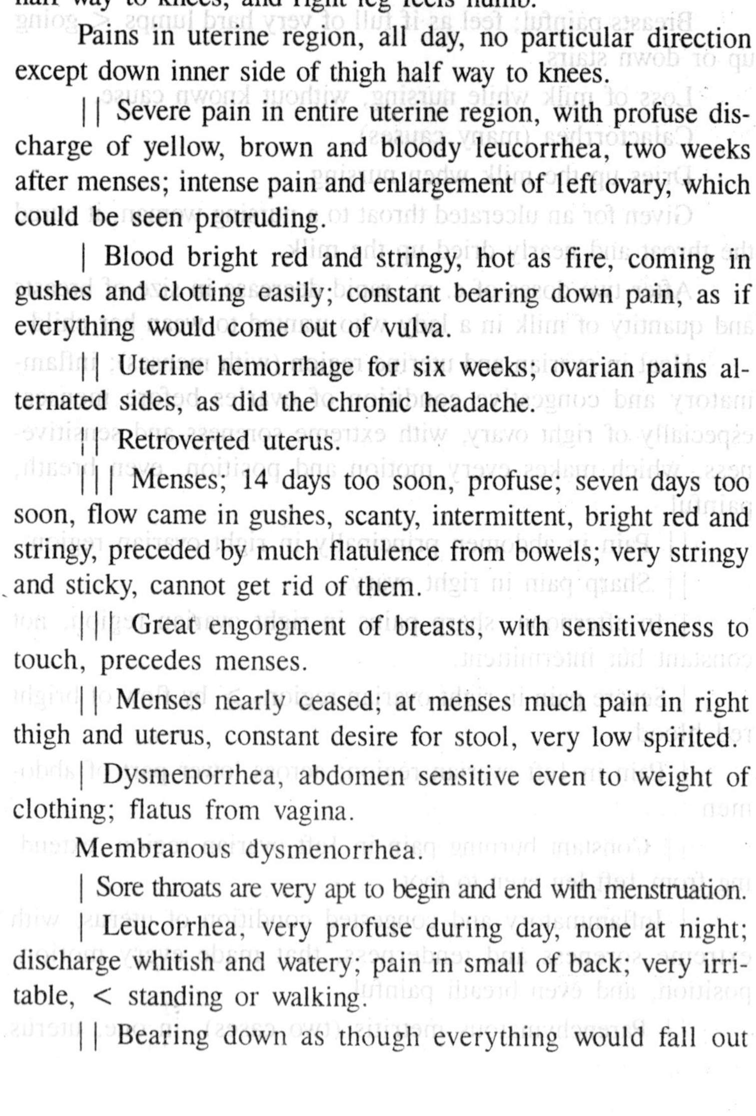

three times as large as natural, round as a ball, and body very hard, cervix obliterated by altered form of body; uterus sensitive.

| | Much pain before and after menses, severe headache and entire prostration for first day or so.

| | Pain in uterine region, passing down inside of thighs, half way to knees, and right leg feels numb.

Pains in uterine region, all day, no particular direction except down inner side of thigh half way to knees.

| | Severe pain in entire uterine region, with profuse discharge of yellow, brown and bloody leucorrhea, two weeks after menses; intense pain and enlargement of left ovary, which could be seen protruding.

| Blood bright red and stringy, hot as fire, coming in gushes and clotting easily; constant bearing down pain, as if everything would come out of vulva.

| | Uterine hemorrhage for six weeks; ovarian pains alternated sides, as did the chronic headache.

| | Retroverted uterus.

| | | Menses; 14 days too soon, profuse; seven days too soon, flow came in gushes, scanty, intermittent, bright red and stringy, preceded by much flatulence from bowels; very stringy and sticky, cannot get rid of them.

| | | Great engorgment of breasts, with sensitiveness to touch, precedes menses.

| | Menses nearly ceased; at menses much pain in right thigh and uterus, constant desire for stool, very low spirited.

| Dysmenorrhea, abdomen sensitive even to weight of clothing; flatus from vagina.

Membranous dysmenorrhea.

| Sore throats are very apt to begin and end with menstruation.

| Leucorrhea, very profuse during day, none at night; discharge whitish and watery; pain in small of back; very irritable, < standing or walking.

| | Bearing down as though everything would fall out

through vagina, with very frequent desire to urinate, and smarting in urethra.

|| Great swelling of left labia and terrible pain while urinating; from gonorrhea.

|| Foul smell from genitals.

|| Pressure on labia causes a slight flow of blood; menstruation commenced entirely normal.

|| Great irritation about vulva and rectum.

| Urination causes intense pain in vulva, when even least drop of urine comes in contact with it.

| Itching of vulva.

| Breasts very sore, sensitive to least pressure; dull, constant aching pain in them all evening.

| Breasts very painful, but no lumps; pains are caused by least jar; has to hold breasts firmly when going up or down stairs; breasts < towards evening, pressure of her arm, in natural position, caused considerable pain.

| Breasts very painful and sore; feel as if full of hard lumps, very painful when going up or down stairs.

|| Soreness and enlargement of breasts.

| Breasts seem very full.

| Constant pain in nipples.

Afterpains very severe, and shooting down thighs.

Knots and cakes in breast, after miscarriage,

Calactorrhea.

Loss of milk while nursing, without known cause.

Serviceable in almost all cases where it is required to dry up milk.

Given for an ulcerated throat to a nursing woman, it cured throat and nearly dried up milk.

Respiratory Organs—

Slight hoarseness, with now and then a change of voice, after walking, but soon passing away.

Cough from tickling in upper anterior part of larynx, < when talking and also when lying.

Cough from tickling under middle of sternum.

Cough with pain and oppression of chest; it jars her all over.

Loss of voice, cannot speak in a whisper (pharyngitis).

Marked soreness on touching larynx (diphtheria).

Sensation as if the breath would leave her when lying down and trying to sleep; has to jump up and stir around for an hour or so every night.

|| Loss of voice.

|| Throat troubles her much if she reads aloud or talks more than usual; it seems almost as though it was stopping up, and she feels very hoarse, but has no soreness; there is a feeling of fulness and choking.

|| Unable to speak loud; distressed feeling while speaking.

|| Respiration was hoarse, crying was whispered and broken, often no sound at all.

|| Excessive hoarseness, and tickling, choking sensation, >moving about.

|| Voice hoarse and husky; interrupted by weakness and hoarseness.

|| Larynx sensitive to pressure.

|| Constriction in lower part of larynx, like a finger across throat; feeling as of a bar across back of throat.

|| Difficult breathing; during evening had severe suffocating spells.

|| Terrible dyspnea immediately after sleep, first on left side of chest; dyspnea compelled her to be lifted upright with violent exertion to get breath; sharp pain in region of heart with each attack.

|| Breathing hoarse and croupy, and at times an entire stoppage of breath, when it would resume with a violent effort.

|| Breathing often snoring only possible through mouth.

|| Short breath.

|| Great difficulty in breathing, could not lie down flat.

|| Breathing very labored.

|| Loud snoring during sleep.

|| Sensation as if breath would leave her when lying down and trying to sleep; has to jump up and stir around for an hour or so every night.

| Tickling sensation in throat, causing cough; in afternoon quite hoarse.

| Cough from tickling in upper anterior part of larynx, > talking and lying down.

|| Cough caused by irritation in upper part of throat, < lying down at night, also after eating and drinking and after talking; with soreness of left side of throat and constant desire to urinate.

|| Cough on taking a long breath, not when swallowing.

|| Hard metallic cough.

|| Croupy cough, a dry, horse bark, penetrating through closed doors all over the house.

|| Cough and dyspnea.

|| Constant cough, accompanying soreness.

|| Expectoration of profuse, sticky, tough, white mucus in masses, with coryza.

Chest—

Terrible dyspnea immediately after sleep, first on left side of chest; the dyspnea compelled her to be lifted upright with violent exertion to get breath; there was sharp pain in region of heart with each of these attacks; after the medicine had but one attack of dyspnea, and all the pain was referred to right side of chest (acute rheumatism).

Lungs feel as though fast to chest, < while writing.

Clavicles sore to touch.

Stabbing pain in right lung just below nipple, preceded by pain in stomach—pit as of a stone or undigested food.

Sharp pain in right breast at 4 P.M.

Feeling of oppression and tightness behind sternum, with desire to draw a deep breath.

|| Sharp, incisive pain between scapulas, passing through sternum, with a sensation of pressure or constriction of chest in afternoon.

|| Trembling, jerking and fluttering through lungs, with numb, prickling sensation all over body, legs and arms.

|| Pulse so rapid it could scarcely be counted.

||Pulse 130.

Palpitation of heart, irregular, causing shortness of breath.

|| Heart beats rapidly from slight causes.

| Pulse quick, full and strong, with pains in chest and throat.

|| Pulse of little volume.

|| Pulse 130, wiry, weak.

|| Pulse: quick and feeble; 100; 149; 170; 130—140; almost gone.

|| Pulse 117.

|| Pulse rapid, quick.

Neck and Back—

|| Neck stiff.

Sharp neuralgic pain under right scapula.

Lameness and cutting pain under left scapula, < turning in bed.

Sharp, cutting pain under left scapula, shooting forwards through lung.

Backache nearly all day between scapulae, < after becoming warm, somewhat > by leaning back.

Pain in sacrum < by stooping, > by leaning back, with weakness; this pain extended around left side of pelvis (leaving the back) to inside of thigh, followed by a bloody leucorrheal discharge after six hours, which came all at once, leaving labia extremely sensitive.

Spine aches from base of brain to coccyx (pharyngitis).

| | Pain in back of neck.

Weakness in muscles of upper part of back.

| | Wandering pains in nape, with stiffness.

Stiffness and soreness of the muscles of the neck.

| | Neck aches, making her want to bend head forwards; entire spine sensitive.

Paralysis of muscles of the neck, causing head to fall forwards, so that it rests on upper part of sternum.

| | Spine aches from base of brain to coccyx.

| | Heat, pain and beating in small of back.

| | Pain in back.

Wakes with severe pain in lower part of back, it is often five minutes before she can straighten; pain leaves her when she has been about work a short time, not returning till morning.

| | Intense, unbearable pain across supersacral region, extending to right natis and down right sciatic nerve; pain so severe as to prevent sleep or rest; at same time diphtheritic sore throat on right side, with sensation of a lump, could not swallow solid food.

Upper Limbs—

Painful swelling and hardness, with suppuration of left axillary gland; menses came on at same time.

Pains down right arm and in fingers, which feel cramped; does not seem to have the same power in right hand.

| From draught in evening, sudden, violent pains in right shoulder, so much that when retiring she could not raise arm to finish toilet, as if disabled by dislocation.

| | Two warts on little finger.

Right wrist lame and painful.

Sharp, shooting pains in ball of right thumb.

Sharp pain round left arm, as of a cutting instrument; felt principally at the vaccination cicatrix; passed from thence to left elbow and disappeared; (forty-five minutes after first dose).

Trembling of left hand as in paralysis agitans.

Woke at night feeling very chilly, with sharp pain in left hand, and sensation in left arm as if asleep; lasting fifteen minutes.

Palms and soles burning hot.

|| Two warts on little finger noticed to be leaving.

Painful eruptions on axilla, like moist herpes, exceedingly painful on washing them.

Veins in hands look bluer than usual, they are swollen.

Sensation as if an insect were crawling on shoulders and neck, occasionally on hands.

Perspiration in axillae, stains linen bright orange colour, no smell.

| Very fetid perspiration in axillae, staining linen brown.

Wrists very lame, especially right which has sharp pains passing from thumb to little finger.

|| Neuralgic pains in shoulders, left then right then vice versa.

|| Pain in one or other shoulder.

|| Shoulders and arms ache.

|| Partial paralysis of left arm, unable to raise hand to head; on attempting to do so was seized with sharp pains in arm below shoulder.

|| Left hand bloats and is numb, with trembling, jerking and fluttering through lungs; numb, pricking sensation all over body, arms and legs.

| Sharp pain in left hand, left arm as if asleep.

|| Trembling of left hand, as in paralysis agitans.

|| Fingers extremely cold but not rest of hands.

Severe pains in all the bones.

Pains in joints of left hand, left ankle, left knee; extremely painful, swollen and red. The day previous, had similar pains and swellings in right ankle and right knee; pain was sharp, darting, erratic, now here, now there and < by any motion.

|| Pain in left shoulder extending across to right; could scarcely move arm.

Lower Limbs—

A few days before menses, inside of both thighs became raw and painful when walking, they then broke out with large, flat, red pimples; the soreness soon left; but the pimples remained.

Varicose veins on outer right thigh, from hip to knee.

Sensation of numbness in left leg with great heat as if burning, but cool to touch; brought on by pressure.

Stiffness through thighs, < on attempting to move after sitting.

Veins of feet and ankles very much swollen.

Feet swollen and very sore, causing considerable pain while walking.

Numbness and paralytic feeling in inner side of both knees, extending to both big toes.

|| Pain in right hip and leg while walking, with a trembling of leg, and slight feeling of uncertainty, especially on going down stairs.

|| Articular rheumatism in right hip and knee joints, especially former; she was seated in an arm chair, unable to move, complaining of bruised, smarting, lancinating pains in both joints and in lumbar region with swelling of affected joints; pains < by slightest motion at night; by touch and by pressure of bed clothes; next day pains and swelling had gone to left hip and knee joints, leaving right almost free; the ensuing day they had almost entirely disappeared from left hip and knee joints and had again attacked right hip and knee; complaining, moaning, and sighing on account of her sufferings and probable termination of her illness.

| Rheumatic pains in left hip and along sciatic nerve; wandering pains in nape of neck, with stiffness; pains in one or other shoulder; pain above left eye and heaviness of eyelids; sensitiveness to light.

Intense, unbearable pain across supersacral region, extending to right natis and down right sciatic nerve; pain so severe as to prevent sleep or rest (sciatica).

|| Partial paralysis of right leg from miscarriage; has to use a cane; leg numb and stiff, but cannot keep it still any length of time; feels > flexing it on abdomen.

Right ovary sore by spells and pain darts down leg sometimes to foot.

Numb pains chiefly in ankles, < while quiet, with swelling; veins of ankles distended; > while extreme heat is applied (rheumatism).

Ecthyma, on right leg.

|| Aching pains in limbs and back.

Staggers in walking.

Rheumatism beginning in soles flying from joint to joint and side to side, < every evening and by movement and touch; numb pains in ankle.

Burning of hands and feet at night (ovaralgia).

|| Cannot walk any distance; trembling through right thigh, and feeling as though entire lower portion of body was giving away; felt as though something was strained across lower part of bowels.

|| Sciatica.

|| Limbs cold to knees.

| Bruised pains in soles of feet, stiffness of ankle, knee and hip joints, and occasionally intense pains which move upwards; pain in ankle joints as of a dull plug pushing; joints stiff and sore, tender to touch; < from heat and least motion; later knees and then hips became involved; at first the left ankle was attacked, and then, after some hours suffering, the right with relief to left, and so on with knees and hips; chest affected, terrible dyspnea coming on immediately after sleep, first on left side; compelled her to be lifted upright with violent exertion to get breath, sharp pain in cardiac region; urine scanty and dark; pain in right side of throat; generally < at 5 P.M.

|| After exposure to cold night air when drunk, sharp, darting pains, < by any motion, with swelling in right knee and right ankle; next day joints of left knee and left ankle and left hand extremely painful, moderately swollen, slightly red; ensuing day, left, ankle and knee better, but right shoulder and elbow similarly affected.

| Numb pains, chiefly in ankles, < while quiet, with swelling; veins of ankles distended; > while extreme heat is applied.

|| Almost constant pain in right hip.

||Ecthyma: a sore breaks out in right leg, excessive itching; inflammation then swelling, blisters form and suppuration sets in; afterwards clear lymph, then discharge of matter; then scabs and scales, turning eventually into a bran-like desquamation; scars have left discoloured skin.

|| Restlessness in legs.

|| Cramps in feet. Pains in limbs as if beaten.

|| Bruised pains in soles making it difficult to walk; in twelve days pains suddenly left soles and appeared in right knee joint, being smarting, lancinating, with light swelling of joint; could not move affected limb, as least motion < pains, as did touch and pressure of bed clothes; on following day left knee joint affected in same way, right >; on ensuing day right again affected, with relief to left; afterwards hip joints attacked alternately with same symptoms, alternating like these in pains and swelling, left joints one day with > of right, and vice versa; also lancinating pains in left side of chest; after four days wrist joints affected, first right, with same symptoms as those of lower extremities, symptoms of one side of body alternating with those of the other; not able to move himself in bed, lancinating pains made him cry out; constipation, sleeplessness, no fever; pains and swelling < every evening, night, by movement, touch and pressure of bed clothes; numb pains chiefly in ankles <.

|| Burning of hands and feet at night.

Cramping pain in calf of right leg at night. Was compelled

to get up and rub it, which <; had this cramping every night for a week.

A knot (objective subjective) in calf of right leg when cramping; sensation as if some one had a stick in muscle and was twisting it around. (Never had cramp except when pregnant several years before.)

Sore aching, with throbbing in the outer side, and along sole of right foot, excruciating pains coming and going by spells; unable to stand on foot during the pain.

LAC DEFLORATUM
(Skimmed Cow's Milk)

Characteristics—

Diseases with faulty and defective nutrition with reflex affections of nervous centers.

Despondent; does not care to live; has no fear of death but is sure he is going to die.

American sick headache: begins in forehead, extending to occiput, in morning on rising (Bry.); *intense throbbing,* with nausea, vomiting, *blindness* and obstinate constipation (Epig., Iris, Sang.); < noise, light, motion (Mag. m., Sil.); great prostration; > pressure, by bandaging head tightly (Arg. n., Puls.); copious, pale urine.

Globus hystericus; sensation of a large ball rising from stomach to throat, causing sense of suffocation (Asaf., Kal.).

Vomiting: incessant, no relation to eating; first of undigested food, intensely acid, then of bitter water; *of pregnancy* (Lac. ac., Psor.).

Constipation: with ineffectual urging (Anac., Nux); feces dry and hard (Bry., Sulph.); *stool large, hard, great straining, lacerating anus* (Nat., San.); painful, extorting cries.

A woman had taken 10 or 12 enemas daily, often passed 4 or 5 weeks without an evacuation; constipation of 15 years, standing.

Menses: delayed; suppressed, *by putting hands in cold water* (Con.); *drinking a glass of milk will promptly suppress flow until next period* (compare Phos.).

Great restlessness, extreme and protracted suffering from *loss of sleep* (Coc., Nit. ac.).

Feels completely exhausted, whether she does anything or not; great fatigue when walking.

Sensation: as if cold air was blowing on her, even while covered up; as if sheets were damp.

Dropsy: from organic heart disease; from chronic liver complaint; far advanced albuminuria; following intermittent fever.

Obesity; fatty degeneration.

Emaciation, both local and general.

Relations—

Antidotes: Ign., Nux.

Compare—

Lac can., Lac vac., Lac. ac., Sac. lac.; Nat. muright, diabetes, albuminuria, headache, constipation, menstrual irregularities and heart affections, especially at cli-maxis; Coc., car or sea sickness and menstrual headaches; Cac., but it lacks the iron hand constriction; Nux in., heavy head but it falls to left; Cal, Kali c., Nat. s., Tub., child takes cold easily, is chilly, the hydrogenoid constitution; CaL, Caps., Fer., Graph., Tub., tendency to obesity; Ars., China, Graph., lod., Lye., Nat. m., Phos., Sil., Stan., Sulph., Tub., general emaciation; Arn., Hip., in traumatism; Con., Phos., suppressed menses.

Aggravation—

Lying down; external heat; motion, especially walking, or extending arms over head (fainting); pressure (fainting); cold water (suppresses menses); sitting down (ever so gently).

Amelioration—

Pressure (pain in eye); bandaging head lightly.

LAC VACCINUM DEFLORATUM

To Dr. Samuel Swan is due the credit of first recognizing the possibilities of this substance when potentized, from reading the reported successful use of it in the crude form by Donkin, in the treatment of diabetes, albuminuria and other affections of the kidneys. He potentized it and began the proving on himself and a lady patient whom he had cured of a chronic ailment with the m. and cm. potencies. Subsequently he induced Dr. Laura Morgan to undertake it, who with her friends made extensive provings, and what is remarkable is that the genuine character of the original work has not only verified many -of the claims of Donkin, but nearly every symptom in the pathogenesis has been clinically verified, especially the peculiar headaches, obstinate constipation and the unusual and irregular menses.

It is well known that the chemical constituents of milk contain an epitome of the salts and tissues of the animal which secretes it, hence we may conclude that its range of action is co-extensive with these tissue salts. Here we find the "mental depression and weeping," the "thirst for large quantities and often," the "periodical headache increasing and decreasing with the sun," the "obstinate constipation and fissure pain" of Natrum muriaticum. And so of other salts.

Grauvogl suggests that hydrogenoid and cold children should not be given milk, and Burnett maintains that a milk diet, even skimmed milk, after the first year renders them susceptible to colds. There is no doubt it prevents nutrition in many persons, both children and adults, developing emaciation in some and obesity in others; in other words, a constitutional diathesis akin to, or that tends toward, the tubercular.

The deep-seated vein of nervous phenomena manifested in its pathogenesis and verified in the care of many obstinate chronic ailments warrants a more careful study of this little known and less used remedy.

Mind—

Loss of memory; listlessness, disinclination for bodily or mental exertion.

| Depression of spirits; don't care to live; question as to quietest and most certain way of hastening one's death.

During conversation, headache and depression of spirits >.

| Depression and weeping with palpitation.

Imagines that all her friends will die and that she must go to a convent.

Profound melancholy.

Does not want to see or talk to any one.

Can remember what has been read only by a strong effort of will.

Vacillation of mind.

Great despondency on account of the disease, is sure he is going to die in 24 hours.

Has no fear of death but is sure he is going to die.

Great depression of spirits, with a strong inclination to weep.

Depression of spirits which is not dissipated by conversation.

Loss of memory, could not remember from one paragraph to another what she had read.

Head light, with throbbing in temples.

Head—

| Vertigo: on moving head from pillow; < lying down and especially turning while lying, obliging to sit up.

Headache preceded by dimness of sight.

Intense vertigo when opening eyes while lying, < when rising up; objects appeared to move swiftly from left to right, at other times moving as if tossed up from below *in every direction* (cured).

| Faintness and nausea when stepping upon floor in morning.

| Pain first in forehead, then extending to occiput, very intense, distracting and unbearable; great photophobia, even to light of candle; deathly sickness all over, with nausea and vomiting, < by movement or sitting up: very chilly, and external heat does not >; frequent and profuse urination of very pale urine.

After injury subject to distress in head; severe pain in forehead just above eyes; breath very offensive; appetite poor, nausea; at times sleeps for hours during attack; great distress across back; urine dark and thick.

Nausea and sometimes vomiting, which >; pain in forehead as if head would burst, with blindness; pain is > by bandaging head tightly; < by light and noise; constipation, stools large; hands and feet cold.

Headache: < during menses; < by speaking; alternating with tonsilitis.

|| Throbbing frontal headache (over eyes), nausea, vomiting and obstinate constipation; especially in anaemic women.

Headache, with pains in eyes; as if full of little stones; < closing eyes; profuse urination.

| Dim vision, as of cloud before eyes; profuse urination; full feeling in head; slight nausea at pit of stomach; face pale; feet cold; coldness in back.

|| Intense pain at point of exit of supra-orbital nerve, diffused thence over forehead; attack commences with chill, quickened pulse, flushed face and belching of wind from stomach (cured).

| Severe headache, with a sensation as if top of head was lifted off, raised about five inches and brains were coming out; head feels hot, motion < pain; face felt as if flesh was off

bones and their edges were separated and sticking out; better in five minutes after taking Lac Defloratum, and next morning was entirely relieved.

| Pain first in forehead, extending through occiput, making her nearly frantic.

| Intense headache in forehead and through head, < in vertex, afterward head felt bruised (cured).

| In morning nausea and sensation of a round ball full of pain in centre of forehead (cured).

|| General sore pain of head produced by coughing.

| At first a sharp pain at apex of heart, as though a knife was cutting up and down; this lasts a few seconds and is followed by a strange feeling in head; forehead feels extremely heavy, with dull sensation over eyes, and considerable throbbing, most marked on each side of head; rest of head feels very light, dimness of vision; can only distinguish light, not objects; at same time great loss of strength; cannot stand, but falls backwards, and remains entirely unconscious for two or three minutes; weakness passes off gradually and is followed by crying, palpitation of heart and great depression of spirits; imagines that all her friends will soon die and that she must go to a convent; she can produce an attack at any time by extending arms high above head, or by pressure around waist; spells come on at 7:3 P.M.

| After light breakfast, pain in forehead, with nausea; very pale face, even lips looked white; vomiting of ingesta and afterwards of mucus and bitter water; deathly sick feeling in pit of stomach, < rising up in bed; profuse urination every half hour; urine colourless as water; great thirst; intense throbbing pain in vertex.

| Periodical pain in forehead, as if head would burst, accompanied by violent effort to vomit, and more rarely vomiting; hands and feet cold; diarrhea alternating with constipation, the latter predominating; loss of appetite; smell or thought of food causes nausea; tongue moist, coated white;

thirstlessness; always < at menstrual period; menses scanty and accompanied with colic.

| Attacks come every eight days; during attack can neither eat nor drink, nor endure light or noise; does not even like to speak; great prostration, < during menstruation; when pains subside inflammation of tonsils appears; tongue white and no relish for food.

| Severe frontal headache; nausea and sometimes vomiting upon rising in morning, or from recumbent position at any time, or upon moving; great constipation; constant chilliness even when near fire; urine profuse and watery, or scanty and high coloured; intense pain throughout whole spinal column; excessive thirst for large quantities; great depression of spirits; sudden prostration of strength at 5 P.M.; skin colour of red rose, with swelling of face, neck, arms and body, generally in morning and during day and evening.

| Severe pain over eyes, with intense throbbing in both temples, eyes feel as if full of little stones; eyeballs intensely painful, and on shutting eyes, pressure of lids increases pain; edges of lids feel contracted, and convey sensation as of a narrow band drawn tightly across eyeball; pain over left hip; constipation and profuse urination during paroxysm.

| Pain commencing in and above inner end of right eyebrow before rising in morning; soon after rising pain passed into eyeball; < until afternoon, at which time it became unbearable; < by walking and particularly by sitting down, though done carefully, also by heat radiated from fire or stooping, > on pressure; pressure on temples disclosed strong pulsation of artery; pain ceased entirely at sunset and did not return till next day. Light did not < it. The eye had no unusual appearance. Lac Fel. had no effect. Partial relief by Sol. and Oxygen (cured by Lac Defloratum cm.).

Pains so severe that she would bury her eyes in her hands and press them into pillow.

| Severe headache for years; severe pain over eyes; intense throbbing in temples.

General sore pain of head produced by coughing.

| Throbbing in temples.

| American sick headache, with gastric symptoms.

Hurting or pressing headache, in different places at different times; generally worse in occiput.

Pain in forehead.

Severe frontal headache, with intense throbbing in the temples, during nausea, passing away with the nausea and heat, leaving a bruised feeling in the head.

Severe frontal headache in the afternoon, passing off during conversation—pain was just above the eyes.

Severe frontal headache above the eyes < by suddenly moving or stooping, with depression of spirits, and strong inclination to weep; passed away during conversation.

Headache all day, worse in the afternoon.

Headache and depression of spirits, head feels heavy with marked tendency to fall to the right.

In the morning the head felt very heavy, and fell to the right side, the muscles of the neck being unable to hold it erect.

Headache in the afternoon and heaviness in the evening.

Constant dull pain just above the eyes.

Pain in the head most marked over the left eye, and in the temples, occasionally extending into the eyes, and causing profuse lachrymation.

Head feels large as if growing externally (cured).

Flashes of heat in head and face.

Pain in left forehead, over left eye.

Severe headache for years, severe pain over eyes, intense throbbing in temples (cured).

Forehead feels extremely heavy.

Heavy feeling in forehead and eyes.

Headache with pressure on vertex; pain over eyes.

Dull, heavy pain all over temples and forehead and extending to occiput.

Burning in the top of the head.

Sensation in base of brain as if pressure would relieve her.

During the headache, feet and hands cold.

Bruised sensation in head caused by coughing.

Intense, awful, mixed-up, aching, drawing, pulling, stabbing pains, with delirium after the 1m.

Vertigo with nausea and vomiting.

Intense aching pain with soreness and heaviness of the whole head; face deathly pale and dreadful weakness and prostration. After 10m. in water, repeated at short intervals, a singular sensation of relief commenced at the head and sensibly passed all through her body, as it were in her nerves, and out through her feet. The next morning, after a good night's sleep, she felt perfectly well, but lazy.

Nose—

During headache, coryza and an apparent tonsillitis. θ Sick headache. 6.

Catarrh in right nostril in afternoon, coming on very suddenly, gone before morning. 3 (11).

Catarrh in afternoon in both nostrils. 3 (12).

Catarrh of both nostrils lasted till 19th day. 3.

° Painful pressure and tightness at root of nose, with catarrh; the tightness was cured, but not the catarrh.

Painful dryness of nostrils.

Face—

° Face very pale and bluish, with dark depressed circle around eyes. θ Sick headache. 7.

° Face very pale, and eyes look heavy. θ Headache from suppressed menses. 8.

During the whole proving, but especially in morning, or when the headache or nausea prevailed, she was extremely pale, a deathly pallor of face. 2.

Flushes of heat in head and face, especially left cheek. 3 (7).

During proving, deathly pallor of face, in morning, so marked as to cause inquiry as to the reason of it. 3.

° Very pale, even lips looked white. θ Sick headache. 9.

° Face pale. θ Sick headache. 9.

° Deathly paleness of face on rising in morning. θ Sick headache. 9.

° Very pale, with vertigo. θ Quininism. 9.

° Flushed face. θ Suppressed menses from putting hands in cold water. 9.

° Pale face in morning; lips and tips of fingers white. θConstipation. 9.

° Face feels as if the flesh were off the bones, and the edges separated and sticking out. θ Headache. 9.

° Pimples on face and forehead. θ Intermittent fever. 9.

° Painful dragging sensation in face, or as if something were dragging down his cheeks. θ Diabetes. A.A.

° Yellow pasty look of face. θ Diabetes. A.A.

° His extreme nervousness, sleepless nights, and general appearance and expression pointed to some deeply-rooted cerebral trouble. θ Incipient softening of brain. 20.

° Twitching of muscles of face. A.A.

° Eczematous eruption in a dyspeptic sallow woman. A.A.

Wasted, thin and excessively sallow, with dark stains beneath the eyes.

Face, neck, arms and body generally flushed, colour of a red rose, with swelling, but no itching or burning.

Lips dry and parched.

Face looked blue during the cold sensation.

Flashes of heat in head and face.

Face flushed, colour of a red rose, with swelling (cured).

Mouth—

Tongue dry and cleaves to the roof of the mouth.

White coating all over tongue. 1 (4).

Tongue thickly coated at first.

° Tongue coated white, moist, no thirst. θ Sick headache. 6.

° Tongue coated white; feels tasteless. θ Sick headache. 6.

Tongue red and devoid of epithelium.

° Bitter disagreeable taste in mouth. θSick headache. 10.

Sweet sickening taste in mouth. 3 (4).

° Mouth very dry. 3.

Breath exhales a sweetish odoright

° Breath very offensive. θ Headache. 9.

° Tongue coated whitish-yellow. θ Incipient softening of brain. 20.

Tongue and lining membrane have a dusky red hue, and covered with aphthae at a later period.

Tongue furred white and rough sometimes. A.A.

Dryness of mouth without thirst.

Dryness of mouth, pharynx and nostrils, with insatiable thirst.

Sweet taste in mouth lasted all day.

Nausea rising from the mouth to the stomach.

Mouth clammy and frothy, especially during conversation (cured).

Teeth—

° Gums spongy and teeth loose. θ Diabetes. A.A.

° Grinding of teeth when asleep, with pain in stomach, headache and vomiting.

Spongy bleeding condition of the gums and teeth.

Looseness of the teeth, especially of the incisors.

Throat—

Painful dryness of nostrils, pharynx, and mouth; with insatiable thirst for cold water, a second goblet-ful being required as soon as the first had been drunk. 2 (after 9 hours, 1st day).

° Globus hystericus; sensation of a large ball rising from a point about lower end of sternum to upper end of esophagus, causing very distressing sense of suffocation. 3.

° Sore throat all around, worse when swallowing, with slight hacking cough.

Painful dryness of the pharynx, nostrils and mouth, with insatiable thirst.

Eyes—

Some photophobia. θ Sick headache. 10.

Pain, with twitching in left inner canthus, worse by reading or sewing. 2 (1).

Pain in eyes on first going into the light, soon passing off. 3 (3).

Objects appeared to move swiftly from left to right, at other times moving as if tossed up from below in every direction (cured).

Pain in eyes on first going into the light. 3 (4).

Great pain in eyes on first going into the light; soon passing off; on θ closing lids on account of the light, pain θ was felt in eyeballs as if from pressure of lids. 3 (15).

° Dim vision, as of a cloud before eyes. θ Sick headache. 9.

° Great photophobia, even to light of candle. θ Sick headache. 9.

° Upper lids feel very heavy; sleepy all day.

° Dim vision; can only distinguish light, not objects. and Faint spells. 3.

° Eyes feel as if full of little stones. θ Headache. 3.

° Eyeballs intensely painful; and on shutting the eyes, the pressure of the lids increases the pain, causing a painful pressure, and the edges of lids feel contracted laterally and convey the sensation of a narrow band drawn tightly across eyeball. θ Headache. 3.

Photophobia for θ sunlight, in both eyes; eyes red, lachrymation; left eye more sore than right 16.

° Great dimness of sight. θ Diabetes. 20. θ Bright's disease. A.A.

° Cannot endure light. θ Incipient softening of brain. 20.

Profuse lachrymation, caused by a pain in the temples extending into the eyes (cured).

Pain in and above the eyes.

Eyeballs sore.

Blurr before sight preceding an attack of headache (cured).

Ears—

° Noise very annoying. θ Sick headache. 10.

° Cannot endure noise or talking of others. θ Incipient softening of brain. 20.

Slight deafness in both ears, 2 or 3 evenings.

Great paleness of ears, face, and lips, principally in morning.

Stomach—

Appetite not so good as formerly, everything tastes alike. 1 (3).

Was unable to go down stairs or eat a particle when brought to her. 1 (4).

Felt hungry and faint, but could not eat from loss of appetite; the thought of food nauseated her. 1(5).

Nausea and gagging after rising, the nausea returning several times during day. 1 (3).

Violent retching and straining to vomit; but cannot succeed; indescribable nausea returning every 6 hours. 1 (4).

Empty retching. 1 (5).

For a long time the nausea and empty retching returned every morning after rising.|

° Nausea, with occasional vomiting which relieves. °—Sick headache. 6.

° Violent retching, seldom vomiting; in last attack could only vomit by putting finger far down throat. θ Sick headache. 6.

° Loss of appetite, the smell or thought of food nauseates. θ Sick headache. 6.

° Can neither eat nor drink during attacks. θ Sick headache. 6.

° Deathly nausea and vomiting, the nausea usually lasting 3 or 4 days. ° Sick headache. 7.

° Sense of deathly sickness, and frequent vomiting of green watery bitter fluid and slime. θ Sick headache. 7.

° Deathly sickness at stomach. θ Diabetes mellitus. 9.

° Vomits some, but retches more; nausea all the time. θ Sick headache. 10.

° Great thirst. θ Sick headache. 9.

° Slight nausea at stomach-pit. θ Sick headache. 9.

° Deathly sickness all over, with nausea and vomiting, worse by movement or rising up in bed. θ Sick headache. 9.

° Nausea in morning. θ Sick headache. 9.

° Great thirst; wants to drink all the time, and takes a glassful at a drink. 3.

° Appetite entirely gone. θ Headache. 9.

° Nausea. θ Headache. 9. θ Threatened premature labor. 9.

° Nausea and sometimes vomiting upon rising in morning, or from a recumbent position at any time during day or evening, or upon moving. θ Sick headache. |

° Excessive thirst for large quantities and often. θ Sick headache. ||

° Deathly sickness, with or without vomiting. θ Constipation. 9.

° Inability to drink milk without sick headache. 9.

° Voluminous tasteless eructations soon after the dose (10 m.). 19.

° Intense thirst. θ Diabetes. A.A.

° Voracious appetite. θ Diabetes. A.A.

° Much dyspepsia, and a feeling as though he would burst after taking food. θ Bright's disease. A.A.

° Indigestion, with distressing flatulency, severe palpitation, difficult breathing, and great giddiness, so that she could with difficulty walk across the room. θ Bright's disease. A.A.

° Invaluable in functional derangements and diseases of the gastric and intestinal organs, especially in certain forms of diarrhea, hypochondriasis and diarrhea; also in cases of catarrh, and ulceration of the stomach. A.A.

° Little or no appetite, but not much thirst. θ Incipient softening of the brain. 20.

° Sour eructations.

° Violent pain in epigastric region and left side below ribs. A.A.

° Incessant vomiting, which had no relation to her meals. A.A.

° Cramps in epigastric region. A.A.

° Violent pain in stomach-pit; seldom lower, brought on by fatigue. A.A.

° Much wind and acidity of stomach, without tenderness. A.A.

° Vomiting, first of ingesta, undigested, intensely acid, then of bitter water, and lastly of a brownish clot; which in water separated and looked like coffee-grounds, without odor, but of bitter taste.

° Deathly nausea, cannot vomit, with groans and cries and great distress; great restlessness with sensation of coldness, although the skin was hot; pulse normal.

° Morning sickness during pregnancy, deathly sickness at stomach on waking, vertigo and waterbrash on rising, constipation.

° Chronic gastro-enteritis with chronic diarrhea and vomiting. A.A.

° During headache, nausea some, retching more.

° Nausea and frequent vomiting of greenish watery bitter fluid, during the headache. 7.

° Bloating in epigastric region, with asthma, so that he could scarcely breathe, followed by hard pressive pain about the 4th cervical vertebra—had only been temporarily relieved by a movement of the bowels. 9.

Great thirst, wants to drink all the time, wants a goblet full at a time; dryness of the mouth (cured).

Insatiable thirst for cold water, a second goblet being required as soon as the first has been drunk.

Sweet taste in mouth.

Nausea, or a deathly feeling of sickness at stomach, recurring every six hours, and continuing about one hour; the nausea rose from stomach to mouth, occasioning belching of bitter flatus which momentarily relieved it; eating did not produce or affect the nausea, the periodical recurrence having apparently no reference to anything else; the periodical recurrence continued for three days; she described the nausea as a deathly sickness throughout whole body; she did not vomit, it being extremely difficult to cause it in her even with an emetic; during the nausea there was great internal heat, also severe frontal headache with intense throbbing in temples; the nausea, heat, and headache passed away simultaneously, leaving a bruised feeling in head. 2 (1).

Nausea was so unbearable that she discontinued the medicine. 2 (2).

Faintness with the nausea. 2 (3).

Great thirst, wants to drink continually, but little at a time. 3(2).

Great thirst, drinking followed by a chill. 3 (5).

Very little appetite. 3 (3).

Nausea during evening. 3 (5).

In morning, faint hollow sensation in stomach, attended with slight nausea; passing off on going into open airight 3 (14).

° Soon after being put to bed, vomited ingesta, and afterwards mucus and bitter wateright θ Sick headache. 9.

° Awful deathly sick feeling in stomach-pit, without retching or vomiting, worse by rising in bed. θ Sick headache. 9.

Great internal heat during the nausea.

During the nausea severe frontal headache, with intense throbbing.

Deathly sickness, without retching or vomiting, so dreadful and unbearable that the proving had to be discontinued.

Nausea momentarily relieved by belching of bitter flatus.

Nausea and vomiting, and a sensation of deathly sickness, < by movement or rising in bed.

Nausea and vomiting, followed by a deathly sick feeling, without either nausea or vomiting, intensified by sitting up in bed. Sickness described as awful.

Dyspepsia (cured)

Indigestion, and a feeling as if he would burst after taking food.

Faintness and nausea when stepping upon the floor in the morning (cured).

Abdomen—

° Bearing down pain in abdomen and back. θ After suppressed menses. 8.

Sensation of weight and dragging in left side of pelvis; worse next day. 3 (9).

Weight and dragging in left side of pelvis, with a burning sensation of pain, relieved somewhat by leaning to right side, increased by pressure of the clothes, or even the hand or arm resting on it. 3 (11).

° Drawing pains, with heat, across lower abdomen and bearing down. θ Sick headache. 9.

° Cannot bear pressure of arm or hand on abdomen. θ Sick headache. 9.

° Great fatigue from walking, on account of heaviness as of a stone in abdomen. θ Sick headache. 9.

° Abdomen very sore and sensitive to touch. 3.

°Pain over left hip. *9* Headache. 3.

° Sensation as if abdomen were full of water, catching the breath like a spasm. 5.

° Drawing pains across uterine region, with heat and pressive bearing-down in both ovarian regions; cannot bear pressure of hand or arm on abdomen; intense distress in lower part of abdomen during menses, not relieved by any position; violent inflammation in ilio-cecal region, with intense pain, swelling, tenderness, fecal accumulation, and violent vomiting.

° Chronic gastritis and enteritis. Symptoms, chronic diarrhea and vomiting.

° Severe pain across the umbilicus with headache.

Flatulence.

Constant pain in frontal region; nausea in morning; deathly paleness of face on rising in morning; aching pains in wrists and ankles; puffy swelling under malleoli; drawing pains, with heat across lower abdomen and bearing down; frequent scanty pale urine; pressing bearing down in both ovarian regions; cannot bear pressure of hand or arm on abdomen; slight yellowish leucorrhea; great lassitude and disinclination to exertion; depression of spirits, does not care to live; questions as to quickest and most certain mode of hastening one's death. For years has been subject to attacks of bloating in the epigastric region, attended with asthma, so that he could scarcely breathe (cured).

Stool and Rectum—

θ No stool for first four days. 1 (1 to 4).

θ Rectum feels impacted with feces, but is unable to eject them. 1 (4).

Bowels partly moved, but with much straining and some laceration of anus θ stool being very large and hard. 1 (5).

Bowels again moved, but with the sime laceration as anus, stool θ being very large and hard; the pain while passing stool extorted cries; passed considerable blood with stool. The constipation was so intense that she took one dose of *Nux vom.* 15m. (Fincke) with immense relief in 24 hours. 1 (6).

° Habitually costive; stools large. θ Sick headache. 6.

° Alternate diarrhea and constipation, the latter predominating. ° Sick headache. 6.

Constipation for 4 days; stool θ dry, θ hard, and passed in small lumps with much pain; θ smarting of anus after stool. 2 (2).

° Constipation. 2 θ Headache. 3 θ Threatened premature laboright 9.

° Great constipation. θ Sick headache. 11.

° Very severe constipation for 15 years; has been in the habit of taking 10 or 12 enemas every day, and often passed 4 or 5 weeks without stool. 14.

In higher potencies it has a very powerful action on the liver, as evinced by the white feces. (Swan's observation).

Causes constipation in most cases of diabetes, rarely diarrhea. A.A.

Constipation set in and lasted a week. Stool dry, hard, and passed in small lumps, with much pain and smarting in anus after stool.

During the constipation was constantly cold, so that she looked blue, hands and chest felt cold as if dead, additional clothing or sitting by a stove failed to warm heright Was awakened in the night by the cold.

Constipation (cured).

Is generally constipated, and when it is most persistent is very chilly and cannot get warm (cured).

Frequent but ineffectual urging to stool, had one natural stool daily without urging.

Constipation with chronic headache.

Constipation with extremely tough salmon coloured stools.

Constipation simply unconquerable by any constant treatment.

Constipation so utterably invincible that neither enemas nor the most powerful purgatives were of any avail.

Stools yellowish or salmon hue after 48 hours.

Violent rectal and sciatic pains following every effort at defecation.

Constipation, feces dry and hard.

Occasional diarrhea.

Diarrhea and borborygm caused by the treatment.

Stool large and hard, passed with great straining, lacerating the anus, extorting cries and passing considerable blood.

Frequent but ineffectual urging to stool.

Constipation, with chronic headache, most powerful purgatives were of no avail; feces dry and hard, passed with great straining, lacerating anus, extorting cries and passing considerable blood; chronic.

Continual, persistent constipation, > only by cathartics and enemas, with violent attacks of sick headache, pain first in forehead, then extending to occiput, intense, unbearable; great photophobia, even to light of candle; deathly sickness all over, with nausea and vomiting < by movement or sitting up; chilly, not > by external heat; frequent and profuse urination of very pale urine.

Frontal headache; deathly sickness, with or without vomiting; pale face in morning, also lips and tips of fingers white; coldness over whole body.

Is generally constipated, and when it is most persistent very chilly; cannot get warm.

Urine—

° Excessive flow of urine, either of high specific gravity, or colourless, watery, low specific gravity, but in both cases strongly impregnated with sugar. 9.

° Urinates profusely every half hour, urine perfectly colourless, specific gravity 1005; Trommer's test showed sugar. 9.

° Frequent and profuse urination (nearly a quart every half hour), colourless as water, odor natural, taste slightly salt, slight acid reaction; Trommer's test showed large quantities of sugar; specific gravity 1010. 9.

Frequent urination, urine scanty and very pale. 3 (5 to 7; more marked 10, 11).

° Urinates profusely every half hour, urine colourless as water; after 1m. during the night the urine became high-coloured and scanty but without sediment; in the morning normal. θ Sick headache. 9 (Mrs. P. aet 71).

° Profuse urination. *8* Sick headache. 9. θ Headache. 3.

° Frequent and profuse urination of very pale urine. θ Sick headache. 9.

° Frequent scanty pale urine. θ Sick headache. 9.

° Urine very light-coloured; has no control over the organs; urine comes away in drops, or gushes out with a sensation of very hot water passing over the parts; involuntary urination, wets the bed every night. 3.

° Urine very dark and thick. θ Headache. 9.

° Urine profuse and watery, or scanty and high-coloured. θ Sick headache. 11

° Frequent scanty urination. ° Threatened premature labor. 9.

° Urine scanty; lowsp.gright and containing 1/3 of albumen; small and large casts of urine, pus cells, epithelium, and oil globules. ° Bright's disease. A.A.

° Sugar in urine; sp. gright from 1035 to 1040; 8 to 10 pints daily. θ Diabetes. A.A.

Produces profuse flow of urine in Bright's disease. A.A.

° Urine intermits in flow, has to strain. 9.

° Urine brown and muddy, quantity nearly normal. θ Incipient softening of brain. 20.

Frequent urination. A.A.

° Albumen in urine; sp. gright of 2 cases, 1014, 1016. A.A.

° Frequent and profuse urination, urine colourless, odor natural, no headache but intense vertigo, worse on opening the eyes or raising up in bed. 9.

° Urine pale straw colour with no sediment on cooling. 9.

° Urine very dark and thick. 9.

Male Sexual Organs—

° Power and function of reproduction suspended. 9.

Frequent and profuse urination of very pale urine.

Albuminuria.

Urine very pale; cannot retain it.

Urine comes away drop by drop, or else gushes out, with a sensation of very hot water passing over the parts; wetting bed at night (cured).

Constant desire to urinate; urine scanty and very pale.

Profuse, very pale urine.

Urinates profusely every half hour, perfectly colourless; specific gravity 1005 (six hours after Defloright 1m. urine became natural in colour and quantity).

Profuse urination during headache.

Frequent urination.

Albumen in urine, several cases cured. Specific gravity of two cases, 1014, 1016.

Frequent and profuse urination; urine colourless, odor natural; no headache accompanied it, but intense vertigo, worse on opening the eyes or rising up in bed. (Specific gravity 1010, taste saltish, slight acid reaction; Trommer's test showed sugar.)

Constant pain in the region of the kidneys, passing round each side above the hips to the region of the bladder, also downward from the sacral region to the gluteal, and from thence down the back part of the thighs. Pain was burning and was not relieved in any position; lying down intensified it.

Females Sexual Organs—

Menses, which are naturally scanty and postponed, came nearer the usual time, and the quantity of the flux was increased for many months.

° Menses always scanty, and attended with colic. θ Sick headache. 6.

° Menses which had just commenced were stopped by wetting from rain. The medicine restored them with some griping pain for a short time; they had previously been painless. 8.

Menses, which had commenced, ceased suddenly and entirely, though they usually last four days. 3 (2).

Menses two days too soon, scanty, and attended with a feeling of intense distress in lower part of abdomen, not relieved by any position or by removing the clothes. 3 (27).

Slight yellowish leucorrhea, with slight itching of vulva. 3(5).

θ Slight yellowish leucorrhea. 3(6,7). *6* Sick headache. 9.

Leucorrhea more marked. 3 (10).

Leucorrhea nearly ceased. 3 (12).

° Pressive bearing-down in both ovarian regions. θ Sick headache. 9.

° Menses irregular, too frequent, scanty. θ Faint spells. 3.

After leaving off proving for three or four months, her husband (physician) said she was pregnant; she became very large, full bosom, later on milk ran out, she felt fetal movement; went a week over what she thought was full time. Examined and found os uteri hard, pointed, strawberry-shaped. Gave one dose of 10m.; she gradually decreased, and the symptoms all disappeared. 2.

° Threatened premature labor; parts tumefied, profuse glairy mucous discharge, os soft and dilated, vertex presentation, occasional irregular bearing-down pains; fetal pulse 158. 9.

° Menses suddenly suppressed by putting hands into cold water to rinse out clothes, with great pain in uterine region, intense headache, aching pains all over, fever, flushed face. 9.

° Irregular menses, sometimes very dark and scanty, sometimes colourless wateright θ Intermittent feveright 9.
Abortion at second month; three cases. 17.

° Menses delayed a week, with congestion of blood to head, coldness of hands, nausea and vertigo; after taking *Lac vaccinum defloratum,* in high potency, flow commenced next morning, scanty, with pain in back, sensation of weight and dragging in left ovarian region. 9.

°Sore pain in left ovarian region. 9 (cm. cured).

Slight exaltation of sexual instincts. 3.

°Menses five days too soon.

Flow bright red.

Morning sickness during pregnancy; deathly sickness at stomach on waking; vertigo and waterbrash on rising; constipation.

Decrease in size of breasts.

Breasts feel sore, worse hanging loose.

||(Has never failed to bring back milk in from 12 to 24 hours.)

Diminished secretion of milk.

Drinking a glass of milk during menstruation will promptly check the flow until next menstrual period (Mrs. B., a medical student, brunette, 33 years of age).

Menses suddenly and entirely cease on the second day, the usual time being four days.

Itching of the vulva.

|| Decrease in the size of the breasts, which after the proving resumed their original size and firmness.

Weight and dragging in the left side of pelvis (ovarian region) with a burning sensation relieved somewhat by leaning to the right, increased by the pressure of the clothes, or even the hand or arm resting upon it.

Drawing pain across the uterine region, with heat, and pressive bearing down in both ovarian regions. Cannot bear the pressure of the hand or arm on the abdomen. Intense distress in lower part of abdomen during menstruation, not relieved by any position. Violent inflammation in the ileo-cecal region, with intense pain, swelling, tenderness, fecal accumulation, and violent vomiting (cured).

Power and function of reproduction are suspended.

Menses suppressed by putting hands in cold water, with great pain in the uterine region, intense headache, aching pains all over, fever and flushed face. After 1m. in water, one spoonful at night, headache left and she slept all night. Next morning slight flow; took another spoonful, and by 10 o'clock flow all right and she was free from pain.

Diminution of the breasts, and diminished secretion of 9

milk in nursing women, never has failed to bring back the milk in from 12 to 24 hours.

Mrs. Y——, aged 42, blonde, sometimes before, at other times just after, this time at about the close of her menses, she has a "hurting headache," involving the whole head at different times. It does not hurt all over the head at once, but in different places at different times. Generally the pressure or hurting is worse when in the occiput, at which time she gets sick at the stomach and feels sick all over. More frequently the pain is in the forehead, but it is only unbearable when in the occiput. She cannot describe the pain; it seems like a severe "hurting" or pressure. It leaves the eyelids sore. Lasts about 24 hours. She knew yesterday that she would have it today, but cannot tell why. She had it this time for four or five hours. Flow bright red. Breasts feel sore, worse hanging loose. Constipation marked. No other pains and not sick in any other way.

Lac vaccinum defloratum dmm., one dose, dry on tongue.

Within a very short time, just a few moments, she "felt big all over," the veins filled up and felt full. Became quite chilly (very characteristic of the remedy). Head very much relieved during the first few minutes, when she arose the head was worse, with immediate relief on lying down. The whole trouble was entirely gone in one and one-half hours. Bowels moved normally about one hour after the single dose. Ringing in her left (deaf) earight No trouble at her next period.

Mammae—

Breasts decreased in size two-thirds, and became flabby, with loss of flesh. 4.

° Diminution of breasts and diminished secretion of milk in nursing women.

Brought milk in the breasts of a full breasted girl.

Larynx and Trachea—

Constricted feeling in throat, causing constant desire to cough. 3 (7).

Constricted sensation in throat, causing constant hacking cough, no expectoration. 3 (11).

° During day, short dry cough with difficult expectoration of a small lump of mucus which relieves the cough.

θApyrexia of intermittent fever. 9.

° Cough caused a bruised sensation in the head. 11

Chest—

Respiration affected on lying down; prolonged inspirations, and short quick expirations. 3 (3).

On lying down, inspirations long, expirations short. 3 (4).

Sudden and violent palpitation of heart, with flushes of heat, caused by the least unusual sight or sound; feels sometimes extremely nervous. 3 (19).

° Palpitation of heart, and flushes of heat, especially in left face and cheek. 3.

° Sharp pain at apex of heart, as if a knife were cutting up and down; lasting a few seconds. θ Faint spells. 3.

° Subject to attacks of bloating in epigastric region, and with them always an attack of asthma so that he can scarcely breathe; then would have hard pressive pain at about 4th cervical vertebra; pressure round the breast (but not like the grasping of *Cactus)* with the dyspnea; always constipated; their symptoms were all relieved by purgative medicines. 9.

Some palpitation of heart, with flashes of heat in head and face. 3 (5, 6).

° Soreness of chest with great pressure.

° In a case of hypertrophied left ventricle, with palpitation of heart, it lowered the pulse and quieted the heart. A.A.

° Tubercular deposit in apices of both lungs. A.A.

Short dry cough, with difficult expectoration of a small lump of mucus, which > cough.

Pressure around heart (not like grasping of *Cactus),* with dyspnea and a feeling of certainty that he is going to die in twenty-four hours.

Sharp pain in apex of heart, as if a knife were cutting up and down; this preceded by a heaviness of head, dulness of eyes, throbbing in temples and palpitation of heart.

Palpitation of heart and flushes of heat, especially in left side of face and neck.

|| Sensible decrease in the breasts which after the proving returned to their original size and firmness.

Pulse rapid and feeble.

Back—

° Chills running up and down between shoulders. θ Sick headache. 7.

° Chills creeping along back and between shoulders.θ Sick headache. 7.

° Considerable pain in back, a little below a line drawn across it from crest of ilium. 10.

Painful aching in small of back; extending up to and between scapulae, worse while sitting, slightly relieved while walking; continued for two days. 2 (12 hours after last dose on third day).

° Coldness in back. θ Sick headache. 9.

° Constant pain in small of back, commencing in region of kidneys, passing round each side above hips to region of bladder; also downward from renal region to gluteal, and thence down back to thighs; this pain is intense burning, relieved by no position, lying down intensified it. 3.

° A symmetrical patch of herpetic eruption on each side of neck, itching and burning after scratching. 3.

° Great distress across back. θ Headache. 9.

Great weakness of the muscles of the neck left side, allowing the head to fall to the right.

° Intense pain throughout the whole spinal column. θ Sick headache. 1

Pain in small of back. θ Threatened premature labor. 9.

° Boring pain, sore as if bruised, and throbbing in right kidney, extending as a dull aching to right hip, to spine, up to right scapula, and across right side of abdomen to bladder; afterwards the boring affected the left kidney also, with a little aching there; backache across sacral region, much worse in the centre, a breaking pain; all the worse from movement. 5.

Hard pressive pain at fourth cervical vertebra; chills creeping along back between scapulae.

Intense burning pain in small of back and sacrum, commencing in region of kidneys, passing around on both sides above hips into groin, also downward from renal region through gluteal region, down back part of thighs; pain, burning, and > by no position.

Dull aching pain in lumbar region of frequent occurrence, with indefinable indisposition.

° During day, back usually feels cold. θ Apyrexia of intermittent fever. 9.

° Dull heavy aching pain over loins. θ Diabetes. A.A.

Constant pain in small of back (cured).

Upper Extremities—

θ During the proving, ends of fingers icy cold and look white, rest of hands warm. 3.

° Aching pains in wrists and ankles. θ Sick headache. 9.

° Ends of ringers icy cold, rest of hand warm. 3.

Sweat on palms, especially right (no name).

Cold hand and feet during headache.

Coldness and numbness of the limbs.

Aching pains in the wrists.

Hands cold as if dead.

Lower Extremities—

Itching of knees at night. 3 (3).

After the weak sick feeling suddenly left, both heels commenced to ache. 3 (13).

Corn on right little toe became very painful and sore when putting on the shoe in morning; soon passed off. 3 (19).

° Feet cold. θ Sick headache. 9.

° Puffy swelling under malleoli. θ Sick headache. 9.

° Pains passing down under side of thighs to heels; pains in top of feet as if the bones were broken across instep; these pains in legs and feet come on as soon as she steps on them in the morning; when she becomes faint and nauseated and has to lie down; has to lie down three or four times before she can get dressed. 9.

° Loss of sensation on anterior surface of things. θ Diabetes. A.A.

Aching pains in wrists and ankles.

° Cramps in legs at night. θ Bright's disease. A.A.

° Legs much swollen. θ Bright's disease. A.A.

After the attack of debility had passed off, both heels commenced to ache.

Weakness and aching in ankles, pumness under the malleoli (cured).

Skin thickened at the edges of the feet (cured).

Numbness and loss of sensation over the outer and anterior surface of the thighs (cured).

Edema of lower extremities (cured).

Anesthesia of the limbs (cured).

Coldness and numbness of the limbs.

Numbness and loss of sensation over outer and anterior surfaces of thighs.

Cold hands or feet during headache.

Fever—

Felt cold all day; sat near the fire, but with no permanent relief. 1 (3).

General coldness of body, and finger nails looked blue as if from ague; a heavy shawl did not prevent her from shivering. 1 (4).

Was cold, and had forebodings all day. 1 (5).

Had a restless night, feet did not get warm the whole night. 1 (6).

The natural warmth returned after several weeks.

° Hands and feet generally cold. θ Sick headache. 6.

° Cold hands and feet. θ Sick headache. 6, 7.

° Coldness and pallor of whole surface of body. θ Sick headache. 7.

°Now and then chilly sensations; hands cold. θ Headache from suppressed menses. 8.

° Hands and feet very cold. θ Sick headache. 10.

During last three days of the constipation is constantly θ cold, so that she looked blue, hands and cheeks felt cold as if dead; during day, she wore a shawl and sat near a fire, which failed to warm her; was awakened in night by feeling cold. 2 (3 to 5).

Chill following drinking.

Two chills during evening; no fever. 3 (4).

During evening felt very chilly, and cold inside body as though it were filled with ice. 3 (14).

° Very chilly, and external heat does not relieve her.θ Sick headache. 9.

° Constant chilliness even when near the fire. θ Sick headache. 11

Constantly cold during the constipation, so that she looked blue; hands and cheeks felt cold as if dead; could not get warm with extra clothing, or by sitting near a hot stove; was awakened at night by the coldness.

° Extremely cold, but no shaking or shivering; could not get warm by extra clothing, nor by sitting near a hot stove. θ Quininism. 9.

° Fever. θ Suppressed menses from putting hands in cold water. 9.

° Coldness over whole body. θ Constipation. 9.

° About 7 or 8 P.M. becomes so sleepy that she cannot resist, and has to lie down; about 9 P.M. a very hot fever comes on; during which she sleeps; the fever continues till near morning, when she awakes in a profuse sweat which stains the linen yellow, and is very difficult to wash out. 9.

Fell asleep after each dose in ten minutes, and woke in an hour in a profuse perspiration. 18.

° Is generally constipated, and when it is most persistent is very chilly and cannot get warm. 9.

° Temperature 100. θ Incipient softening of brain. 20.

Alternate flashes of heat and cold (no name).

Feverishness and thirst (no name).

° In malignant typhoid. A.A.

°Rhazes recommended it in all hectic fevers. A.A.

Hot fever 9 P.M., continues until near morning, wakes in profuse sweat, which stains linen yellow, difficult to wash out.

Hectic fever; malignant typhoid.

Sensation as if the sheets were damp.

Flushes of heat in the head and face, especially the left cheek.

Burning sensation in pelvis with sensation of weight.

Great internal heat during the nausea.

Sweat in the palms of the hands, especially the right.

Pulse rapid and feeble.

Chilliness.

Extreme coldness of the tips of the fingers which looked white.

Sleep—

° Feels sleepy all the time, but is much disturbed by unpleasant dreams. θ After suppressed menses. 8.

° Sleeps but little. θ Sick headache. 10.

Falls asleep while going upstairs or standing up. 4.

° Sleepy all day long. 3.

° At times sleeps for hours during attacks of headache. 9.

Most absurd dreams. 12 (1st week).

θ Dreamed that he had to go on a journey and was in danger of losing the train. 5 (4th and 5th night).

° Dreamed that herself and daughter started for the Grand Union Depot, a mile and a half distant, and were told they had only ten minutes to get there; that they ran most of the way, and arrived in time to see the train moving off, and awakened as much fatigued as if it had been a real experience. 9 (This, based upon above symptom, was the keynote of a case cured).

° Sleepless, restless at night, from incessant intolerable thirst. θDiabetes. A.A.

° Sleepless at night, and drowsy by day. Diabetes. A.A.

° No sleep at night, but occasionally slept towards morning. θ Diabetes. A.A.

° Almost complete loss of sleep. θ Diabetes. A.A.

° Quite nervous and sleepless. θ Incipient softening of brain. 20.

Intense sleepiness. A.A.

Sleepiness well marked for two weeks. A.A.

Sudden waking, wide awake without cause, soon went to sleep again. (No name.)

Sleeplessness in the first part of the night, little sleep near morning.

θVery sleepy all the time, can with difficulty keep awake. (No name.)

Great somnolency. (No name.)

Wakened by a sensation of coldness.

At times will sleep for hours (cured).

Great restlessness and extreme and protracted suffering from loss of sleep at night (cured).

Skin—

° Skin the colour of a red rose, with swelling of face, neck, arms, and body generally, in the morning, and during day and evening, no itching or burning. θ Sick headache. 11

° Sensation as if the sheets were damp. 9.

Sensation as if cold air was blowing on her, even when covered up warm. 9.

° Parched skin. θ Diabetes. A.A.

° Sallow complexion, with eczematous eruption disappeared, leaving a perfectly pure clean spotless skin; she was dyspeptic, but was well after eruption left. A.A.

° Wasted, thin, and excessively sallow, with dark stains beneath eyes. A.A.

Skin became beautifully clear after use of skim milk.

Itching of both knees at night.

Itching of the vulva.

Corn on the right little toe was very painful and sore every morning during the proving.

A symmetrical patch of herpetic eruption on each side of the neck, itching and burning after scratching, disappeared during the proving (cured).

Dry, parched skin.

Numbness and loss of sensation over the outer and anterior surfaces of the thighs.

Nerves—

|| Great lassitude and disinclination to exertion.

| Great restlessness and extreme and protracted suffering from loss of sleep at night.

| Feels completely tired out and exhausted, whether she does anything or not; great fatigue from walking.

| Great loss of strength, commencing with a sharp cutting pain in apex of heart; forehead feels heavy, with a dull sensation over eyes and throbbing, principally in temples, rest of head feels light.

Generalities—

Some of the symptoms lasted upwards of six weeks after the cessation of the medicine. 1.

° Formerly slender, became stout after the medicine. θ Sick headache. *6.*

° Feels so tired and languid that she is hardly able to turn over in bed; limbs almost tremble on trying to use them.

θHeadache from suppressed menses. 8.

Inclination to lean continually to right side. 3 (10).

In evening, suddenly felt very sick, could not sit up, no particular pain, but felt very weary. 3 (12).

In evening at 8 P.M., the same weak sick feeling came on as on 12th day, but did not last so long, and ceased suddenly. 3 (13).

At 8 P.M., the same symptoms of weakness appeared as on 12th and 13th days. 3 (15).

About 7:3° P.M., feels a tired weary sensation creeping over her, gradually increasing till it results in complete exhaustion, so that it is impossible to stand or sit up; at the same time, head feels very heavy, and falls to right side; she also wants to lie on right side with the body straight; when it commences to pass off, it does so very rapidly in an hour, leaving no disagreeable sensation whatever, but she feels perfectly well and strong. 3 (17 to 26).

During the proving, loss of flesh, most marked in the *shrinkage of the breasts, which have since resumed their natural size and firmness. 3.

° Cannot lie on left side. 3.

° Feels completely tired out and exhausted, whether she does anything or not. 3.

° Faint spells from one to three times a week, at first irregular as to time of day, now coming on at 7:30 P.M.; can produce an attack any time by extending her arms high above head, or by pressure round waist. 3.

° Great loss of strength; cannot stand, but falls backwards, and remains entirely unconscious for two or three minutes;, the weakness gradually passes off in half an houright θ Faint spells. 3.

° Sudden prostration of strength at 5 P.M. θ Sick headache. | |

° Aching pains all overight θ Suppressed menses from putting hands in cold water. 9.

° Cannot walk more than one-fourth mile without resting.

θ Diabetes. A.A.

° As soon as she steps on feet in morning, she becomes faint and nauseated, and has to lie down; must lie down three or four times before she can get dressed. 9.

° Languor, lassitude, impaired sensibility. θ Diabetes. A.A.

° Loss of energy, and fatigue on exertion; always feeling dull, heavy, and languid. θ Diabetes. A.A.

° Coldness and numbness of limbs. θ Diabetes. A.A.

° Flabby and inclined to obesity. θ Diabetes. A.A.

° Great fatigue on the slightest exertion. θ Diabetes. A.A.

° Very stout, with much difficulty in breathing. θ Bright's disease. A.A.

° Very anemic. θ Bright's disease. A.A.

Great lassitude and disinclination to exertion.

Great fatigue from walking.

Felt cold and chilly inside of the body, as though it was filled with ice.

Loss of flesh during the proving, particularly of the breasts, but they resumed their natural size after the proving.

Great depression of spirits, with strong inclination to cry.

Twitching of the muscles of the body.

Occasionally felt extremely nervous.

Loss of weight in various cases.

Great loss of strength, commencing with a sharp cutting pain in the apex of the heart, followed by a strange feeling in the head; the forehead feels heavy with a dull sensation over the eyes, and throbbing, principally in the temples—rest of the head feels light—dimness of vision; can only see light, not objects. Loss of strength, falls backward and is unconscious. Attack soon passes off, followed by weeping, palpitation of the heart and great depression of spirits. Attack can be brought on at any time by raising the hands above the head, or by pressure around the waist. In a young girl of 17 whose menses were irregular (cured).

Indefinable indisposition, not usually associated with local suffering, except a dull aching pain in the lumbar region.

Great debility or prostration of muscular power, as well as of nervous energy.

Fatigued and exhausted after moderate exertion, unable to walk even a short distance without being obliged to take a rest.

Listlessness and disinclination for either bodily or mental exertion.

Great restlessness and extreme and protracted suffering from loss of sleep at night.

Increased emaciation which ultimately becomes extreme.

Perverse and deficient nutrition.

Loss of energy.

Enormous obesity in a lady (cured).

Ability to walk a long distance without rest or fatigue.

A woman who could not drink milk without its causing sick headache (cured).

Recommended by Hippocrates in phthisis, in gouty affections, particularly where the articulations are involved, also in sciatica and leucorrhea.

Considered the best and surest remedy in all dropsies, in asthma when the result of emphysema and pulmonary catarrh, in obstinate neuralgia, when its cause lies in the intestinal canal, in diseases of the liver, simple hypertrophy and fatty degeneration, and generally in diseases when there is faulty nutrition, often a consequence of obscure subacute inflammation of the stomach or intestines, followed by affections of the nervous centers.

Found to be a sovereign remedy in dropsical cases, with hypertrophied liver and following intermittent fever.

Marked improvement had been seen in cases where the dropsy is the result of organic heart disease, or of old standing liver complaint, or of far advanced Bright's disease.

Noise very annoying.

| | Pain commencing across the upper sacral region, passing around either side over the hips down to groins and down thighs inside, sometimes to the feet—cured several cases.

Bell Barnum, age 13, dark hair: For the last year has had severe headache at times, and great pain across the umbilicus; also pains passing down the under side of thighs to the heels. Pains in the top of feet as if the bones were broken across the instep.

These pains in the legs and feet would come on as soon as she stepped upon them in the morning, upon which she would be faint and nauseated and have to lie down. Would have to lie down three or four times before she could get dressed (cured). Three or four months after the headache returned, and was again cured by Defloratum.

Judge Martin for years has had a bloating, at times in the epigastric region, and with it he would always have an attack of asthma, so that he could scarcely breathe; then he would have a hard pressive pain at about the fourth cervical vertebra. These symptoms were only relieved by taking pills, which would cause a free evacuation of the bowels. Was always constipated (cured).

Caroline Betz, German, aged 18: About 7 or 8 P.M. becomes so sleepy that she cannot resist and has to lie down about 9 P.M. A very hot fever comes on during which she sleeps; the fever continues till near morning, when she wakes in a profuse sweat which stains the linen yellow and is very difficult to wash out.

During the day her back usually feels cold; short dry cough

with difficult expectoration of a small lump of mucus, which relieves the cough. Irregular menstruation, sometimes very dark and scanty, and sometimes colourless wateright Pimples oh face and forehead. Nov. 8, gave Deflor. 1m. Was entirely relieved of all the symptoms after the first dose. Nov. 14. The menstrual period is not yet due.

"Sore aching," with some throbbing in the outer side, and partly along the sole of right foot, very excruciating pains coming and going by spells; walking did not seem to affect it. The pain would come quite often, perhaps every half hour, last a few moments, then pass away. It gave her a good deal of trouble and caused her to suddenly drop to the floor to hold the foot; she could not stand on the foot during the pain. The pain would come on suddenly and go away rather suddenly, but leave the part sore for a short time. Lac caninum cmm. in water, a spoonful every three hours, relieved.

After the first dose a decided aggravation, pains going more to the sole of the foot, and much more severe. Shortly after the second dose there was entire relief. She took but two doses and continues entirely free from the trouble.

Skin—

Sensation as if an insect was crawling on shoulders and neck, occasionally on both hands.

| Herpetic eruption in both axillse, with light brownish scab, extremely painful when washing; eruption most in right axilla, and in both instances appeared previous to pain in labia, which was followed by a discharge of blood from vagina.

Every scratch gets sore.

Ichthyosis, with branlike desquamation of skin.

I Shining, glazed, and red appearance of ulcers on shin and wrist.

Crusts on skin, under which greyish yellow matter formed and was squeezed out.

Slight roughness of skin of forehead, as of numerous pimples.

| | On face, hands, neck and chest, bright scarlet eruption exactly like scarlatina.

Throat full of large foul, grey yellow patches; deglutition especially painful after sleep and from swallowing fruits (acid); lumpy sensation felt in the middle of the throat; unrest, delirium with undefined fears; considerable bright red, fine eruption on face and chest; itching with dry skin.

| | Bright scarlet redness on chest and around neck; next day all over body except legs, which were, however, covered that night; skin in large patches assumed dark red colour bordering on purple, as seen in malignant cases, while body seemed swollen.

| | Diphtheria with or following scarlatina.

| | Ichthyosis, with branlike desquamation of skin.

Very small blotches like flea-bites.

| Small blotches on chest, wrists and right knee.

| | Several boils on left side.

| | Crusts on skin, under which greyish yellow matter formed and was squeezed out.

Sleep—

| | Great desire to sleep.

| | Cried out and talked in sleep.

| Cannot find any comfortable position in bed; there is no way that she can put her hands that they do not bother her; falls asleep at last on her face.

| | Dreamed a large snake was in bed.

| | Got to sleep late; profuse sweat during sleep; felt feverish all night; in morning > in every way.

| | At night lies with leg flexed on thigh, and thigh on pelvis; restless; < after sleep.

Symptoms < after sleep.

| | Sleeplessness from emotional strain, with entire nervous debility.

Very restless at night; very difficult to get into a comfortable position; generally goes to sleep lying on back with hands over head.

| Sleep disturbed, very wakeful; limbs cold all night.

|| Sleep prevented by being very cold for one hour after retiring, with great nervousness.

Very restless all night, could not keep clothes over her.

|| Sleepless and crying continually.

|| Restless sleep at night, bad dreams.

Got to sleep late; profuse sweat during sleep; felt feverish all night; in morning > in every way.

| Dreams frequently that she is urinating, and wakes to find herself on point of doing so, requiring immediate relief.

|| Dreams of going on a journey, and was separated from party, and had to walk a long distance, and arrived at station just in time to see train start off.

|| Aggravation of symptoms after sleep.

Fever—

Chilly feeling lasting all day.

Internal chilliness with external warmth.

Cold chills run down back, hands as cold as ice (on entering house 4 P.M.; 6:30 entire > after a good dinner).

||Fever and chills for a few days, and up and down every few hours.

Intense fever on waking in morning, with perspiration.

Dry, hot skin.

| Exhausting sweats; after sleep.

Wakes at night in cold perspiration, with fearful foreboding.

Perspired considerably through night, sweat having a rank smell.

|| Severe chills.

| Feels feverish.

||Fever and bathed in warm perspiration, especially about face, neck and hands.

|| Intense heat.

|| Moderate fever.

|| Fever

|| High fever

|| Dry, hot skin.

|| Fever returning every afternoon.

|| Temperature, 102, 102¾, 103, 103¼.

|| Sweat all over

|| Skin clammy.

|| Wakes in night in cold perspiration, with fearful foreboding.

|| Perspired considerably through night, sweat having a rank smell.

Feverish in evening.

Flashes of heat, commencing in chest and extending up over face and head, when she would break out in sweat, which would dry up in a short time; face would become moist first, and become dry first.

Sensation over whole chest as if dripping with sweat when only slightly moist.

Nerves—

Restlessness.

| No inclination for least exertion, would like to do nothing but sleep; much lassitude.

|| Heaviness, weakness, general languor.

|| Profound depression of vitality.

| General weakness and prostration very marked.

|| Great exhaustion, with 'poisoned' feeling.

|| Profound prostration, to extent of refusing to make effort to take a dose of medicine.

|| In morning so much prostrated that she could not turn in bed; so tired.

|| Very weak.

|| Sinking spells every morning, attended with great nervousness.

| | Often feels as if she would lose use of limbs.

| | Child partially paralyzed after diphtheria; could not walk; pain all over, cough, aphonia, loss of appetite, emaciation.

| | When walking seems to be walking on air; when lying does not seem to touch bed.

| Suffering from very unpleasant nervous symptoms; not in low spirits, but weak, and nerves so thoroughly out of order that she cannot bear one finger to touch the other, and often feels as though she should lose use of her limbs; sensation as if throat were closing, sensation is between throat and nose; feels as if something in throat was either enlarged or relaxed, and has a desire to keep mouth open; talking difficult; disposition to talk through nose; sometimes cannot swallow, because there seems to be a kind of muscular contraction in throat; sleep restless, frequently wakes with sick headache, which seems to commence at nape; wakes with severe pain at lower part of back; pain leaves when about work a short time, does not return until next morning; nerves very much overwrought, afraid of being unable to perform duties.

The prejudice held by many honorable men against the use of this remedy, like that meted to Lachesis—because they could not obtain the tincture—would soon yield to gratitude for its excellent work if given bedside test in some terrible left sided headaches. Two remedies in the materia medica excel its eye pathogenesis in symptoms of eye strain, in asthenopia and ciliary neuritis. It vies with Onosmodium in affections of eye strain in children and with Spigelia in neuralgias of the left orbit.

It was introduced and proved by Swan with the 17th, 30th and 200th potencies. Its complete pathogenesis was published in the *Medical Visitor* in Aug., 1893, and in the *Homeopathic World,* Vol. 18, p. 151, from which this record is taken.

LAC FELINUM (Cat's Milk)

Mind—Great depression of spirits.

Very cross to every one.

Fear of falling down stairs, but without vertigo.

Morbid concientiousness; every little fault appeared a crime.

Mental illusion that the corners of furniture, or any pointed object near her, were about to run into eyes; the symptom is purely mental; the objects do not appear to her sight to be too close (asthenopia).

Head—

Dull pain in forehead in region of eyebrows

Heaviness in forehead.

Heavy pressure in sides of head and vertex.

Pulsations in head, with sensation of heat in forehead, and constriction across bridge of nose.

Acute pains on vertex.

Acute pains in frontal region.

Intense pain early in morning on vertex, and left side of head; it commences just in front of vertex, with a flush of heat which extends front about an inch, and is followed by the intense pain; the heat and pain then spread, never crossing median line, down left side as a veil, taking half the nose and jaws, and entering ear, causing her to close the eyes from its intensity; during the pain, head drawn down so that chin pressed heavily on chest, and her agony was so great that she had to hold the head firmly in her hands, and rush through the house from room to room screaming (from the 17th potency).

Acute pain over left eye and temple.

Pain in head < from reading.

Sharp lancinating pains passing zig-zag down left side of head about every ten minutes from vertex toward left ear.

Pain commencing with a chilly sensation at root of nose; also a cold pain passing up median line to vertex, and passing up to ear (like the previous symptom).

Headache over eyes (1).

Pain in forehead, occiput, and left side of head, with rigidity of cords of neck (splenius and trapezius), and heat in vertex; the pain in forehead is heavy pressing down over eyes (headache).

Intense pain from head along lower jaw, causing mouth to fill with saliva.

Crawling on top of brain (asthenopia).

Weight on vertex (asthenopia).

Terrible headache penetrating left eyeball to centre of brain, with pain in left supra-orbital region extending through brain to vertex (headache).

Burning in left temple near eye, < at night (keratitis).

Eyes—

Sharp lancinating pain through centre of left eyeball, leaving it very sore internally, and causing profuse lachrymation (from the 1m.).

Heavy pressure downwards of eyebrows and eyelids, as if the parts were lead.

Inclination to keep eyes shut.

Eyes feel as if sunken in head, and left eye occasionally waters.

Twitching of outer end of left upper lid, inside.

(Twitching of eyelids right and left)

(Ciliary neuralgia.)

Sharp lancinating pain in centre of right eyeball extending externally to temple and frontal region over eye, with intense photophobia, redness of conjunctiva, and lachrymation; < by reading or writing; the pain appears to be in interior of eyeball, and extends thence to posterior wall of orbit, and then to the temples with throbbing; dim sight when reading; also constipation, loss of appetite, lassitude in legs (choroiditis).

(Have had great success with it in eye cases, especially where there is severe pain in back of orbit, indicating choroiditis.— Swan.)

On looking fixedly, reading, or writing, darting pain from eyes nearly to occiput; much < in right eye (asthenopia).

When reading letters run together, with dull aching pain behind eyes, or shooting in eyes, the confused sight and shooting being < in right eye; symptoms excited by catching cold or by over-fatigue (asthenopia).

Pain in eyes, back into head, extremely sharp, with a sensation as if eyes extended back; great photophobia to natural or artificial light; any continued glare results in this pain (improved).

Darting pain going backwards in centre of right eye, < at night (keratitis).

If she lies on left side, right eye feels as if it were moving about and too heavy, with great pain.

(Ulceration of cornea).

Photophobia.

[Left eye feels hot and adheres in morning.

White spot on outer edge of left cornea, with red vessels running up to it from conjunctiva, and shooting pains from the spot to occiput.

Pain in right lower orbital border as if sore, with tenderness there on touch, and shooting in right eye.

Right eye inflamed with shooting backward where the white spot is; left eye also inflamed, but without shooting.

Stye on left upper lid.

Two styes on right lower lid.

Eyes get bad ever September.

Eyes ache by gaslight.

(Cured in various cases of ulceration of cornea.)]

Whitish ulcer in right cornea over pupil; right eyelids red and swollen; lachrymation of right eye. Darting pain going backward in centre of right eye, < at night. If she lies on left side, right eye feels as if it were moving about and were too heavy, with severe pain. With the right eye everything seems in a white fog. Photophobia of right eye. Always feels weary.

Mright E., aged 28, chronic iritis; in the last three years had six attacks alternating in either eye. First attack lasted five weeks; intervals between attacks from five to eight months. Had been told he was incurable.

March 26, '88. Right eye much inflamed; dull aching pain at night; shooting from right eye to temple and eye-brow; worse between 3 and 5 A.M. Sight very hazy. Iris looks red. A black spot before right eye, moving with the eye when in sunlight. Lac felinum cm. Gradual and certain improvement, sight less hazy, eye looks clear; sensation of sand in right eye on waking; black specks have disappeared; can read print now.—Berridge.

Right eye inflamed; dull aching pain at night.

Shooting from right eye to temple and eyebrow, < between 3 and 5 A.M.

Sight very hazy.

Iris, red.

A black spot before right eye, moving with the eye when in sunlight.

Sensation of sand in right eye on waking.

Nose—

Cannot bear the smell of clams, of which she is naturally very fond, and cannot eat them.

Teeth—

Pains in all the teeth as the hot pain from head touched them.

Mouth—

Sensation as if tongue were scalded by a hot drink.

Redness under tongue, on gums, and whole buccal cavity.

Soreness and sensation of ulcers on tongue and roof of mouth.

The parts of mouth seem to stick together, requiring an injection of air or saliva to separate them.

Loss of taste.

Brassy taste in mouth.

Salivation, tongue enlarged and serrated at edges by teeth.

Small white ulcers covering tongue and whole buccal cavity.

Elongation of palate.

Very sore mouth.

(Dryness of mouth.)

Throat—

Tough mucus in pharynx.

Stringy, tough mucus in pharynx, cannot hawk it up and has to swallow it; when it can be expectorated it is yellow.

Mucus in pharynx between head and throat is thick, yellow, tough, stringy, expectorated with difficulty, and has a sickish sweet taste.

Posterior wall of pharynx slightly inflamed, with sensation of soreness.

Stomach—

No appetite.

After eating feels swollen; has to take off her dress and. loosen clothes.

Great desire to eat paper.

Stomach sore all around just below the belt, < left side.

Occasionally very slight nausea.

Heat in epigastrium.

Great soreness and sensitiveness of epigastric region.

Abdomen—

Pain in abdomen and back, as if menses about commencing.

Pain in bowels.

At midnight, sensation of a cold bandage over lower part of abdomen.

Great weight and bearing down in pelvis, like falling of the womb, as if she could not walk; < when standing.

Pain in pelvis through hips on pressure, as when placing arms akimbo.

Stool and Rectum.—

Natural stool, but very slow in passing, at 2 A.M.

Stool long, tenacious, slipping back when ceasing to strain; seeming inability of rectum to expel its contents.

Urinary Organs—

Frequent desire to urinate, urine very pale.

(Obstruction in urinating, has to wait.)

Female Sexual Organs—

Leucorrhea ceased on third and reappeared on fourth day.

Furious itching of vulva, inside and out; yellow leucorrhea.

(Dragging pain in left ovary.)

Respiratory Organs—

Dryness of rim of glottis.

Chest—

Very much oppressed for breath, continuing for several days; it is a difficulty in drawing a long breath, or rather that requires the drawing of a long inspiration, for it seems as if the breathing was done by upper part of lungs alone.

Upper Limbs—

Pain in right side of left wrist when using index finger.

Lower Limbs—

Left foot feels cold when touched by right foot.

Legs ache.

Sleep—

Dulness, sleepiness, gaping.

Heavy, profound sleep, not easily awakened.

Dreamed of earthquakes.

Fever—

Cold and heat alternately, each continuing but a short time.

Generalities—

Entire right side from crown to sole felt terribly weak, heavy, and distressed, so that it was difficult to walk.

(Constant nervous trembling, especially of hands, as in drunkards.)

LAC VACCINUM (Cow's Milk)

Introduced and proved by Dr. J. C. Boardman, of Trenton, New Jersey, who used Swan's 200th. Many persons are very intolerant of milk, in whom it produces headache, "biliousness," intestinal flatulence and obstinate constipation. These effects of milk were developed in the proving, especially the characteristic headache and constipation, and have been clinically verified. It is also well to remember that it develops or aggravates the uric acid diathesis, thus increasing the rheumatic tendency, while the thirst and polyuria should call our attention to it as a remedy to study in diabetes.

In some highly sensitive women the effect on the function of the sexual organs is pronounced; the menstrual flow being suppressed by putting the hands in cold water; drinking a glass of milk will promptly suppress flow until the next period, mark the idiosyncrasy. Burnett remarks as a clinical fact that children who drink much milk after their teeth are fully grown become very liable to colds.

Like Natrum muriaticum, the potentized remedy will produce its characteristic symptoms, even when the prover is using it in the crude form at the same time.

Mind–

General nervousness, with depression of spirits, feeling as though about to hear bad news.

Mental confusion, lasting a long time after proving.

Mental prostration, came on so suddenly, was unable to collect her thoughts or write her symptoms.

Mental confusion, could not express her thoughts.

Dull, weak, confused, with trembling of whole body.

Head—

Vertigo: falls backwards if she closes her eyes.

A creeping sensation, or screw-like or vertical motion, began over left eye, and continued upwards to vertex, next the same motion or feeling began two inches behind left ear, and likewise went upwards to vertex; also a pressure on vertex, with a sensation of heat when hand was applied (1 h.).

Sensation like a fire-ball in each temple simultaneously (20m.).

All these symptoms passed away except pain on top of head, which feels as though something heavy were laid there, and occasionally a sharp pain simultaneously (3½h.).

Woke in morning with an aching pain all over head, most severe in occiput.

Fullness of head as if too large and heavy.

Vertigo.

Eyes—

Dull pain over right eye, and very slight dull feeling over left eye.

Eyes have a blur, or dimness, or obscurity of sight, off and on for a few moments at a time.

Blindness of both eyes, which came on three or four times in succession, lasting only a second at a time, then passing entirely away, leaving a pain in each temple, on top of head, left ear, and below left ear in the neck (2½h.).

Ears—

Ears felt stopped up; felt deaf in both ears, although she could hear as before.

Mouth—

Had a dirty, yellow-coated tongue, which felt parched.

Sour taste.

Acid saliva staining handkerchief yellow.

Ulcers on tongue, flat, white, sunken; tongue swollen, exceedingly sensitive, covered with white, slimy mucus on the parts not ulcerated; breath extremely fetid; sores extend to inside of cheeks and tonsils; deglutition painful.

Throat—

Sensation of plug in throat or larynx.

Appetite—

Thirst for cold water in quantities; drank three tumblerfuls during evening.

Stomach.—Had a swelling or bloating of stomach (3d d.).

At 10:30 A.M. sour taste; nausea, but no rising or vomiting (1 h.).

Contractive, pressing pain in stomach-pit, > by external pressure.

Eructation

Abdomen—

Pain proceeding from sternum, extending across abdomen about an inch below umbilicus.

Constant intolerable flatulence, begins an hour after drinking milk for lunch and lasts all the afternoon.

Borborygmus, with loud, noisy rumbling (200).

Stool—

Obstinate constipation; stool hard, dry; inimpacted balls; can be passed only with great straining.

Passage of stinking flatus, in large quantity, which relieves.

Urinary Organs—

Urine was not increased in morning, but was dark red, without sediment.

Filled a large iron spoon with the urine and boiled it for twenty minutes; it left quite a mass of albumin, about a quarter of the whole; specific gravity 1030.

Yesterday the urine turned blue paper red; to-day it turns the red paper blue (13th d.).

In afternoon was obliged to urinate every fifteen minutes, in large quantity each time; was afraid to go across the street to a store for fear it would overtake me before I could return; it all passed off the same night.

The density of urine varied during a few days from 1,018 to 1,028, colour clear, odorless, acid reaction.

Frequent discharge of clear urine, nearly colourless, no sediment.

Female Sexual Organs—

White watery leucorrhea; pain in sacrum.

Drinking a glass of milk will promptly suppress the flow until next menstrual period.

Menses, suppressed, delayed by putting hands in cold water.

"Nausea of pregnancy with desire for food > by drinking milk."

Respiratory Organs.—

Sensation of plug in throat or larynx.

Chest—

A sharp pain appeared in a spot the size of a shilling on each side of sternum and about middle of chest, with a sense of suffocation.

Later a burning sensation in same region.

Same pain extends across abdomen about five inches lower down (about an inch below umbilicus); it did not seem to involve the bladder; no rumbling or passing of flatus.

Sharp pains in left lower chest, or in region of lower lobe of left lung; the pain was momentary and did not return (5th d.).

Sharp pain began in right chest, about three inches below clavicle; it passed upward to top of right shoulder, then down arm and forearm to thumb, and then passed off.

Back—

Pains in sacrum.

Severe, dull, aching pains in lumbar region; prover often exclaims, "Oh, how my back aches !

Upper Limbs—

Fingers of both hands, especially when stretched out, tremble and quiver as from extreme weakness.

A clammy sticky coldness in both hands and both feet simultaneously.

Sharp pain under left scapula, about three inches down from top; it then passed upwards to top of left shoulder, then down arm and forearm and hand to the four fingers of the left hand, and then passed off.

Soon afterwards an aching pain was felt in left hip-joint, which soon passed off.

Lower Limbs—

Piercing or lancinating pain in each hip-joint, not severe.

Aching pain along both thighs on outer side and terminating in both knees.

Aching pains in both knees like a rheumatic pain; they began simultaneously in both knees, but the right was most severe (5th d.).

On going up stairs the knees trembled or quivered or were extremely weak, so as to be unable to take a step forwards.

Aching pains in bones from both hip-joints to both feet simultaneously; also burning sensation in both feet.

All the joints of the body, especially knees, feel weak and powerless, as when half drunk.

Short rheumatic pains in knee and tarsal joints when walking.

Sleep—

Slept well all night, and woke in morning free from. pain (8:30 A.M.).

Head feels all over heavy, dull, aching, drowsy, wants to go to sleep.

Gait is unsteady.

Must force herself to keep awake.

Must force herself to keep her eyes open, for if she shuts them she cannot avoid falling backwards and down to the floor.

In seven hours said she still felt sleepy, and could have fallen asleep in a minute at any time during the whole day.

General restlessness and bad dreams.

Dreams of trying to lay out a corpse, etc.

Fever—

Hands became hot and dry, a decided fever heat of hands.

Also pain on left side of head, extending from neck to top of head, and a chilling sensation with it.

A slight fever over the entire body with a moisture in both hands, and aching in legs from thighs to knees, both sides simultaneously.

Fever at night, followed by profuse sweat all over; the fever was preceded by chilly feeling, commencing at shoulders, and then running up from feet to head; headache.

Skin—

Brown crusts, having a greasy appearance, especially in corners of mouth, similar to what are called "butter-sores."

Miss H. took one dose 1m (Fincke). It caused frequent profuse discharge of clear urine, no sediment, and nearly colourless. White, watery leucorrhea; pains in sacrum; sensation of plug in throat or larynx; sour taste in mouth; acid saliva staining handkerchief yellow; contractive pressing pain in stomach-pit, relieved by external pressure.

Generalities—

The pains in chest, abdomen, hips, thighs, and knees were all felt on right and left sides simultaneously.

She was so suddenly prostrated mentally and bodily that she was unable to collect her thoughts or use a pencil to write her symptoms; I was therefore compelled to witness and ask questions and record them; after the proving was nearly over she said she had so much mental confusion that she could not get mentally clear enough to feel her thoughts or express them;

she could only give direct short answers to questions; as for writing her symptoms, she had no physical power to do it. In two hours all symptoms subsided gradually, but still there was a general trembling or quivering of whole body as well as the fingers. In six and a half hours nearly relieved, except great physical prostration; mind is again normal.

LYSSIN (Hydrophobinum ; Saliva of a Rabid Dog)

Introduced and proved by Hering in 1833, fifty years before the crude experiments of Pasteur with the serum.

The toxic or non-toxic property of animal saliva has long been a question of scientific discussion. Trevinarus found that the human saliva became red by the addition of tincture of iron; and Gmelin discovered that this colour was caused by Sulpho-cyanate. The question in dispute appeared to be that Cyanic acid being a poison, Sulpho-cyanate also must be one, and of course its combination with alkalies, and being poisons, they could not be in the saliva. Years before this discovery, Oken had declared that "saliva is poison." But the discoveries of Liebig and other chemists have demonstrated that Sulpho-cyanic acid is to be found in sheep, dogs and many other animals.

The experiments of Bernard and others, in *Virchow's Archives,* 1858, have decided that Sulpho-cyanate of Potash found in saliva of animals, acts as a poison under certain conditions. Bernard considered that it acted only by application to cellular tissue. In this he was, no doubt, in error, being misled by the analogy of the snake poison. But, Weir Mitchell in his "Researches on the Venom of the Rattlesnake," page 34, says, he "could not discover any in the rattlesnake poison, notwithstanding repeated experiments."

Livingston, the African explorer, has reported the bite of the lion as poisonous; and the same claim is made in the East Indies regarding the bite of the tiger. From time immemorial it has been known in every country village that the bite of an angry cat is poisonous, and the effects often severe, even fatal. This is also true with the bite of all other animals, human beings included, when in a fit of passion.

Hering reports a case taken from a French journal in which a healthy farmer, aet. 19, while holding a duck in his lap was bitten on the lip by the angry drake. The same day he felt sick, grew rapidly worse, and a few weeks after died. He also says, that "after the bite of a dog not rabid difficult healing ulcers will follow." It is further known, that after the bite of a rabid dog not only the wounds made by the teeth heal in an unusually short time, but several physicians have observed that even the usual cauterizations are not inclined to inflame, rather more inclined to heal quickly. We may take this for a pathognomonic symptom of the slumbering poison of Lyssin; the same thing is true of leprosy before it breaks out.

Now comes the work of Pasteur, in 1878, 1879 and 1880:

His experiments furnished evidence that the malignant disease, splenic fever, was caused by bacteria.

An animal inoculated with a few drops of a liquid containing this bacteria, develops the disease with astonishing rapidity and dies within one or two days. But, he claims that chickens are an exception to this rule, because when similarly inoculated they remain in perfect health. Pasteur's explanation of this strange fact is based on a higher bodily temperature of birds than any other warm blooded animals. The temperature of animals most readily affected by splenic fever ranges from 33 to 35C., while the blood temperature of chickens is from 42 to 43C. degrees. Now, by reducing the temperature of the chicken after inoculation, Pasteur found it had died of splenic fever, the same as any other animal. Further experiments by Pasteur convinced him that propagation of bacteria is arrested by a temperature of 44 or more degrees. These facts called Pasteur's attention to radiate heat as the best local application to prevent the generation of bacteria. And the same principle has been applied in domestic practice for the cure of a snakebite by killing a chicken, cutting it open and applying the warm surface to the bitten limb, replacing it as soon as it became cold by another, and in this way it is claimed that on the plains of the West, where the bite of the rattlesnake is so common, that nearly every case has been cured; the 10 degrees of greater heat seemed to be sufficient in the bite of the rattlesnake as well as of the bacteria of splenic fever.

In June, 1831, Hering published a letter in Stapf's *Archives,* Vol. 10, which was dated June 18th, 1830, in which he says: "The proving of snake poison might pave the way to the prevention of hydrophobia and variola by the proving of their respective morbific poisons." And on page 30, of the same volume, he says: "Same is said of psora."

It will be remembered that Hering's immortal proving of Lachesis was begun in 1828, and experimented with for three years, when it was finally published; hence the experience which Hering obtained in the proving of the serpent poison was evidently the inspiration for his suggestion that the proving on the healthy of Lyssin, Variolinum, Psorinum and other nosodes would form valuable remedies in the treatment of many of our obstinate diseases. Hering no sooner became firmly convinced of the truth of his suggestion than he at once set to work to put it into execution.

But, the first thing to do was to find a mad dog. The opportunity occurred on the 27th of August, 1833, when a German baker invited him to come to his house to examine a dog. The following description of his capture of a rabid dog and obtaining the saliva for a proving is taken from a paper by Hering in the *North American Journal* of 1878:

It was a middle-sized, chestnut-brown terrier, not more than two or three years old, a female, with puppies of two or three months old. It had been bitten ten days before (with August) in the street by a running dog, which was biting all around, and had been killed soon afterwards as mad. The owner, in trying to save his terrier, had beaten the strange dog with a stick after it had killed one of the puppies, and had already taken hold of another. The mother, in defending her young ones, had received three bloody wounds. She carried the dead one in her mouth from the street home into the yard. Since that she was somewhat changed, but continued to nurse the remaining puppies, one of which had received a bite. She had been otherwise true to her nature until the previous day (Aug. 26th), when she had commenced snapping and biting her young. The master had then suspected her, and kept her in the yard, tied by a rope; and several times she had been biting and trying to loosen herself. She soon grew worse and commenced to bite at everything. Her voice was entirely altered. On the 26th of August, in the evening, she had commenced to howl in a peculiar, way and to run against the doors. She shook her head a great deal, and scraped the ground with her fore feet; and afterwards turned her head in a strange way. She put her mouth into the water placed before her, as if she was trying to swallow but could not.

When seen on August 27th she was furious; snapping and biting, had a wild look, injected red eyes, frothy saliva around the mouth, and seemed evidently to be in the last stage of the disease. An empty flour-barrel was, from behind, put over her; and, in order to make it possible to secure some of the saliva, the barrel was lifted on one side until the dog, in trying to escape, put out her head, between the edge of the barrel and the ground. She seemed to be in convulsive motions, as from anger or fury; but while a quill was used to get as much of the saliva as possible out of her mouth and from her teeth (part to be put into milk sugar and part into alcohol), the motions lessened and the dog lay quiet and exhausted, breathing quick and short, with eyes closed. While the quill was still held in her mouth, and while the baker had hold of the barrel, the dog suddenly sprang up, snapping and trying to get on to its feet; but the owner prevented its escape. After enough had been collected, the dog was allowed to withdraw its head; and by a heavy weight was secured under the barrel. After a box had been prepared, the dog was brought into it by means of the rope, and thus transported, with both puppies, to my house.

Next morning the mother was dead, and no permission given by the inmates to make a post mortem. Both the young ones were returned to the master; and even the bitten one remained well. They were given to inhale in the evening some of the 6th centesimal potency, just prepared. Of course, a true Hahneniannian never draws his conclusions, as the slanderers have said: *post hoc ergo propter hoc,* nor even the equally foolish; it followed, but could not have been caused by it.

The saliva obtained in the aforesaid way was on the same day triturated; one drop with one hundred grains of milk sugar, and, exactly according to Hahnemann's method, carried to the 3d centesimal; and, by the aid of some water and alcohol, further by alcohol alone, up to the 6th centesimal, and later to the 30th.

From the tincture of the saliva put in alcohol, some weeks after, one drop was also potentized in the usual way for the purpose of comparative experiments. All the rest, collected on split pieces of quill for inoculation, was one night clandestinely taken by the lady of the house and thrown into the fire.

All this has been related in its particulars as an advice to others who may have a chance to get saliva from another dog. It might be of some use to get it from a male for comparison.

Symptoms were observed during the hours of trituration, as there had been triturating the Lachesis poison, and they were afterwards corroborated by provings with the lower; the very peculiar feelings of apprehension became so intolerable that the higher were preferred ill further provings. Nothing was written for publication in the *Archives* until May, 1834. This was printed in the beginning of 1836, *Archives,* 15, left, p. 33.

To the provings of Schmid and Behlert* were added those of John Redmond Cox, in 1853, when a suggestion was made that, in order to remove the stigma of cowardice in the profession, their shrinking from their first duty of proving remedies on themselves was made in a public meeting. Dr. Cox not only offered to prove it on himself, but on his entire family and his friends besides, and furnished us perhaps the best provings that have ever been made of Lyssin; he also furnished the day-books in which the symptoms were recorded.

Many of the most valuable symptoms were from provings by Hering, on himself, but he was prevented from continuing by the most terrible feelings of apprehension.

Dr. Knerr made some valuable provings, in 1869, on a woman bitten by a dog in the fleshy part of right arm.

Dr. Lippe cured an important case in which he was guided by a symptom produced only from bites, but never observed any provings. But Lippe's observation was confirmed by many other good observers. Some symptoms from bites of rabid dogs have been added:

Pasteur's method of administration is very different from that employed by homeopaths, but he is working on homeopathic lines in seeking to neutralize a virus in the system by introducing a modification of the same virus. His experiments led him to produce the rabic poison in a highly intensified form in the spinal cords of rabbits. He then modified its intensity in different degrees by exposure to air for a longer or shorter period. Patients who come to the Institute are inoculated first with the least potent, and later with the most potent 'vaccin,' after which they are pronounced 'cured.' The 'cure' is, however, extremely uncertain, as the degree of susceptibility to the poison is unknown in any case, and many hundreds of the patients subjected to the inoculations have died of the disease. Pasteur's first method was admitted to be too strong, and was soon modified; a number of patients having died from the inoculations. One of these cases I investigated, and the symptoms were sufficiently striking to deserve recording.

The patient was Arthur Wilde, of Rotherham, aged 29, and received the account from his mother, who nursed him through his illness. He had been bitten severely by a man suffering from hydrophobia, and was persuaded, much against his wish, to go to Pasteur. This he did a few days, after the bite, returning on October 19, 1886, after undergoing the course. On Saturday, October 30th, he complained of a pricking sensation below the ribs in the right side, in the part where the injections had been made. Pressure relieved the pain somewhat. That evening he vomited, and the vomiting continued, and he became very prostrate. On Monday the prostration was intense, vomiting continued; restless; skin cool, perspiring; quite conscious. The spots where the inoculations were made were dark and livid. Twitching occurred every few hours, sometimes more violently than others; most marked on the abdomen. From Monday through Tuesday he was making a peculiar loud noise, something like a waggoner driving horses, 'bis,' 'whoo,' though he had never had to do with horses. He seemed completely helpless. On Tuesday night vomiting ceased and he began to froth a great deal. Early on Wednesday morning he began to talk thick. His breathing, which had been peculiar all through—he would hold his breath for a long time when making the noise, and then breathe rapidly for a few breaths—became very bad at 3 A.M. on Wednesday. He died shortly after 12, having been apparently conscious to the end, though unable to speak for the last houright The frothing had increased up to the time of his death and he seemed to choke with it.

This case was paralleled by that of Goffi, an attendant at St. Thomas' Hospital, who was bitten by a cat and sent to Pasteuright On his return he was taken ill, and his case was at first diagnosed as Landry's paralysis, but finally proved (by experiments made with his spinal cord) to be 'paralytic rabies,' the result of inoculation. It was after the occurrence of these and similar 'accidents' that the intensity of the 'vaccins' was reduced.—*Clarke.*

Thus, nearly fifty years after the experiments of Hering with the virus of hydrophobia, Pasteur's work began. But, on account of the crude preparation, like Koch's experiments with Tuberculin, many of Pasteur's cases were fatal. No better illustration can be found in medicine of the scientific accuracy and its successful clinical demonstration than is to be had in the results of the labors of these two men. The homeopathic methods have been demonstrated to be not only accurate and scientific, but safe and efficacious.

The following case is from *El Siglo Medico:*

Finally swallowing was impossible, restraint had to be used to prevent him biting his nurses in the hospital, when, as a last resource, a piece of Agave was offered to the boy by the doctor in attendance, cut from a hedge of the plant with which the hospital grounds were fenced. To the astonishment of all, the boy reached for it and ate it greedily, almost without chewing. By evening a decrease in the violence of the nervous attacks was manifest, though they remained as frequent as before. The improvement was slow but continued. On the fourth day he took some nourish ment, but also continued chewing Agave and swallowing the juice. On the fifth day he recovered consciousness, but still demanded Agave. On the eighth day he said he did not want any more, as "it tasted too bitter and caused a burning in the mouth."

Fagus: Dread of liquids; profuse salivation; swelling of the mouth; intense frontal headache; trembling; convulsions with periodic spasms; stiffness and coldness; pointing to the same kind of nerve irritation as caused by the poison of rabies.

Lachesis is closely allied (< from sun; bluish discolouration of wounds and ulcers; irritability; < from warm, damp air; from touch and a pressure; < after sleep; and Clarke adds, "though the late evolution of Lyssin is in striking contrast with the lightning like rapidity of the effects of snake venom").

Characteristics–

The sight or sound of running water or pouring water aggravates all complaints.

Lyssophobia; fear of becoming mad; exceedingly apprehensive.

Bluish discolouration of wounds (Lach.).

Complaints resulting from abnormal sexual desire (from abstinence, Con.).

Mental emotion or mortifying news always makes him worse (Gels.).

Cannot bear heat of sun (Gels., Glon., Lach., Nat.).

Convulsions: from dazzling or reflected light from water or mirror (Stram.), from even thinking of fluids of any kind; from slightest touch or current of air.

Headache: from bites of dogs, whether rabid or not; chronic, from mental emotion or exertion; < *by noise of running water or bright light.*

Saliva: tough, ropy, viscid, frothy in mouth and throat, with constant spitting (Hydright).

Sore throat, constant desire to swallow (Lac c., Mer,).

Difficulty in swallowing, even spasm of esophagus from swallowing liquids; gagging when swallowing water.

Constant desire to urinate on *seeing running water* (Canth., Sulph.); urine scanty, cloudy, contains sugar.

Prolapsus uteri; many cases of years' standing cured.

Leucorrhea, profuse, running down the legs (Alum., Syph., Tub.),

Sensitiveness of vagina, rendering coition painful.

Relation—

Compare: Agave, Bell., Canth., Fagus, Hyos., Lach., Stram., in hydrophobia.

Antidote: For overaction of potencies, Agave, Coc., Nux.

Lyssin antidotes effects of bite of non-rabid animals.

Agg. stooping; heat of sun; slight touch; draft of air or electric fan; warmth, damp air.

Lyssin is an analogue of many animal and nearly all the serpent poisons, especially Lachesis and Vipera.

Compare: Apis, Bell., Gels., Glon., Nat. c., Lach.; heat of sun or summer, Lach.; bluish colour of wounds or ulcers; sensitive to pressure or touch; rapid, lightning-like action, Coc., Con., Gels.; symptoms of ascending paralysis; Adren., Bell., Gels., Sol. n. m., paralysis of respiration; Coc., Sanic., bad effects of car, carriage-riding and sea-sickness; Canth., Sulph., desire to urinate on seeing running water; Strain., convulsions from dazzling light; Helon., consciousness of a womb; Hell., Hep., Hyos., hurried speech and drinking; Gels., mortifying news; Agaright, Arg. n., Lil., Sep., prolapsus uteri; internal coldness, Camp., Helod., Ver.

It follows well: Arg. n., Con., Gels., Hyos., Stram., Lach.

Is followed by: Gels., Nat. c., Nat. m. and serpent poisons.

Aggravation—

Sight or sound of water; bright, dazzling light (Stram-); carriage-riding (Coc., Sanic.; better from, Nit. ac.).

Amelioration—

Bending head backward, > pain in neck; heat, hot steam or hot water; warm bathing; cold air > headache.

Mind—

Loses consciousness for a moment.

Loss of consciousness sometimes at an early stage, but not generally until a short time before death.

Does not see nor hear persons around him.

| Memory for single words much improved.

Strange sensation in head, with loss of memory.

Does not converse as well as usual, but plays chess better; more inclined to reflect than talk; not at all lively.

Thoughts of something terrible going to happen come into his mind against his will; feels impelled to do reckless things, such as throwing child, which he carries in his arms, through the window, and the like.

Could not get rid of the indescribable tormenting feeling that something terrible was going to happen to him.

Fits of abstraction, takes hold of wrong things, often does not know what he wants, says wrong words which have but a remote similarity of sound.

They appreciate the formidable character of the disease

and speak frequently with a remarkable quick and sharp articulation of the impending fatal results.

During the tranquil intervals responded correctly to questions put to him, recognized those around him, and with a presentiment of impending death begged them to pray for him and not to leave him alone.

The majority of patients have no adequate conception of real origin of their malady, and affirm in decided terms that the scar is of no significance whatever and causes them no pain.

Most commonly the mental faculties are in a superior state of excitement, shown by quick perception, amazing acuteness of understanding and rapidity with which they answer questions.

Is astonished in his dream at the readiness with which he can express himself in elegant Latin.

It seems to her as if two entirely different trains of thought influenced her at the same time.

A certain confusion, unsteadiness, weakness of mind.

It is very difficult for him to think, sometimes impossible.

Weary and incapable of mental exertion; school tasks, which before had been a pleasure to her, had to be laid aside.

Range of ideas extremely limited, if left to himself is occupied continuously with the same thing, bringing frequently forward same ideas within a short space of time and always in same manner.

Dulness and stupidity; at night restlessness.

During convulsions, mental illusions and hallucinations; in intervals of consciousness mental faculties are retained.

Believe that they are reduced to their present wretched condition by the instrumentality of those about them.

Imagine that they are being abused, and energetically defend themselves against attacks and insults, which in reality are products of their own fancy.

Fancies he is being blown at by several persons, some of whom are not present.

Raved about the dog that had bitten her; imagined it to be near her and fought as if to drive it away.

Thinks he is a dog or a bird, and runs up and down chirping and twittering, until he falls down fainting.

They fancy that they see objects, animals and men that are not present.

Complains bitterly that a fire has been lighted and that the stove is smoking, although there is no fire; another continually directed a window to be closed, which was not opened.

Strange notions and apprehensions during pregnancy.

Slight fits of delirium occur (in advanced state); patients frequently forget their friends and relatives; delirium attended with constant talking.

Some delirium and illusions; fancied doctors were two young girls who had come in to see her.

During night delirium <.

Makes speeches in his delirium; thinks he is a man of great authority.

Insane ideas enter his head; for instance, to throw a glass of water, which he is carrying in his hand, into some one's face, or to stab his flesh with the knife he is holding, and the like.

His mania takes a gloomy character.

| Mania spermatica; stallions.

Inclined to use insulting language, scold his friends, beat and abuse those near him.

| Inclination to be rude and abusive, to bite and strike.

A kind of savageness in his temperight

A strong and uncontrollable impulse to do certain acts; to spring at and bite any moving object that came within reach; dog.

Is continually tempted to bite her pillow at night.

Deny, with great obstinacy, that they have ever been bitten.

Incessant talking during night.

Speech, labored, short and pathetic.

Wrote to doctor: I am waiting with impatience that you give me and my young ones something to eat.

After fainting spell he wrote on paper: I am forsaken by all; even the birds of heaven, they do not look at me, do not feed me if hungry; I hunger with the young ones and am thirsty with their she ones; my nest is made out of dirt, not gotten by my own exertions, but by driving them out of their nests and sitting there with the females and the young.

Sang more than usual, but involuntarily; she did not feel at all happy or cheerful.

Goes about house all day singing; moves with greater alacrity and precision than ordinary.

Sighing: with oppressive breathing; with pain in heart.

Declares amid violent sobs that she is suffering the torments of hell.

Lament with greatest anxiety their inability to relieve thirst which afflicts them, and by various contrivances endeavor eagerly to drink.

Had a good cry before going to bed.

Weeps bitterly on account of headache.

Before and after as well as during paroxysms, shrieks or inarticulate sounds expressive of utmost despair.

During fits, snapping motions of the jaws, of an involuntary and spasmodic character.

Quiet patients spit into provided vessels, more excited ones discharge saliva upon all sides.

Biting, snapping, with convulsions.

Ordered her husband to go away, as she wanted to bite him, and joining act to threat, she bit herself in arm.

Pieces of carpet put into kennel for dog to lie upon were torn up until they became heaps of loose wool.

Desperate efforts were made to break chain; dog.

Break out of their stables furiously and run and jump over ditches and fences. Lyssa of sheep.

He cautioned people around him not to inhale his exhaled air, it was spoiled, stinking like rotten eggs, worse than cholera, and could injure.

Does not answer questions.

Disinclination to change position of head; two distinct trains of thought existing at one time in her mind, the idea that she was unable to move her head (when lying down), with the positive conviction that she has only to make up her mind that she will do it to achieve it.

Not afraid of dogs, but dislikes to see them because their sight renews her fearight (Lissophobia, after bite by non-rabid dog.)

Cannot bear to hear others sing, or eat apples.

Exhilarated, felt as if he had received joyful intelligence.

Occasionally exhilarated, then again morose, both feelings, going off very readily upon conversing.

Pain in head makes him very uneasy.

Feels depressed and very weak all day.

Depressed, as if something would happen.

An attack of mental depression and indifference quite strange to him; feels as if he could do nothing; if he forces himself he lacks mental power.

To such as had continual apprehension respecting their safety it appeared a shorter time since bite.

Feels as if something disagreeable would happen; when thinking the matter over, the feeling passes off.

He feels as if he had heard unpleasant news, or would soon, hear it; until 4 P.M.

Felt as if she was going to get a fit; at 11 P.M.

||Lyssophobia; fear of becoming mad.

| Feels as if he cannot physically endure his fears much longer, and shall be compelled to go into an insane asylum. Lyssophobia.

Mary M., aet. 17, had been bitten several years previously by a dog, and reading of several cases of hydrophobia as reported in papers, was found in following condition; crouched in corner of sofa, dark red bloated face, expression of terror in face, eyes glistening, conjunctiva injected red; was brought into this condition by endeavoring to take a drink of water, and could not hear water mentioned without a shudder of fear, could not swallow, pulse very high, tongue dry and coated red; Lyssin 200 one dose; she was better next day, but had several slight attacks afterwards, always induced by running of water, but always yielding to remedy; has not had an attack in nearly a year.

Felt as if she was going to die; as if she was going to sink away.

She has been unable to sleep a wink for several nights; is driven from bed by indescribable anxiety; can but sit and walk, or find momentary peace in prayer.

Anxiety of mind; restlessness, with great prostration; with pain in heart; with headache; fear of being alone.

| A musician received a bite from a small pet dog in calf of left leg while walking through a dark entry; the bite was very slight, scarcely wounding skin; the animal was in a healthy condition and remained so; a pain in bitten place kept return ing from time to time independently of mind dwelling on it, until it finally grew to a burning which extended through entire body, causing an indescribably strange sensation; in night trembling, and a tormenting fear that he would have hydrophobia; was thirsty and drank water freely; it was two years after the bite when these and the following symptoms appeared; frequent spitting of saliva all through day, only ceasing awhile after taking strong tea in evening; disturbed dreams at night; finally could not partake of food or drink, and complained of pricking stitches under tongue; mental excitement now as all his life, affects him badly; hot vapor relieved burning pain in bite, and Lyssin 2C. (Jenichen) improved all symptoms rapidly; in three weeks he considered himself cured, and started on a journey.

Indecision even in small matters. .

Ill humor.

Fretful, hypochondriac mood in evening.

Feels nervous and irritable.

Very cross, so much so that his children expressed great surprise; he took offense at veriest trifles, scolding his wife and children, felt wretched, could not concentrate his attention on anything; sullen, does not wish to see or speak to any one.

After attacks of fury, evinces great regret at his behavior, making earnest apologies, warning those about him not to allow him to bite them.

Implacable hatred against owners of dog that bit her, with inclination to utter maledictions which, by reason of her careful bringing up and sobriety of her parents, shock her dreadfully.

Hit oeser piyesnvessnfall the senses.

Exalted state of smell, taste and touch, with a feeling of anxiety and a fear of being alone.

Everything affects him more powerfully; also tobacco.

He knew exactly where his nurses, his doctors and acquaintances were, if at any distance from him.

On a watch held to scorbiculum he sees the hour and minute hands.

He says he can see hands on dial plate of church clock.

He could hear what was spoken in next room, and counting coppers in a room below him.

He knows every one, and answers questions, also is in mesmeric rapport with his physicians. Linen dipped in sugar water, put on pit of stomach, gives a sweet taste in mouth.

Copper, if in his room, makes him restless and full of pain.

Felt same rheumatic pain his brother complained of. Lyssophobia.

Before every spell of somnambulism he crowed like a cock.

Very uneasy; mental disquietude, with headache.

Driven incessantly about without any definite aim.

Restlessness, driving him hither and thither, although weak enough to lie down.

Restlessness and anxiety at precordia, frequent change of posture and sighing.

| Restless, constant bleating in a hoarse voice. Lyssa of sheep.

| Sometimes he could control inclination to stool by a strong effort of will, but effort caused much nervous irritation.

Showing him a bird, he got frightened and thought it was a mouse.

Was much frightened during attack, and began to pray; her husband had to sit up with her and hold her hand; did not get entirely over attack until 3 A.M.

She feels as after night watching and great anxiety.

Unusually exhausted.

While reading and thinking, headache.

Worse while reading or writing; headache; aching in lower jaw.

Severe headache and noseache upon going to bed, after writing all her symptoms.

| Attacks of nervous headache become awful and insupportable if he hears water run out of a hydrant.

Pressing headache, < while reading and thinking.

|| When he hears water poured out, or if he hears it run, or if he sees it, he becomes very irritable, nervous; it causes desire for stool and other ailments.

The mere sight of a drinking vessel containing water is intolerable; they turn away their faces, shriek out loud, beckon anxiously with hands to have the water removed, for voice and breath fail.

Mental emotion always makes him worse.

Mortifying news affects him very much.

A certain wildness of humor.

Disposed to get angry; flying into a passion.

Every offense she feels very much.

Excitability prevents sleep.

Frequent gaping without being sleepy, most when he has to listen to others.

Thinking of fluids of any kind, even of blood, brings on convulsions.

The mere idea of drink, fluids, pouring out fluids, may cause a paroxysm.

Hyperesthesia, current of air, bright light, sight of any shining object, slightest touch, even conversation in vicinity of patient, may throw him into a most violent agitation and bring on severe convulsions.

The mere thought of fluids, of drinking, of swallowing, or offer of anything to drink, is sufficient to bring on severe convulsions; the same effect is produced by other sources of irritation, such as a simple breath of air, the attempt to touch the sick, every hurried approach towards him, the light of shining objects.

Even the sight of water, or other fluid, or of anything having the least resemblance to it, such as a looking glass or white substance, whereby an occasion will be given for renewal of idea of their former pain, occasions greatest distress and a return of convulsions.

Such as were afflicted with grief from any cause were much sooner affected with the disease.

A sudden fright starts convulsions.

Nose pains from thinking.

Had no symptoms of disease for four months until after receiving ill usage.

Head.—Peculiar lightness in head; lightness after nausea.

Singular sensation in vertex, as if he momentarily lost consciousness, but only in that place; or as if a habitual feeling had disappeared from there; it is no fulness, no motion, but it causes a vacillating motion of head; in evening.

| | Dizziness: as if something was drawing around in a circle, and as if she could not hold her head straight; after lying down, like a shock in upper part of brain; with inclination to fall to right when stooping; towards evening in upper part of head, as if she would fall, while walking; frequent and transient; with dim sight while walking and sitting; and nausea; with cramps in abdomen; temporarily > by return of diarrhea; < by teaching, spelling, or being obliged to notice letters; after lying down in bed, shock in upper part of brain; dimness of vision on rising from stooping; on rising from chair, staggers; while sitting; on rising, cannot walk straight.

A slow vacillation or wavering of head, from something being loose in upper part of head.

Surging towards head is felt inwardly, deep in brain.

Dulness: of head; in forehead, more to right side; in middle of brain, where it surges; and stupidity at night, with restlessness; amounting to pain in occiput.

Violent vertigo during morning, accompanied by a chill and an intolerable snappish headache.

Headache: with dizziness, lasting all day; in morning, violent, with vertigo (> by Tabac.); over eyes; in temples; very severe in afternoon; < from writing; > by cold air; from noon until evening; from 3 to 9 P.M., < from writing; > by cold air; alternating with hot flushes in face; with shooting pain in upper face; toward noon, with increase of saliva; and sore throat all day; < on seeing water or hearing it run.

Sensation as if a small leaden ball was rolling about in brain.

| Rush of blood to head: while lying down; from chest upward, with toothache; during pregnancy; when rising.

Throbbing headache in forehead, vertex and occiput, down to neck.

Burning, surging towards head.

Pain above left eye before going to bed.

Pain in a small spot above right eyebrow < while writing.

Pressing inward, throbbing or drawing above right eye.

Sharp pain above eyebrows, followed by burning in lids.

Sharp pain above eyebrows and up nose five minutes after walking, with headache.

Severe shooting pains in head, above eyes and temples.

Headache extending into right eye.

Aching in bones above eyes, particularly right; < by stooping.

A sensation in forehead as of something moving.

Dull pain in forehead, with a stupid feeling afternoon and evening.

Pressing or burning pain in forehead.

Tearing from middle of forehead towards left side.

Two P.M., intense pain in head, extending back of forehead to organ of firmness; soon after to whole top of head and to eyes, lasting all day.

Dull heavy pain in forehead and sharp pricking in left temple, alternating at times with throbbing and jerking.

Pressing in vertex and in forehead, particularly when stooping or moving head; afternoon.

Slight frontal headache in morning on waking. < after rising.

Passes hand across forehead.

Maddening outward pressing pain in forehead; he presses his head against the wall.

Pressing pain in forehead and top of head, returns 4 p.M., seventh day, with uneasiness of mind when reading or thinking.

Continual dull pain in forehead, principally on left side, with Stupefaction, in afternoon and evening.

Throbbing pain in forehead, vertex and occiput, extending into nape of neck.

Pressing in forehead, with slight sensation of heat, 6 P.M.

Headache at times very severe in right temple.

Severe headache in both temples and above eyes, beginning at 9 A.M., so unbearable that he cries bitterly; violent jerking in limbs.

Violent headache from temple to temple.

Tearing pain: in right temple; from jaw to temple.

Occasional stitches in right temple.

Sharp pricking pain in left temple, alternated with throbbing and punching.

Boring in right temple very short, 5 P.M.; repeats every other day; but on fourth day in left temple, and in morning when getting awake.

Beating, throbbing headache; most severe in right temple and above right eye; each bone feels shattered and sore; from temple to temple.

Violent headache, most in temples and forehead, < during day and from stooping and stirring about. Uterine disease.

Severe pressing pain in left side of head, occasionally boring stitches from without in, later pressing extends to left side of forehead and left orbit; 10 P.M.

Dull weight, first on left side of head, then on vertex.

Pressing weight on right parietal bone.

Dull pricking pain in left side, from head to waist.

Left side of head is now, and has always been, most severely affected.

Headache most severe one and a half inches above left ear, in evening.

Piercing pain in right side of head, with sensation of stiffness, or as if part would become insensible.

Woke in morning with a burning, aching headache in left side of head and down neck.

In vertex: dulness and tensive sensation; stupefied feeling; vertiginous shocks; a peculiar sensation; pressing weight; pressing stinging; right side: pressing shooting; pressing beating; pressing heaviness, right side; strange pulsation; burning surging; throbbing.

Pressure in upper part of head and forehead; < stooping or moving head; at 4 P.M., while reading and reflecting, with mental restlessness.

Frequent pressure on vertex, as if a cast, which fitted top of head, was pressing it down.

Severe headache, extending from behind forehead to organ of firmness, soon after spreading over vertex and to eyes, at 2 P.M., lasting all day.

Pressing from forehead to vertex and jaws.

Pain on top of head and in teeth running into each other.

Painful pressure, most on upper part of head, < when moving head; later also in forehead, with considerable heat and prostration.

In occiput: painful dulness; pressure in left side; tearing and stinging as if in bones; < after rising; aching; burning; pain in left side, < during wet weather; dreadful pains running up neck and down spine, < when lying down.

Sharp pain across eyebrows and up nose, while walking out doors; exceedingly fatigued and weary after a short walk.

Intolerable headache extending to ends of nose and into teeth; some pressure on head, and for a moment a feeling as of an invisible hammer striking upon back of head (relieved by Tabac.).

Frequent attacks of headache, in which head, nose and teeth appeared to be soldered together.

Feeling of tension in head; much pressing pain in head.

Head feels as if it would split with severe pressure on vertex.

Pain as if head would burst.

At 3 P.M.; headache very severe; dull heavy pain in head.

Afternoon, pain in head; sick headache.

Headaches from bite of dogs, rabid or not.

In rare cases serous effusion in opaque subarachnoid tissue and lateral ventricle, and also increased adherence of membranes of brain to convolutions.

All morning severe headache which makes him impatient.

At noon slight headache, lasting all day.

Dull heavy pain in afternoon in head.

Painful rush of blood to head after moving, turning around, or stooping.

Unbearable headache for three days making her snappish, harsh and irritable; trifles annoy her; lower jaw feels stiff and aching, hands numb.

Crying bitterly during headache.

A peculiar sensation in head all day, as if something drew the head towards shoulders.

Headache with nausea and sore pain in heart, in afternoon; > in cold air.

Pain from mouth up through head and down back of neck.

Burning aching from left side of occiput down neck. Violent headache and backache.

Painful pressure on top on moving head, with fever and prostration.

Horrible headache, accompanied by general weariness.

Headache in bones of skull.

On top of head, pressing heaviness, same in right parietal bone.

Tearing and stinging in occiput, as if in bones, < after rising.

Beating pain in forehead, parietal bone, occiput and nape of neck; > in neck when bending head backwards.

Irritable headache, touching head makes it ache; very sensitive scalp.

Right side of head feels stiff, as if it would become numb.

Numbness of left side of head.

Very annoying headache, more outside, near vertex, > by gentle scratching, or by rubbing, but it must be done by hands of others, thus by a kind of mesmerizing.

A darting from within outward to scalp, on right side of vertex, followed by itching.

Itching in locality of acquisitiveness.

Small pustule, painful when touched, on left frontal eminence, later same on right.

Hair which is usually dry has become very oily.

Scalp feels contracted and pinched.

Eyes and Sight—

Sensitive to light.

Left eye exceedingly sensitive to light and water.

Sight of water: agitation; renews idea of pain; causes convulsions (pregnancy).

Sparks before eyes.

Something moves to and fro before eyes while sewing, but always a little farther off the point at which she is looking.

False vision, dulness of sight, together with dilatation of pupils, sometimes actual blindness.

Great weakness in eyes, without pain.

I Since five years could not read longer than a few minutes at a time, when she would see letters double and would read something else than the right words; had tried all sorts of spectacles without benefit, was often ashamed because she could not sign her name properly.

On looking up eyes are very weak.

Dimness of vision with vertigo; dizziness when walking and sitting.

Vision much impaired or absent; lasts twelve hours.

Vanishing of sight.

I Could not see or hear.

Drawing, beating pain over right eye, extending into eyes.

Aching over eyes, as if in bone, < right side and stooping.

Pain over right eye, pressing inward.

Pressing sensation in upper part of right orbit.

Drawing, beating pain over eyes and into balls.

Throbbing over right eye.

At 9 P. M.: severe shooting pains in head, over eyes and in temples; also very violent aching pain inside of and all over chest.

Pain over left eye previous to retiring.

Sharp pain across eyebrows, afterwards burning in eyelids.

Pain in small spot over right eyebrow, < writing.

Soreness in eyes and above them, pain in forehead.

Pressing sensation in orbits.

Headache extends into right eye.

At 9 P.M. felt a curious stinging pain in left eye, extending to forehead, over right eye, painful.

Eyes feel very bad, severe pain in them and in all his joints.

Eyes ached intensely; feeling of soreness.

Burning of eyeballs.

Eye draws heat from nape of neck.

Itching heat in eyes.

If mental anxiety is great, pupils are in some cases dilated, while face and conjunctiva are injected.

During period of tranquility, in last stage, pupils are contracted or of unequal size, eye fixed, strabismus.

Pupils were a little dilated and eye had a somewhat wild and restless appearance.

Eyes are wild, rolling, staring and livid.

Disturbed look, or eyes firm and penetrating.

Lachrymal glands evince increased activity.

Eyes red and cornea somewhat inflamed.

Eyes congested and painful.

Sore eyes and some fever after a bite in nose.

Dulness and inflammation of eyes; dogs.

| Inflamed, dim, watery, staring eyes, with very much dilated pupils, upper lid drawn up, and diminished sight.

Eyes somewhat red and inflamed (cornea).

Eyes bloodshot and painful.

Eyes slightly red, and occasional stitches in right temple.

| Great inflammation in an eye from which gushes foamy pus; pustules around eye; in morning lid puffed up like an eggshell, small pustules on one fingeright Dog-bite.

Eyelids fly open involuntarily.

Pressure in left side, shooting to eyes in evening.

Burning in lids.

Eyelids feel paralyzed on awaking in morning, and appear to be more firmly closed, as if glued together.

Swelling of eyelids after bite of dogs. In sheep. Extreme ulceration of eye, lids closed and puffed up by pus. In sheep.

Ears and Hearing—

Conversation in vicinity of patient may throw him into a most violent agitation.

Ringing of church bells makes him anxious, and causes a sharp, salty taste, with stitches in heart.

Water poured into a basin, with splashing noise, caused paroxysm to be reproduced, with convulsion and agitation.

Sudden noise causes involuntary startings.

Hearing water poured out in next room makes him very irritable and nervous.

On crossing ferry, soon after eating, noise which water made caused unspeakable torture in her back.

Convulsions excited by barking of dog, from great sensibility; any other sudden noise, shutting a door or a blast of wind, produce the same.

During his attacks of chronic headache, which come after mental emotion or excessive mental exertion and last a day or two, he cannot bear to hear running water; if hydrant is allowed to run in an adjoining room, or even if water is poured into a basin, his headache increases to an insupportable degree.

After the pain following an evacuation had lessened, and he was sitting at open window, the large street waterplug was opened to cleanse the streets, and as soon as he noticed water running down gutter in front of his house, he was seized with violent pains and had to go at once to the watercloset. Dysentery.

If, during night, or in morning before rising, he heard pouring out of water in next room, he was immediately obliged to rise and have an evacuation. Chronic camp diarrhea.

Hearing water poured out brought on convulsions.

Sensation as if blood rushed to right ear, then a pressure as from a dull knife, interiorly and superiorly.

Sound as of rushing water in left ear.

Buzzing in right ear.

Hears various noises in night.

Temporary stoppage of right ear; about two hours afterward while thinking upon it, ear commenced aching; pain extends into teeth and through head.

Tearing pain from lower jaw into ear.

Bending pain in right ear.

Shooting stitches in right ear, from without in.

In morning, pressing in forehead and drowsiness, with stitches passing inward in both ears.

Stinging pressure behind ears; afternoon.

Rush of blood to right ear; after pressure like from a dull point.

Pressive burning in right external ear.

Burning and heat in ear.

Earache extends into teeth.

Tearing pain a few inches from right ear.

Pressing from nape of neck into ear.

Above left ear, headache most severe.

Pressing burning in right concha, in evening.

The ears feel stiff.

Ear tickles, after rubbing pain.

Itching in a small spot in upper part of both ears, disappears after scratching.

Nose and Smell—

Strong odors may start spasms.

During three days her sense of smell, which is always extremely acute, became painfully so, particularly in reference to unpleasant effluvia; action of nostrils extremely painful.

The greatest sensibility to smell of tobacco; taste of snuff while box is one foot distant.

Frequent bleeding from nose; repeatedly some clotted blood in nose.

Tickling in nasal cavity causes sneezing.

Itching in nose all day.

Repeated sneezing, which stops on being interrupted.

Frequent sneezing, mostly early in morning or late in evening, as if a coryza would begin; also when looking at something bright, and from every little dust.

Fluid discharge from nose.

Coryza, with tickling in roof of mouth and in front of nose (relieved by Phosphorus).

Thick green mucus runs out of nose (horse).

Pain in nose.

Sensation of stiffness in nose, in right side of neck, and principally in jaws.

Nose feels bruised.

Nose, right neck and side feel very stiff, more about jaws.

Nose extremely sensitive to touch.

Headache extends into nose.

Nose itches all day.

Face—

Jawbones feel quite sore.

Both jaws feel stiff; tingling in cheek bones.

Gnawing and crawling sensation in right zygoma.

Transitory drawing in left side of face, from cheek bone toward nose, as if in muscles, in evening.

Tearing in right upper jaw extending into ear, same in temple.

Shooting pains in upper jaw and violent headache.

Darting pains in right side of face.

Burning neuralgic pain down left side of face.

A sensation moves about in right side of face and goes across forehead.

Slight twitchings in face and hands.

Quivering in face.

Facial muscles become variously contorted, countenance changes its aspects frequently.

Spasmodic affections take place in muscles of face, occasioning violent contortions and most horrid assemblage of features; in muscles moving lower jaw, inducing involuntary gnashing and a grinding of teeth, which some have construed into a desire of biting; during convulsive attack expression of face indicates great anxiety and alarm.

Disturbed look with dyspnea.

Expression of face quite variable; reddening countenance often exhibits reflections of utmost mental and physical misery, of most horrible agony.

Face flushed; complained of his head, said they were running needles into his brain.

Heat in right side of face and right ear, followed by headache in vertex and forehead; as soon as headache gets >, heat returns; heat comes from within and spreads from back of neck to ear and into eyes and face, accompanied by constant pain in nape of neck, which increases after heat and headache disappear.

A feeling of heat and soreness in middle of left cheek.

Heat in face, with soreness of left cheek, from thinking.

Heat in right side of face, and particularly in eye, where it causes a tickling; returns after drinking coffee.

Face sweat; with sensation of heat; with flushes.

In morning (6 A.M.), tickling in left cheek.

Heat and redness of face.

First heat in right side of face and in ear, then a quiet aching in front of upper part of head; this headache lessens, the heat increases.

Heat in face in morning, with redness; at times very deep.

Complexion pallid and cyanotic, and expression stupid.

Flushes and headache alternately.

Pale face with squeamishness and nausea.

Face pale and yellowish, almost brownish.

Appearance peculiar; skin sallow, pale or anemic; bloated all over, but no 'pitting.' Chronic camp diarrhea.

Sensation as if she had been bitten in left side of face near mouth.

Tickling on left cheek, at 6 A.M.

The scratches on cheek became red, thirty-three days after bite, and on following day looked quite fresh, as if they had been made only a few hours before, but were a little darker in colour than newly made abrasions.

Pimple on eminence of forehead, painful to touch; later one on right cheek.

On left cheek near nose, towards eye, a pain, < when touched; a pimple with soreness around.

Painless hard nodules on cheek, where a pimple seemed to have appeared; on ninth day a little scurf on it and redness; if picked or pricked, a very disagreeable kind of pain, but not violent, is felt in cheek even a distance from nodule, and here and there deep in upper part of jaw; cheeks bluish red and soft; discharges after the scurf is scratched off, lymph and blood.

Slow maturing bluish pimples on face.

Pain in left cheek near nose, from fifth to seventh day; followed by a hard, painless swelling of size of a pea, turned redder on thirtieth day, and became covered with a small scab; on thirty-second day it grew soft and turned bluish red, particularly around edges; on puncturing, a disagreeable yet not severe pain at some distance from swelling and more inside of cheek; a small quantity of blood and matter was discharged; on fortieth day the place ceased to discharge and healed.

The jawbones feel sore; aching in lower jaw.

Violent jerking pains in lower jaw.

Tearing in right lower and upper jaw up into earight

When reading or writing, felt a pain in lower jaw; the longer she read the < it got.

Masseter muscles not affected by spasms.

During phrensical fits, snapping motions are made with jaw of an involuntary or spasmodic character, bearing some resemblance to motions of biting.

Attempted to bite her fingers before death.

Biting snapping with convulsions.

Jaws feel stiff; crawling in zygqmatic arch.

Lower jaw stiff and painful; with inclination to yawn; with headache; imagines he cannot open mouth.

Jaws feel sore and stiff; a great disposition to press hand against lower jaw.

Sensation as if she would have mumps.

A chilling, biting, burning sensation on inner side of right upper lip, as if a corroding acid had touched spot; sensation passes up and back, in a lesser degree, to right nasal cavity, where it produces tickling and sneezing; subsequently increase of saliva; after several hours.

Lips cracked on inside of middle line.

Spasms with froth before mouth.

It seldom happens that froth is observed around outside of mouth.

Teeth and Gums—

Grinding of teeth.

Painful sensation of coldness shoots into teeth, it passes from lower posterior part upward and into jaw.

Teeth hurt more on right side, it is a kind of aching dulness.

Sensation in right lower jaw, in bone as it were, it shoots into root of a decayed tooth.

Shooting pain in right eyetooth, preceded by burning, passing down esophagus.

Frequent shooting pain in teeth; all the teeth ache.

Aching in carious root of a molar.

Toothache and other complaints during pregnancy, with internal ebullition of blood from chest to head; head feels as if filled with air to bursting.

Teeth very sensitive; feel as if on edge.

Headache and earache extend into teeth.

Chilling painfulness starts in teeth of right side behind and below in bone of lower maxilla and passes upwards.

Neuralgic pain in gums, principally in front. Aching in swollen gums on right side.

Drawing in gums, most in front.

Taste and Tongue—

Food does not have right taste.

Scrapy taste, with much saliva.

Bitter taste in morning, on awaking.

Salt victuals tasted too strongly of salt, other food seemed to lack salt.

Speech is labored, short and pathetic.

Difficult, incorrect speech.

Impediment in his speech, would begin a sentence with difficulty after several fruitless attempts; some palatal vowels he could not pronounce, others but incorrectly.

A cool feeling on tongue like after peppermint.

Pain in root of tongue and left side of throat.

Peculiar pain at root of tongue as if it was swollen.

Tickling, queer feeling in throat and root of tongue.

Tongue usually moist and clean; frequently slightly coated, more seldom dry and thickly coated.

Tongue coated with thin layer of yellowish white fur.

Tongue coated with foam.

Tongue dark red on sides, coated in centre.

| Tongue large, pale and flabby. | Pricking sensation under tongue.

Ranula returns periodically, with dryness of mouth, < in afternoon, soreness when chewing; with hemorrhoids and constipation.

Mouth—

Feeling of coldness, like essence of peppermint.

Severe pain passing from mouth upward through head and down into neck.

Constant sensation of intense dryness of mouth and throat.

Dryness in mouth: in afternoon; with thirst.

Sore mouth, feels as if there were lumps in it.

Much tenacious mucus in mouth and throat.

Tough, short frothy phlegm in mouth (horse).

Frothed at mouth, attempted to spit out with much difficulty (before death).

Saliva more viscid, constant spitting, feeling of general malaise.

Saliva runs together in mouth, without occasion; flows back and is swallowed.

Saliva in back part of mouth like after sugar, or when liquorice is swallowed.

Mouth full of saliva, total disinclination to drink.

Great flow of saliva and difficulty in swallowing liquids.

Accumulation of foaming saliva, with inflammation of throat.

Saliva more plentiful, but thin and of yellow colour.

Secretion of a thick and frothy saliva, but without any morbid repulsion toward drinks.

Ejected saliva is frothy, slimy and ropy.

Much tenacious saliva, with sore throat.

Large quantities of tough saliva in mouth, with constant spitting.

Saliva is not ejected, but runs from open mouth.

Quantities of saliva are collected in and about mouth; presents a frothy appearance; patient is constantly endeavoring to get rid of it by wiping it with a handkerchief, or spitting it out with great force.

Spits all the time small quantities of a frothy saliva; with pain in limbs.

Frequent spitting.

At 10 A.M. began to spit a great deal, continuing all day till supper.

Dark, coffee coloured fluid oozed from mouth (before death).

Much mucus in throat and nose; hanging in posterior nares.

Scraping sensation on palate where cool sensation had been, slight coughing does not reach spot, hemming and hawking does occasionally.

Fauces and pharynx pervaded by an equally diffused purplish scarlet blush, no pain in throat, except when patient attempts to swallow.

Follicular enlargement is common, involves also pharyngeal follicles and lymphatic glands in neighbourhood of jaw; similar swelling upon inner side of epiglottis, pretty firm and characterized by abundance of lymph corpuscles found in gland substance.

Hyperplasia and recent swelling of tonsils and follicular glands of tongue; flat, roundish swellings at root of tongue, in middle of each one of which was seen dilated opening of a follicle.

Sensation as if uvula was too long; it is slightly inflamed but not elongated.

Mucous membrane of pharynx and epiglottis of a deep red colour and injected; soft palate frequently reddened and swollen.

Entire mucous membrane of mouth and pharynx was of an equally distributed pink without any swelling.

Throat—

Slight redness of palate and throat, with spasm of esophagus and difficult speech.

Sore throat, as after swallowing red pepper.

Quite a sore throat, constrictive sensation much < when attempting to swallow liquids, which he could not do without pain; solids not painful.

At 11 A.M.: soreness in throat till noon.

Sore throat: very severe; all day; in forenoon; > at 6 P.M.; after supper (7 P.M.); not able to swallow without great pain; as if swelled; as if raw; aches; on right side; with headache; with soreness in eyes; with increased tenacious saliva.

Cooling sensation in esophagus.

Throat quite sore, headache in both temples, numbness in both arms, slight pain in lumbar region all day.

Fauces and pharynx as far as one can see are slightly inflamed, there is inclination to swallow, and increase of saliva.

Painful sore throat, throat much inflamed, headache <, tenacious mucus in mouth and throat; great weakness with aversion to move.

Inflammation of throat with foamy saliva.

Violent spasm in throat as if he would suffocate, from 2 P.M. to 9:30 P.M.

Great heat in throat and about heart.

Sudden jerks going from esophagus to heart.

Sore throat, constant desire to swallow; much saliva and feeling as if beaten.

Periodical spasm of esophagus, continual painful inclination to swallow without being able to swallow anything; constriction is most severe when taking water into mouth, if he tried to swallow it forcibly, he had burning and stinging pain in throat, cough and retching which forced fluid from his mouth; difficult speech.

Difficulty in swallowing; particularly fluids.

Dryness in throat and difficult swallowing, with slight erysipelatous redness in pharynx.

Stinging sensation when swallowing.

Sore throat at 2 o'clock; with difficulty in swallowing fluids; felt as if epiglottis was paralyzed.

Sore throat with great inflammation, could only swallow with difficulty, fluids returned through nose.

A peculiar sense of constriction in back of throat at 3 P.M., < at 4 P.M., could not swallow without pain; disappeared at 6 P.M., but returned at 7 and lasted until bedtime.

Sore throat with constriction, particularly when attempting to swallow fluids, which is painful.

Terrible pain in throat, particularly when swallowing.

Constant inclination to swallow, or remove phlegm which seems to stick between nose and throat.

Constant desire to swallow, painful and ineffectual.

Some will drink water without difficulty.

Activity to drink is restored before sudden death.

Warm drinks, milk, soups and wine are often more easily taken than water.

Imagines that he cannot swallow anything.

Difficulty in swallowing can, at first, be overcome by firm resolution.

Declared he could not swallow for something in throat that interrupted the passage.

Swallowing more difficult at 5 P.M. than in the morning (after Bellad.).

Solid food sometimes consumed with great difficulty.

Absolute impossibility to swallow anything; whenever attempt is made, attacks of suffocation and spasms of respiratory muscles as well as of muscles of face, neck and rest of body, with great mental disturbance.

After some days patient equally abhorred solids as well as fluids; when importuned to eat, he was thrown into convulsions. Any attempt to swallow bread occasioned greatest agony.

Often happens that they succeed in drinking after those who were around them have retired, or when attempt is made with closed eyes and with aid of a straw.

No disgust for fluids until difficulty in swallowing came on; when fluid touched fauces it seemed at the peril of his life.

At 3 P.M. felt a strange constrictive sensation in back part of throat, never experienced before, < at 4 P.M., could not swallow without great pain; went off at 6 P.M.; returned in an hour, lasting until 10 P.M.

When taking water into mouth, constriction was greatest.

Periodical spasms of esophagus. Attempt to drink water starts convulsions.

Had difficulty in speaking; a connected sentence could only be uttered after making several fruitless attempts; palatic letters could not be pronounced at all, all were pronounced wrong.

At 10 A.M. felt a soreness and suffocation in back of throat.

Violent spasms of throat at 2 P.M., feeling as if he was about to be suffocated; went off at 9 P.M.

A ball, as it were, rises from stomach up to throat, seems to threaten suffocation.

Sensation of a lump in throat with desire to swallow.

A terrible pain in throat all day, and great pain on swallowing.

Pain extended upwards from wounded arm toward throat.

Stitching sensation when swallowing.

Burning stinging in left side of chest, with palpitation in afternoon.

Burning stinging in throat.

Trying to swallow water forcibly, it caused burning and stinging in throat, besides cough and gagging, which forced out contents of mouth. Spasm of throat.

Burning down esophagus.

Great heat in throat and around heart.

A slight redness of affected parts.

Intense and deep seated inflammation of mucous membrane of mouth, gums, throat and larynx, with smarting pains on swallowing.

Feels as if he had swallowed a small quantity of red pepper.

APPETITE, THIRST, DESIRES, AVERSIONS.— Appetite good, but digestion deficient; a portion of nearly everything he ate passing bowels in an undigested state. Chronic camp diarrhea.

Voracious appetite; swallowed wheat without chewing.

Little appetite in morning; want of appetite, headache, depression.

Want of appetite. Hydrophobia of sheep.

Could take no nourishment (with spitting), could not remain at table.

Symptoms of digestive organs extremely variable; excessive thirst, vomiting, constipation.

Thirst and disinclination for food.

| Felt very thirsty and had no aversion to drink, on contrary drank large quantities of water.

Thirst much increased, complains of burning pains in throat.

Thirst and desire to drink, but is prevented from doing so

by spasmodic constriction of throat, attempts excite most disagreeable sensations, even spasms.

Had not been drinking any water for some time, only some hot tea.

Drank some strong tea at supper, after which salivation discontinued until 8 P.M., then commenced again.

No appetite, except for sour things.

Called for burnt brandy and drank it; next day a strong rising in his stomach and an impossibility to drink.

Excessive desire for salt.

First days, smoking unpleasant; after first week, a crazy, insatiable desire to smoke, he does not allow pipe to cool.

Picked up bits of cotton and shreds of cloth; bits of chips and coal were devoured whenever getting near; anything that was within reach and could be grasped by the jaws was gnawed away very quickly; a dog.

Urine and feces were frequently devoured as soon as they were voided; a dog.

Abnormal cravings during pregnancy.

Aversion to water; imagines he cannot swallow; says he is thirsty, but cannot look at water or hear it poured out.

Aversion to water of place he arrived at.

Aversion to drinking water, but can take small quantities of chocolate.

Aversion to fluids; great sensitiveness to every breath of air and reflection of light.

Since bite she has a frightful aversion to water; at first she could wash herself by dint of great self-control, but later not at all.

Wine tasted poorly and affected him more than usual.

Aversion to fat food and drink; there remains a long greasy aftertaste, < after mutton.

Eating and Drinking—

Before dinner a very strange sensation, a strangeness of whole body.

Warm drinks, such as milk, soups and wine, are more easily taken than water.

Inability to take solid food, or else it is consumed with greatest difficulty.

At times ability to drink is restored before death.

After supper, 7 P.M., feels >, less sore throat, no difficulty in swallowing.

After eating: all cooling, burning, wavelike sensations disappear, also congestion; pressing inward in epigastrium; lasciviousness with sexual excitement; lewdness with a sensation of weakness in parts, but inclined to an emission of semen; increased lassitude and drowsiness, slept an hour without making it any better.

After meals very ill disposed, every noise irritates him; if others eat apples, or hawk, or blow their noses, it brings him beside himself; passes away after siesta and coffee.

After dinner and in evening disinclined to think.

After supper: pressing in spleen.

Nausea after eating eggs or fat food.

After coffee: more frequent beating of pulse; heat in face.

Tobacco affected him more than usual.

Hiccough, Belching, Nausea and Vomiting—

Squeamish sensation; a want of appetite in evening, followed by great lightness of head.

Nausea: with giddiness, headache and pale face; with pale face after diarrhea; food does not taste right; and loss of appetite in evening; at 10 to 11 P.M.

Hiccoughing.

Continual belching of wind; convulsive eructations.

Belching in afternoon; sour, in afternoon.

Gagging when he forcibly attempts to swallow water, forces it out of his mouth.

Rising of bile into throat during day, at same time an unusual quantity of tenacious saliva in mouth and throat.

Nausea and vomiting, after diarrhea.

Vomiting: of food; of fluid while drinking, followed by faintness; of what was eaten at supper, at night in sleep.

Nausea and vomiting of a foamy, mucous, dark coloured substance resembling coffee grounds.

Scrobiculum and Stomach—

Pressure in epigastrium after eating.

Suffocating pain at pit of stomach.

Distress in epigastrium and precordial region with dyspnea.

In epigastric region sensation half coldish, half burning.

Pain in epigastric region, deep in, as if in or behind duodenum.

Aching, with coldness in stomach.

A cooling pain in stomach, with here and there a sharp and pointed pressure.

A sensation of motion in stomach.

Loud gurgling in left side of stomach, becomes more continuous, like water from a bottle.

A loud cooing noise in stomach, to left, and after a while repeated as a quick croaking.

Great oppression in stomach, has to open her clothes.

A slightly hot, quiet, aching sensation below chest, sometimes lower down, often in entire abdomen, as if in intestines.

Stomach empty, or may contain a dark, opaque substance, frequently resembling coffee grounds; in mucous membrane of stomach and intestines, decided injection of blood-vessels; upon former frequently hemorrhagic erosions.

Hypochondia—

A pressing pain: in right side, near last ribs, with breathing; in hypochondria, after quick walking.

Shooting in right side of abdomen.

Pain in region of liver and right kidney.

Pain from within outward in right side.

Fatty degeneration of liver.

In upper part of abdomen, left side (region of stomach and spleen), a continued gnawing pressure in forenoon.

Aching from below waist to feet.

Pain in left side at 8 A.M.

Pressing pain in region of spleen when walking fast.

Painful throbbing as if an abscess was forming in region of spleen, but very deep in, exact locality is half way between median line and outline of left side; it lasted eight days; with it departed remnant of a similar affection in this locality, against which eleven years of allopathic treatment had proved of no avail.

Under mamma hot sensation, quietly aching, sometimes same lower down or in whole of abdomen, as if in intestine.

Tearing from left hypochondriac region to right.

Abdomen—

A rending pain across abdomen from left to right, in evening when in bed.

Pain in right side of abdomen proceeding from uterus.

Pain down left side of abdomen.

Pressing in abdomen.

A drawing in abdomen below navel.

Cramp in lower part of abdomen.

Painful sensation deep in upper portion of abdomen, as if behind duodenum; in forenoon.

Colicky pain in abdomen; when it subsides, stinging in small of back.

Severe bellyache, lasting an hour, awoke from sleep at 11:30.

Violent bellyache.

Sticking: in right side of abdomen, when taking a breath; in abdomen above hip; with feeling of motion in lower part of abdomen.

Stitches: in right side of abdomen; in belly, an inc from crista ilea.

Shooting in abdomen.

A sense of motion, with slight stinging in middle of abdomen.

A burning, waving and surging, proceeding from abdomen, spreads through entire chest to head.

After cooling sensation and scratching in esophagus had subsided, there appeared a half cooling, half burning sensation in entire upper part of abdomen.

| General soreness in whole of lower abdomen.

Distension of abdomen; every evening.

Rigidity of muscles of abdomen.

From both loins a drawing downward, followed by cramps in lower abdomen.

Aching: in loins; into back; down to feet.

Dull pressing pain above right inguinal region on a deined place.

Pain in right groin, with some swelling.

Drawing, dragging pain in groins; heavy, bruised feeling in highs.

Drawing from groins downward, then cramps in abdomen, accompanied by dizziness.

Aching from groins to feet, in evening.

Pain in both groins; in right, two small kernels under skin, very painful.

Inguinal glands very much swollen, they pain for two hours.

Stool and Rectum—

Tenesmus during and after stool.

Dysenteric stools with tenesmus; renewed as soon as he hears or sees water run.

When in morning some water was poured out from pitcher into basin, pain and desire to stool returned. Dysentery.

When he sees or hears running water, violent pain and tenesmus return; in a case of dysentery in Summer, of six weeks' standing, in which stools were most frequent in night, consisted of bloody mucus and were followed by pains in rectum and small of back, which forced patient to walk about in spite of great weakness; could neither stand nor lie down; had drank no water whole time, only hot tea occasionally.

Stools watery and profuse, with severe pains in lower bowels; frequency of stools not uniform, some days five or six, others fifteen or twenty, usually more frequent in morning. Chronic camp diarrhea.

Diarrhea: with much pain, most during day, eighteen hours after dose, lasting twenty-four hours, with pain in lower part of bowels; < in morning; followed by nausea as if she would have to vomit; attended with violent pains early in morning; after stitches in side.

| Chronic diarrhea contracted in Southern camps.

Difficult passage of flatus as if anus resisted expulsion.

|| Stools of bloody mucus.

Involuntary stools.

Straining to evacuate, causing a violent pain in small of back and in rectum, afterwards compelling him to walk about, although weak.

Bowels constipated; stool very dark in colour.

Stool became dark and thickish in appearance, mingled with shreds of wool or cotton, bits of wood and coal that had been swallowed; a dog.

Passage of bright red blood from anus, with terrible burning and pricking in it as from thorns.

Difficult stool, piles protrude.

Hemorrhoidal troubles, passes blood from anus during catamenia.

Throbbing in anus externally.

Darting into anus causes contraction.

Urinary Organs—

Dull pressure in region of left kidney.

Flying pains increase, seize urinary organs; create a difficulty and heat in discharging urine.

Some pain about neck of bladder in evening.

A cooling, burning, congested feeling in region of bladder, in evening.

Profuse watery urine, in evening.

In morning and evening urine is yellowish brown, turbid and diminished in quantity; reddish sediment.

Urine dark, brownish, with whitish sediment, visible when urinating upon snow.

Brighter coloured urine and in larger quantities, but not more frequent.

Urine scanty or muddy, often of a dull, greenish yellow colour; dog.

A whitish yellow sediment in urine.

Urine scanty, no albumin; dark, cloudy, frequently contains sugar, evidently the result of lesions in medulla oblongata.

| Urine too scanty and high coloured,

Urging to urinate after a slight accumulation.

| Constant desire to urinate on seeing running water; urinates a little at a time.

Tickling burning in urethra near orifice after urinating.

After passing feces and urine there is an urging to urinate again, it moves slowly several times from above downward without succeeding in passing a drop.

Prostatic juice passes after urinating.

Since fourteenth day after bite says she has passed no water; passes daily from time to time a little dark blood from uterus, differing in quantity and quality from menstrual flow.

If he passes but a small quantity of urine his sense of weakness is increased; weakness after urinating as if he passed his strength away.

Male Sexual Organs—

Inclined to lascivious ideas, although there is not much sexual desire.

Lasciviousness: after eating, with feeling of weakness in parts; with erections in afternoon.

Erections with but little desire.

| Strong erections, without sexual excitement or thoughts, in evening while undressing in cold room.

Sexual indifference with erections, even during act of coition, which is perfectly performed.

| Increased sexual desire. (Dropsy of spine with sheep. Hydrophobia of sheep.)

Priapism, with frequent seminal emissions.

| Satyriasis in a stallion; hot breath streamed from nostrils.

Insufficient seminal discharge.

Semen is discharged too late or not at all during coition.

During a very strong and warm embrace excitement diminished at its height, and there followed no emission.

No emission during coition, but afterwards semen escaped unconsciously in sleep.

A seminal emission with dreams, quite unusual.

Without being preceded by an erection there is a discharge of prostatic fluid, smelling salty and musty; the glans penis is dry.

Feeling of weakness around and in sexual parts.

After coition, with difficult and tardy emission, there is a sensation of emptiness and discomfort in parts, lasting all of next day.

Painful urging in penis, as after excessive coition, accompanied by lasciviousness.

Itching and burning on corona glandis, with tickling and discharge of greenish pus, in afternoon.

Glans is dry and sticks to foreskin.

Burning and tenesmus as if in prostatic gland and in urethra; in afternoon.

Itching on os pubis, left side, extending to root of penis.

Increased peristaltic motion of scrotum, all afternoon and evening; motion of testicles also increased.

Scrotum tightly drawn up for two or three weeks.

Hanging down of scrotum on eighth day, while before and after it was contracted.

Painful sensation in testicles.

Pain in testicles on day after an embrace, particularly felt towards noon and first afternoon hours.

| Hydrocele.

| Atrophy of testicles; testicles diminish in size, first left, then right.

|| Complaints resulting from abnormal sexual desire.

FEMALE SEXUAL ORGANS.—Aphrodisiac sense deficient.

Pain extending from uterus into breast and right side of abdomen.

Insatiable heat; with cows.

Pain in left ovarian region, uneasiness there.

Bearing down in uterine region.

Sharp pain in uterus, shooting down to labia.

Occasional acute pain in and below uterus; at times a violent shooting pain in left of vagina, extending upward, so severe as almost to cause her to scream.

Increase of uterine sensitiveness, conscious of having a womb.

| With a painful sensitiveness of womb, slight degree of prolapsus, so that after any considerable effort there would be a strong conviction that it was prolapsed.

| Considerable pain in lower part of back, with a soreness felt through pubic region, which was clearly proved to be in neck of womb by an increase of pain from pressing finger on neck; principally at point where finger came in contact with womb.

| Womb high up in abdomen, enlarged in fundus.

| Abrasion about os tincae (treated with caustic) some tumefaction of cervix and walls of vagina remained, showing a low degree of inflammation.

| Speculum showed os tincae of size of a small goose quill, smooth and normal, except that there was a string of bloody mucus of size of os hanging from it, so tough and viscid that it was difficult to wipe it away with a sponge.

| Swelling of womb in all its parts, extending somewhat into vagina. Prolapsus.

Bright redness of vaginal portion of womb.

| After menses found that prolapsus uterus, a case considered incurable, was in its proper position, and continued so after an interval of two months, though she has done much to test the cure, lifting a heavy child in and out of bed at night, when she was necessarily without her supporter.

| Prolapsus uteri of seven years' standing.

Metritis, prolapsus or induration of uterus; in cows.

A girl, aet. 14, and another aet. 21 took the 30th after their catamenia had ceased for three days, next day it reappeared.

Catamenia appeared (after a few globules of 30th) two weeks before time, and very copious.

Menstruation, with hemorrhoids, pulsations in anus and weakness of back.

Menses rather frequent, protracted, dark, and at times fetid.

| During interval of menses 'a show' that seemed quite obstinate.

| Anemia in consequence of disturbed sexual function.

Continual discharge of offensive mucus from uterus for several months.

White discharge like leucorrhea, which weakened her; never had leucorrhea.

Slimy leucorrhea.

Severe leucorrhea, with pains in back and lower part of bowels; sore vagina.

|| Sensitiveness of vagina rendering coition quite painful.

| Menses too profuse, at times a little too frequent.

Discharge of blood from rectum during menses.

| Weakness in back, with copious catamenia.

| Tearing, followed by pressing downward, could not make a hard step during catamenia.

Pregnancy. Parturition. Lactation—

|| During pregnancy: strange notions, desires or cravings; rush of blood from chest upward; toothache, backache and other complaints; great sense of bearing down; intense pain from inflammation of os and cervix (formerly treated with Caustic.); great soreness in lower part of back and bowels.

| All changes of position that tilt or rotate to a moderate extent the os uteri cause much pain.

| Spasms excited whenever she attempts to drink water, or if she hears it poured from one vessel into another; sight or sound of water affects unpleasantly, even though desiring water.

| Since childbirth more pain with coition and a dislike to it.

Since cessation of lochia a severe leucorrhea; pain in back and lower part of bowels; soreness of vagina.

Both breasts swollen when waking in morning, she can hardly get up; three mornings in succession; same swelling of breasts at night when opening her dress.

Voice and Larynx. Tracheachea and Bronchia—

Voice altered in tone; tones much suppressed; hoarse; rough; harsh and weak (last stage); shrill, inarticulate sounds; shrill sounds of utmost despair, or occasioned by violent expirations; very shrill and piercing bark, changing near its termination into a distressing, continuous howl (dogs).

Epiglottis crisp and dry.

Inflammation or redness in superior part of trachea.

Pain next to larynx, on right side, felt on turning neck and on pressure.

Respiration—

The breath is hot; sulphurous.

Hot breath streams from nostrils. Satyriasis in a stallion.

On inspiring: a cooling sensation; stinging on left side.

Can scarcely speak from weakness.

Weakness of chest; tired from talking or reading.

When breathing, stitches in right side of abdomen.

Breathing accelerated or rattling in last stage.

Asthmatic sensation, air going through larynx makes a kind of wheezing.

Sighing and groaning respiration, may be occasioned by violent expiration.

Frequent sighing and sobbing.

A general feeling of discomfort in chest forces him to deep breathing or to emit sighs, which alleviate.

| | Sighing with pain in heart.

Now and then he has to take a deep breath, with coldish feeling far back and deep in throat, followed by great relief.

At 9 A.M. suffocating feeling in chest, had to sigh several times, lasting till 10:30 P.M., when he fell asleep.

Breathing laborious and difficult, quickly repeated, and attended with a constant and peculiar kind of hawking, in order to expel breath, which has been taken for an imitation of bark of a dog.

| Dyspnea: with flatulency, cough and rattling in chest; with sighing, groaning respiration; from cardiac pain; <, lying down.

Constriction about breast and difficulty in breathing become so extreme, that on a blast of air blowing on them they are seized with greatest distress, cover their mouths, seem ready to expire, as if struggling for breath.

On attempting, at request, to drink a little water; a violent spasm of muscles of neck and throat came on, preceded by a deep sigh or gasp, as if she might just have plunged into cold water.

Difficult breathing and spasmodic sensation in trachea.

Suffocative spasm in throat.

Convulsive breathing and spasm in muscles of throat, either come together or breathing precedes throat spasms.

The convulsive breathings during paroxysms are very similar to those produced by a sudden cold water bath, and are always combined with spasms in throat muscles.

Oppression in breathing before a severe suffocative attack occurs, induced by spasmodic contractions of respiratory muscles, combined with spasmodic, alarming constriction of pharynx.

Breathing during paroxysm gasping, irregular and usually quite rapid, often with decided dyspnea.

Cough—

Barking like *a* dog, with a sort of noisy cough; headache.

| Coughing when attempting to swallow water forcibly, forces it out of mouth.

| Cough and gagging.

Inner Chest and Lungs—

Chest and abdomen feel expanded; expanding chest seems to invigorate him, though usually it fatigues.

Pressing in chest; between tenth and eleventh ribs, right side.

Rheumatic pain across chest when drawing her breath.

Pain as if in nerves, from side of chest up to throat.

Cramplike pain and stitches in left side, followed by diarrhea and afterwards nausea and inclination to vomit.

Pinching pain: at fourth rib on right side.

Stinging in lower part of chest.

Stitches under left mamma, going towards left.

Shooting between left mamma and last ribs.

Shooting, flying pains through left chest.

Burning, surging through chest.

Burning stinging in left side of chest when taking a deep breath.

Burning like heartburn in right side of back, in region where ribs end.

Blood mounts from chest to head.

Extending to chest, pain in uterus.

Great weakness in chest, particularly when walking and reading aloud, chest feels fatigued; some deep pain in left side.

Upon pleura is often seen a soaplike deposit, as in case of cholera.

| Gangrene of lungs, caused by pneumonia and sexual excitement. Satyriasis in stallion.

Heart Pulse and Circulation—

Pain in left chest on a small spot in region of heart; more backward and to left in chest.

Dull pain in heart all day, with a pinching pain about fourth rib, right side.

Constant pain in lower part of heart.

A very strange and unusual feeling in heart, something like bands compressing it, in middle of chest, and as if needles were sticking in it, a dull kind of stitching pain, very painful, alarming and disagreeable.

Pain in heart entirely gone, but every two or three hours has a twitch there.

Painful shock or jerk from lower or hind part of esophagus to heart and front chest.

7 P.M., slight, dull shooting pain in heart, lasting till he went to sleep at 10:30 P.M.

Considerable pain in heart, and a corresponding pain in right side; a severe sticking and shooting pain, producing shortness of breath and sighing.

At 11 A.M. two or three stitches of a shooting kind in heart, lasting a few minutes.

Stitches in and around heart.

Pricking sticking pain in heart.

Stinging, sharp pain in heart.

Sticking pains at intervals in heart.

Sharp, shooting pains in region of heart, lasting four hours.

At 9 P.M., violent pain of a sticking character in heart and to left of it.

Stitches in heart from ringing of church bells.

Stitches in heart, more while walking; they would kill him if they continued.

Heart had for three months not been free from a sticking, drawing, squeezing pain, result of an attack of rheumatism and cold, together with a palpitation and difficulty of breathing.

Violent pain in heart, as if it would burst or had needles running into it.

Heat and burning in heart.

Burning pain around heart and in forehead.

Pain in heart: with headache; with sore throat and heaviness in legs.

Sensation going from heart through to back, with sinking.

| Pain in cardiac region, to which he is subject, is < half an hour after, but much > in several days.

While writing, a burning ebullition and gurgling from upper part of abdomen through chest and head, at first followed by a pain in ear; now a pressing stinging in inner upper vertex to right; as if a hot, wavelike stream was moving on and spreading outward, but not extending to spine or limbs.

Heart palpitated violently and felt as if it was coming up into throat; drank several mouthfuls of water, which relieved.

Palpitation causes anxiety.

Feels beating of pulse through whole body, and from time

to time like a slow rising wave through throat into head, followed by a sensation of a momentary rush of blood.

Pulse: steady, but rather full and hard, about ten beats above normal standard (80); slightly accelerated and hard, being more frequently small than full; quick and irritable; 160; becomes gradually weaker and quicker, especially after paroxysm, 120 to 180; frequently irregular, becoming variable in its rate, and this variation takes place with great rapidity; unequal, some beats stronger, some quickened; weak, quick, intermitting; very small, irregular and very rapid (last stage); weak, quick and intermittent (latter period); becomes constantly more rapid and smaller, until at length it is threadlike, and finally no longer can be felt.

Outer Chest—

The clavicles feel as if they would slip from their sockets; has to place arms akimbo.

Quivering about sternum.

Spasmodic tearing under left ribs; at same time it runs to anus, where it causes a constriction; also at same time a tearing between skin and flesh down thigh to knee.

Pressure: on sternum between mammae; between last ribs on right side.

Stinging in left breast (between mamma and last ribs).

Chest as if beaten, in evening.

Soreness across chest, both breasts swollen; when waking in morning can hardly get up; three mornings in succession.

Neck and Back—

Constant pain in neck.

Going to neck: pain from head and from back.

Pressing in neck and up back of head.

From neck heat passes to ear and face.

Pressure and drawing pain in neck.

A stitch in nape of neck.

Muscles of neck and breast, frequently entire muscular system, contract spasmodically.

With inward heat, pains in neck, < if headache is >, or heat in right side of face.

Burning pain in neck.

Throbbing pain extending into neck.

Neck feels stiff; right side of neck stiff; muscles felt stiff in morning.

Tearing, stinging and stiffness in neck.

Stiff neck with rending and shooting.

Pain in cicatrix and also some stiffness in muscles of neck and throat.

Pain in muscles of neck and along cervical portion of spinal column.

From nape of neck a heat draws over right ear into right eye and face, seems to pass from within outward.

Neck feels stiff, held himself more erect than usual.

All day difficulty in moving head.

Stiffness in joints of neck; if she allows her head to hang awhile, it is difficult to raise.

Neck feels more comfortable when, in sneezing, she throws head back.

Emphysetnatous swelling of subcutaneous cellular tissue of lower part of neck; may extend along upper portion of breast and into mediastinum.

Sterno-cleido mastoid muscle on each side stands out like a thick cord; a look of mingled anxiety and terror on countenance.

Head feels lopsided and as if something was drawing it toward shoulder.

At 2 P.M. laid down, found his head twisted to left side; under ordinary circumstances would very soon have changed position, but to his surprise found it quite comfortable and fell asleep; woke at 4 P.M., felt a numbness in left side of head, and flesh of lower part of body looked like goose-flesh.

As if head was being drawn to shoulders.

Cramplike pressure under right shoulder-blade and between scapulae.

In back, near right shoulder-blade, a pressing with heat, draws into nape of neck, thence into muscles of left upper arm.

At 2 P.M., severe pain across back between shoulders and waist.

A pain or ache in and between both shoulders, as if a heavy weight was there, lasting two hours.

Pressing, running from between shoulders to occiput and across right ear, in morning.

Below right shoulder-blade a pressure; not pressing from out inward or > by bending backward.

Pressure in back, five inches below point of right shoulder, one inch from spine; had same sensation during each of her pregnancies, always on right side, inward from lowest rib to breast bone.

Stinging: below right shoulder-blade; in cervical vertebra.

Severe backache all day, and numbness of hands.

Spine aches; right side of throat sore.

Backache and headache.

Pain in back across hips, lasting all day.

Pain in back and both groins.

Burning in back near last ribs, right side, like heartburn.

Pressing in region of kidneys; dull pressure in region of left.

At 4 P.M. violent pain in right kidney, lasting an hour.

Pain from 4 A.M. till evening in both kidneys and across hips, severe and a little burning, > at 9 P.M.

Back extremely sore; as if beaten, in evening.

Pains with cutaneous hyperesthesia along vertebral column.

Could not bear least touch along whole vertebrae; slightest touch produced an irritability akin to convulsions.

Sheep turn and wriggle their backs because they cannot bear heat of sun; increased sexual excitement; symptoms pointing to madness; scratching their backs appears to be agreeable to them, as they remain quiet and make a peculiar motion with their mouths, which does not express pain.

Going to back from heart, sensation with sinking.

Want of strength in back, must lean against back of chair in sitting.

Weakness in region of kidneys, loins and sacrum.

| Great weakness in back, as if it would split and fall apart.

| A sore lameness in back, with some degree of soreness in lower abdomen.

Pain in lower part of spine severe.

Considerable pain in lower part of back, with a soreness felt through the pubic region; pressing finger on neck increased it.

Pressing pain in sacrum, right side; later it moves to middle of back (repeated eight times).

Shooting through small of back.

Disease peculiar to sheep, termed the 'gid;' dropsy of spine.

Upper Limbs—

Pain on top of right shoulder joint.

Pain in left shoulder joint, as if beaten and paralyzed; lameness in left axilla.

All day a tearing, then a stinging in left shoulder joint, as if in middle of bone, down arm and into finger; and after getting up from bed, for one hour in right arm, then all day in left.

1 P.M., slight pain in right shoulder joint; also in head.

Has a lump in right axilla.

Rheumatic pain, first in right then in left shoulder.

Feeling of great weight on shoulders all day.

Stinging tearing pain in shoulders, passing down through bones of arm to fingers.

Sudden sharp, darting pain, in bitten hand, extending up arm to shoulder and base of brain.

Pain down wounded left arm; generally in afternoon and evening, < 10 o'clock.

Arm aches and is swollen.

Aching in right arm (the left is bitten); feeling as if weather was going to change.

Slight twitching in right arm.

A sting in sore arm once in a while, which makes her start all over (dogbite).

Felt two shocks down wounded arm as from a galvanic battery, clear to finger ends.

Cramp in arms.

The pain up arm was followed by cramps and drawing in back and limbs of bitten side.

Numbness in right arm at 4 P.M., lasting till bedtime.

At 10:30 P.M., soon after taking last dose, numbness in right arm.

Weakness in arms.

Right arm becomes so heavy and inactive that writing is too great an exertion, and he allows arm to drop.

After some pain in arm (finger had a small wound exposed during dissection of a mad dog, forty days ago), feeling of malaise and fatigue, followed by death.

In left upper arm, about axilla, pain as if beaten and lame; the same near elbow, several minutes after in wrist; in evening.

Her arm has felt very sore, although wound is almost healed.

A cold flush goes down arm as if ice water was being poured upon it.

Feels a chill strike her right arm when she goes into open air.

Burning pain down wounded arm.

Felt as if fleas were running over right arm.

Arm itches all over; itching on arms appearing suddenly.

Pain in right elbow as if paralyzed, at noon; same at 2 P.M. in left, > in a horizontal position and when allowing forearm to hang; soon after in left knee.

To right of right elbow a black and blue spot.

Throbbing pain in right forearm on flexor side.

Muscles of forearm, as far as hand, painful when pressed, or taking hold of anything.

Blueness in streaks down right forearm.

Wrists have felt some time as if strained; < in morning. Lame feeling in wrist.

At 10 P.M., straining pain in right hand.

Soreness in right hand.

Quivering in hands.

Hand trembles so much he can scarcely write.

Trembling of left hand when taking hold of anything or pressing it; muscles hurt most on upper side of forearm down to hand.

Trembling of left hand.

Right hand numb for a long time, clumsy, stiff.

Hands numb with headache.

Right hand swollen.

The ball of right hand hard, cramped and swollen.

After counting copper coin, violent pain in right hand, between third and fourth metacarpal phalanx, in some motions and on pressure.

Smarting in palm of right hand.

Intense pain in forefinger of left hand.

Pain in first joint of right ring finger, as if it was going to gather.

Stiffness of fingers and hand.

Woke at 5 P.M. with stinging in forepart of right index finger, nail turned quite blue.

Lower Limbs—

A pressive pain in right hip bone, goes from there to middle of sacral bone.

Left hip aches in bone.

Felt as if hip bones would slip out of their sockets; had to rest with hands on hips to > the feeling.

Something runs round and round several times in flesh, in region of hip, then down leg to knee.

Pain in thighs, particularly in anterior portion; as if fatigued, after going up stairs; < after sitting down.

Along left sciatic nerve a dull pain, returning periodically; < when rising from sitting.

Pain in anterior part of right thigh, as from a bruise.

Twitching in right femur, as if some one was pulling from below; not painful, comes and goes.

Cramps in thighs.

Biting and itching on thighs.

Laming pain inside of left thigh above knee joint, and extending into it.

Tearing pain from middle of anterior portion of right thigh to knee.

Tearing in left thigh to knee.

Knees ache; tearing, drawing pain.

Stinging in right knee.

Knees tremble at every step.

Laming pain in right knee joint when getting awake in night; next morning same in left knee.

Aching and heaviness in legs below knee.

All day a feeling of weight in legs below knee, seemed as if there were several pounds of lead in tibia of each leg.

Numbness in right leg below knee.

Pain in all joints of feet, like pressure with a dull point, now here, now there.

Pain in legs very troublesome, not able to walk.

Legs feel as if he had rheumatism.

Pain going down left leg.

Twitching in legs.

Legs tired and aching; feel as if beaten, in evening, feel sore and very heavy.

A pain in legs, as if thighs were too heavy, went off at night.

Right leg falls asleep; after seven hours.

After sitting awhile, lower limbs go to sleep; prickling sensation.

Weakness in legs when going up stairs.

Ulcers on legs, with emaciation and coldness, left side; contraction of hamstrings and relaxation of ligaments of ankle joint and flexors of toes.

A curious feeling in legs, as if calf was heavier than usual.

Cramp in right calf.

Cramp in calves of legs at night in bed; < from stretching out limbs.

Calf of left leg ached as if it had been cramped, after waking. The pain in calf came even when he was not thinking of bite at all; lately much < and quite severe.

Sharp, biting pain in left ankle.

Painful lameness in left ankle joint in night while lying in bed.

Heavy feeling in lower limbs, as if a weight was attached to ankles.

Pain from heel into thigh.

After going to bed, intense pain in back of right heel.

Pain in right heel and in toes of left foot.

Balls of heels so sore that it is painful to walk.

| Great swelling in heel of a cow from dogbite; very restless.

Pain in sole of right foot extending to ankle. Lyssophobia.

Severe pain in right instep; < after being in bed during

catamenia; at times extremely painful to move foot; does not pain much when walking upon side of foot; left slightly troubling at times.

Extending to feet, pain from groins.

Pain extends from ankle bone to great toe.

Shooting from fourth toe to foot.

Some pain in toe next to little toe of left foot; shooting into foot.

Tearing in first joint of left little toe.

Toes of both feet troublesome, as if nails were too long and broken; pain in small of back and right temple.

Each dose he has taken has made him feel as if he was getting corns on every toe, his real corns felt remarkably well and did not pain him at all.

Her corns have troubled her but on one occasion since the proving; where she felt as having corns, she had twinges.

Pain like rheumatism; shooting and stinging from knees down; stinging in palm of right hand to finger ends, as though she had fallen on it.

Aching in knees and shoulders.

Shortly after pain in shoulder joint, afternoon third day; pain goes into knee joint of same side.

Feeling of pressure on shoulders and weight in legs.

Pains or aches in all his limbs; feeling of languor and extreme fatigue.

Weight and heaviness of legs and shoulders.

Heaviness of limbs.

A convulsive trembling of limbs during attacks.-

When lying in bed, an unusual morbid contraction and tossing about of limbs.

Severe twitches in arms and legs, much resembling chorea.

Shaking or convulsive trembling of limbs.

He felt a severe, bruiselike pain in shoulders, chest, back, arms and legs.

All muscles feel bruised in morning, can neither sit nor lie down.

Loss of power in limbs; gait unsteady, at times some stiffness of hind legs; dog.

Rest, Position, Motion—

Moved quite briskly, though feeling fatigued.

After moving, turning, or stooping, feels as if head would burst.

Very little exertion wearies him, and he feels quite languid.

All day had a disposition to straighten herself up.

Had to rest with hands on hips to > feeling as if hip bones would slip out of their sockets.

Horizontal position: pain in elbows >, also when allowing forearm to hang.

Lying down: thinks she is unable to move head; like a shock in upper part of brain; rush of blood to head; pains up neck and down spine; impossible, pain in rectum and small of back; dyspnea; impossible in dysentery; could not sleep.

Lying in bed: contraction and tossing about of limbs.

Parts on which he lies: burning heat.

Does not wish to rise.

Can neither sit nor lie; all muscles feel bruised.

Sitting: dizziness; must lean back, want of strength in back; pain in thighs <.

After sitting awhile: lower limbs go to sleep.

On rising from a chair: staggers; cannot walk straight; dull pain along sciatic nerve.

When rising: rush of blood to head; tearing stinging in occiput <.

Stooping: inclination to fall to right; aching in bones above eyes <; pressing in vertex and forehead; violent headache <; painful rush of blood to head; aching over eyes <; dizzy on right side of head.

On rising from stooping: dizziness and dimness of vision.

Turning neck: pain in larynx.

Bending head backwards: pain in neck >.

If she allows her head to hang awhile it is difficult to raise.

Throws head back: when sneezing.

Bending backwards: does not > pressure below shoulder blade.

Standing: pain in rectum and small of back; impossible, dysentery.

Standing still: on waking, head fixed.

Change of position: disinclination to change position of head; continual change (dog); that would tilt or rotate os uteri would cause much pain.

Stretching limbs: cramps in calves.

Can hardly bend fingers; stiffness.

Turning around: painful rush of blood to head.

Taking hold of anything: muscles of forearm painful; trembling of left hand.

Least motion: all joints cracked.

Moving: head < pressing in vertex and forehead.

Aversion to move: great weakness.

At every step: knees tremble.

Could not make a hard step: during catamenia.

Walking: as if she would fall; dizziness, with dim sight; five minutes after, sharp pain above eyebrows and up nose; quickly, causes pressing pain in hypochondria; pain in region of spleen; enforced by terrible pain in rectum and small of back; great weakness in chest; stitches in heart; impossible on account of pain in legs; painful on account of soreness of heel; on side of foot, instep not so painful.

Going up stairs: pain in thighs; weakness of legs; very weak.

After a short walk: exceedingly fatigued and weary.

Stirring about: violent headache <; painful rush of blood to head.

Swallowing: difficult, particularly fluids; stinging sensation; causes constriction of throat; causes terrible pain; bread causes greatest agony; stitching sensation.

Nerves—

Until dinner time he felt so strangely in his whole body as never before, without being able to define the feeling.

In all motions of her body and in her looks is expressed a peculiar erethism.

All things affect him more, tobacco included.

Irritability; violent agitations.

| He could neither lie down nor stand up for any length of time.

Great restlessness, anxiousness, distress; tossing about.

In afternoon whole body trembles, she can scarcely speak; stinging in one of cervical vertebra; when stooping feels dizzy on right side.

Afternoon tremulous, in whole body and very weak, can hardly talk.

| Continual trembling sensation through whole body.

| The strange feeling changed during night into a trembling, and he is full of fear.

Twitching of muscles throughout entire body (last stage).

Twitching of tendons, with tendency to general convulsions.

Severe nervous twitches in whole body all day.

Felt quivery all over.

If during great restlessness she attempts to sit down and work, she has alternately twitching in arms and legs.

Nervous twitching, with trembling of right hand.

Starts now and then.

Muscular contractions appear with various degrees of intensity, from slightest convulsion to those of most severe and clonic form; frequently tetanic convulsions.

Spasms of individual muscles, as well as of muscular system in general, clonic, rarely tetanic.

The spasms have the character of reflexed spasms; their proximate causes are: attempts to swallow; speaking; a current of air; sight or idea of fluids; sight or sound of running water; coming in contact with another person; a bright light; sight of shining objects or of some strange person; a loud noise or strong odors.

Sensation of convulsive actions in different parts; distress of epigastrium; heaviness of limbs and general prostration.

Exertion is frequently succeeded by convulsions.

|| Attacks returned every few minutes, for five hours, until they were arrested; pain passing down spine to loins and hips, and from thence to knees.

Convulsions conjoined with an exalted state of sense of smell, taste and touch.

Spasms of legs and arms, occasionally very severe.

Clonic convulsions; decided tetanus or trismus not observed; opisthotonos in rare cases.

In quick succession violent epileptic attacks.

Spasms so violent that four strong men could hardly hold him and prevent him from hurting himself.

Every day at [illegible] P.M., convulsive startings.

She struck, snapped and bit at everything and every person.

Pain commencing in cicatrix of bitten thumb, producing slight spasm, and still greater disposition to snap and bite and to grind teeth, which were entirely beyond his control, causing him to fall on floor.

Suddenly a severe pain in bitten thumb, after nine days, instantly passing up spine and thence into brain, producing a violent, nervous convulsion for a few moments, with a disposition to snap and bite; passed off in two or three minutes.

Convulsions came on and lasted for a short time, then perfectly placid for some time before death.

|| Convulsions daily; rolls head from side to side; winking and rolling eyes; attempts to bite others; pelvis and legs are turned to one side as far as possible. Child, aet. 2, after scarlatina.

Feels as she did when she got up from a nine day's illness; feels so heavy and sore.

Great debility and disinclination to move about, lasting till 2 P.M., gradually diminishing.

Feeling of malaise and debility at 8 P.M., great disinclination to move.

Does not wish to rise.

Very soon a sensation of weakness, a kind of flabby lassitude, like days after great exertion, or after a fever or other disease.

Great weakness and restlessness, does not know where to turn, would prefer to lie down, but it affects his breathing.

Such weakness that knees tremble at every step, and she feels as. if she would fall.

Weakness: with sore throat; after urinating; of sexual organs.

During exhaustion more nimble and active.

Fatigue and heaviness in legs.

Great physical relaxation; whole body feels fatigued; tired all over.

Felt irritable, tired and nervous.

With numbness of paralytic symptoms the violence of all others increases.

| At times a singular sensation, a kind of "die away" feeling, quite instantaneous, cannot describe it; seems to extend through heart to back; accompanied with quivering around breast bones and pain in nerves, from left side of chest to throat and left jaw; fluttering about heart.

Felt stiff and tired; required an effort to draw his breath.

After singing, suddenly falls down as if dead, with eyes shut, face red, quick breathing, pulse 100.

A stage of general paralysis; an abatement of most distressing symptoms; a freer respiration; a diminution of reflex excitability; less impediment to deglutition; a rapidly increasing debility and prostration before death.

Sleep—

Inclination to yawn, with stiffness of lower jaw.

Felt inclination to gape and stretch.

Felt drowsy; in afternoon; irresistable drowsiness, 9 P.M.

Sleepy after a meal, slept one hour without relief.

Frequent yawning, without sleepiness, particularly when hearing others yawn.

Did not sleep more than thirty minutes until after 2 A.M.

Insomnia; sleepless in spite of narcotics.

Passed most of his nights sleeplessly, walking up and down in despairight Lyssophobia.

Restless night, with stupefaction in head.

Sleep fitful, position continually changed; dog.

Excited, cannot sleep.

Felt as he did some years since, when sitting up with a sick relative three nights out of five, unable to sleep during day from nervous anxiety.

When lying down could not sleep, eyes open, unless he purposely closed them, when they reopened involuntarily.

Went to bed at 10:30 P.M. (as usual), could not sleep (a very unusual circumstance); dozed and heard various noises till 3 A.M., which caused him to get out of bed to ascertain what they were; started frequently; slept soundly from 7 to 8:30 A.M.

Went to bed at 10 P.M. in great pain all over; woke up at 11:30 P.M. with very severe pain in stomach, lasting one hour.

After 10 P.M., while in bed, all symptoms more severe.

Had a restless night, woke repeatedly and felt tired.

Woke several times at night with pain in wounded arm.

Starting in sleep, afternoon.

Has to scratch whole body, and has no sleep for it all night.

Became more restless night before death.

Dreams: of influential persons to whom he occupies position of servant or subordinate; of a Latin debate with students of law, astonished at facility and fluency with which he spoke Latin, it being far greater than he was capable of in a waking state; of dogs all the time, but they are different dogs from the one that bit her; of fighting, of high places, of insane asylum, of churches; disagreeable, when she falls asleep, night or day; only in first half hour.

Jumped up in bed.

| During night slept but little; was disturbed by disagreeable, disconnected dreams; felt strangely. Lyssophobia.

On waking stands perfectly still for a time; head fixed as if gazing at some distant object; a dog.

Sleepiness when unable to sleep, and sleeplessness when she might otherwise have slept; generally restless at night.

On waking is morose, inclined to be angry.

Late getting awake, and difficult to recover from sleep.

Slept from 4 to 6 P.M., woke up and felt dreadfully nervous; had a great fear as if something was going to happen.

In morning, after exciting dreams, much fatigued, feels tired in sacrum and back.

If inclined to sleep, it is short, disturbed, with frightful dreams, and on awaking is apt to fall into slight convulsions.

On awaking from siesta, numbness in head.

Time—

2 A.M.: did not sleep more than thirty minutes until after.

3 A.M.: became cold in bed for one hour.

Morning: violent vertigo, with chill and headache; after rising, slight frontal headache <; when getting awake, boring in temples; woke with burning, aching headache; severe headache; lid puffed up like an eggshell; on awaking lids feel paralyzed before rising; on hearing water poured, obliged to have an evacuation; pressing in forehead early; frequent sneezing; (6 A.M.) tickling in left cheek; heat in face; bitter taste; swallowing less difficult; little appetite; stools more frequent, diarrhea, with violent pains; urine yellowish brown; both breasts swollen; muscles stiff; pressing across right ear; wrists as if strained <; pain in left knee; all muscles feel bruised; much fatigued.

8 A.M.: pain in left side.

9 A.M.: severe headache begins; suffocating feeling in chest lasting till 10:30 P.M.

At 10 A.M.: began to spit a great deal; soreness and constriction in throat.

At 11 A.M.: soreness in throat till noon; stitches in heart for a few minutes.

In forenoon: sore throat; belching; gnawing pressure in left side; painful sensation in upper part of abdomen.

Towards noon: headache with increase of saliva; pain in testicles <.

At noon: slight headache, lasting rest of day; pain in right elbow.

Until dinner time: felt strangely in his whole body.

After dinner: disinclined to think; headache very severe; pressing in epigastrium; sexual excitement.

Afternoon: very severe headache; dull pain in forehead, with stupid feeling; pressing in vertex and forehead; dull pain in forehead; sick headache; dull heavy pain in head; headache, with nausea and sore pain around heart; stinging pressure behind ears; ranula, with dryness of mouth <; stinging in chest, with palpitation; sour belching; 'erections; itching and burning on corona glandis; burning and tenesmus as if in prostatic gland and in urethra; increased peristaltic motion of scrotum; first hours pain in testicles <; pain in wounded left arm; pain in shoulder joint; whole body trembles; drowsy; starting in sleep; fever.

1 P.M.: slight pain in right shoulder joint.

2 P.M.: intense pain in head; sore throat; violent spasm of throat; laid down and found head twisted to left side, found it quite comfortable; felt numbness in left side; severe pain across back; pain in left elbow.

3 P.M.: headache very severe; peculiar constriction in back of throat; feeling of malaise and debility.

Until 4 P.M.: feels as if he had heard or would hear unpleasant news; pressure on upper part of head.

4 P.M.: constriction in throat <; violent pain in right kidney lasting one hour.

5 P.M.: swallowing more difficult; woke with stinging in forepart of index finger.

During day: rising of bile in throat; diarrhea, with pain <; unable to sleep from nervous anxiety; disagreeable dreams when falling asleep, only first half hour.

All day: felt depressed and weak; spitting of saliva; headache with dizziness; sore throat; intense pain in head; violent headache <; a peculiar sensation of head; itching in nose; spitting; very severe sore throat; slight pain in lumbar region; terrible pain in throat; sensation of emptiness and discomfort in sexual parts after coition; dull pain in heart; difficulty in moving head; severe backache and numbness of hands; pain in back across hips; a tearing and stinging in left shoulder joint; weight on shoulders; feeling of weight in legs; severe nervous twitches in whole body; had to lie in bed, with severe pain in all bones.

Evening: fretful, hypochondriac mood; vacillating motion of head; dull pain in forehead; pain above left ear; shooting in eyes; pressive burning in right concha; late, frequent sneezing; drawing in side of face; disinclined to think; want of appetite, followed by great lightness of head; when in bed, rending across abdomen; aching from groins to feet; pain about neck of bladder; cooling, burning, congested feeling in region of bladder; profuse watery urine; urine yellowish brown; strong erections without sexual excitement or thoughts; increased peristaltic motion of scrotum; chest as if beaten; back extremely sore; pain in wounded left arm; pain in left arm and wrist; legs tired and aching; late, less inclinjed to chilliness.

After supper: pressing in spleen; lewdness, with weakness of parts but inclined to an emission.

6 P.M.: sore throat >.

7 P.M.: sore throat; slight, dull shooting pain in heart till 10:30 P.M.

8 P.M.: salivation recommended.

9 P.M.: severe shooting pain in head; curious stinging pain in left eye; spasm of throat >; violent pain in heart; irresistible drowsiness; a dripping, warm perspiration from wrist to nails of right hand.

10 P.M.: pressing pain in head; pain in wounded left arm <; stinging pain in right hand; pains severe until that time.

After 10 P.M.: while in bed all symptoms more severe.

10:30 P.M.: numbness in right arm; went to bed, could not sleep; dozed and heard various noises till 3 A.M., started frequently.

11 P.M.: as if she was going to have a fit.

11:30 P.M.: awakes from sleep with severe bellyache.

After going to bed: intense pain in back of right heel; pain in heel.

Night: delirium <; tempted to bite her pillow; incessant talking; disturbed dreams; stupidity with restlessness; on hearing water poured, obliged to have an evacuation; hears various noises; vomiting in sleep; stools most frequent; swelling of breasts; laming pain in right knee joint when getting awake; pain in legs goes off; cramp in calves of legs; while lying in bed, laming pain in joint of left foot; painful lameness in left ankle joint; strange feeling changed into a trembling, generally sleepless; walking up and down in despair; stupefaction in head; woke several times with pain in wounded arm; sleepless on account of scratching of whole body; more restless; disagreeable dreams; itching quite severe; intolerable itching in lower part of body t'o feet; stitches in heart; pain in back; itching on lower half of abdomen.

Temperature and Weather—

| Burning sensation in bitten place > by hot steam striking against it. Lyssophobia.

| Unbearableness of heat of sun. Dropsy of spine with sheep.

The damp, warm weather oppressed him.

Expressed a desire to go into bath; after warm bath more irritable to external air, the most distressing symptom that occurs.

Great sensitiveness to every breath of air.

A very gentle stream of air projected from lips on to patient's forehead, and continued only for a few seconds, brought on a violent spasm.

Asked her mother to beg him not to breath upon her face again, as it distressed her so much (after Bellad.).

Air, of agreeable temperature, feels cold and disagreeable.

Continually directs a window to be closed which is not open.

Draft of air, or opening or closing door, brings on spasms.

Extreme sensibility to cold or least variation in temperature of air.

Heat of sun: cannot bear it.

Warm drinks: more easily taken than water.

As soon as he gets warm in bed: itching in inner sides of thighs and knees; compelled to scratch.

Open air: headache >; feels a chill strike right arm.

Breath of air: sensitive to.

Blast of air: causes greatest distress.

Wet weather: aching in left side of head <.

In cold room, while undressing: strong erections.

Cold air: > headache; headache, with nausea and sore pain in heart >.

Fever—

Paroxysms of intense coldness with pain in spine.

During paroxysm, limbs cool and livid.

Attacks of vertigo, chilliness, sometimes chills; at least one a day for several days, not always accompanied by vertigo, though always accompanying it.

Late in evening less inclined to chilliness.

Chilly feeling, more down right (bitten) arm.

Felt chilly and cold all over; shaking.

"Desire for heat marked".

Became cold in bed at 3 A.M., although covered with four blankets; lasted about one hour.

Chills intermixed and followed by cold sweat.

A fever, sometimes preceded by slight shiverings, generally very mild.

Face sweats, with flushes.

Temperature of body 100 to 104° Fahrenheit, seldom rises to 105 or 106.

Cannot bear heat of sun.

Fever in afternoon.

Slight fever, with flushes of heat.

Fever every evening, commencing at dusk and lasting until bedtime (midnight).

Sensation of burning heat in parts on which he lies.

He feels the pulse's beat through body; from time to time there is a surging through throat into head, like a slow wave.

Great fever, no chill; pulse 160; no appetite; thirst, drinks cold water very often; stupid and sleepy.

Feverish heat, with headache.

Sensation as if a hot wave, fine, like vapor, surged through body, taking an outward course, yet not reaching surface or extending into limbs.

Heat, with pressure in forehead and back.

After drinking some coffee, a strong heat in right side of face, followed by aching in front of upper part of head; after this again heat from nape of neck up head over ears and right side of face; with heat in eye from within outward and tickling in ear.

Sensation of heat felt internally and externally through entire body, no external warmth, it forces perspiration out on face as from weakness, and is accompanied by lassitude and aching in legs.

At 9 P.M., a dripping, warm perspiration from whole right hand, from wrist to nails; afterwards hands and fingers stiff, she can hardly bend them.

Skin covered with clammy sweat (last stage).

Skin moist, even covered with sweat; during spells, limbs cold and livid.

Much better after perspiring.

Intermittent fever.

Attacks, Periodicity—

"Other diseases, when poison is absorbed, have their periods: the canine poison depends on climate and constitution and different periods, from first day till nineteen months."

Took several drops of 300, after having been bitten in nose; symptoms next day and the following, and well the third day, first symptoms returned on the twelfth day.

First day >; next day <; on third day salivation returned. Lyssophobia.

Irregular fits of backache and chills, increasing steadily.

Paroxysm, combined with a feeling of suffocation, almost produces strangulation.

Sudden convulsions of a paroxysmal character.

| Periodically since two weeks. Spasms of throat.

Attacks every few minutes, for five hours: pain down spine to loins and knees.

Periodical: ranula; spasm of esophagus; dull pain along left sciatic nerve.

Alternating: of heat and headache; twitches in arms and legs.

Repeated eight times: pain from sacrum to middle of back.

For one hour: pain in right arm.

For two hours: pain in and between both shoulders; pain in inguinal glands.

Every two or three hours: has a twitch in heart.

For four hours: sharp shooting pains in region of heart.

After seven hours: right leg falls asleep.

From noon till evening: headache.

From 2 P.M. to 9:30 P.M.: violent spasm in throat.

From 3 to 4 P.M.: headache.

From 4 A.M. till evening: pain in kidneys and across hips.

From 4 P.M. till bedtime: feeling of numbness in right arm.

Daily: passes from time to time a little dark blood from uterus.

Every evening: distension of abdomen; fever commencing at dusk and lasting until midnight.

Three successive mornings: soreness across chest, both breasts swollen.

First days: smoking unpleasant, after first week a crazy, insatiable desire to smoke.

Day after embrace: pain in testicles.

Every other day at 5 P.M.: boring in temples.

During three days: her sense of smell painfully acute.

Lasted eight days: painful throbbing in region of spleen.

After nine days: severe pain in bitten thumb, thence to brain, nervous convulsion for a few moments, passes off in two or three minutes.

Forty days ago: small wound exposed during dissection of mad dog, feeling of malaise and fatigue, followed by death.

Two weeks before time: catamenia.

For two or three weeks: scrotum tightly drawn up.

In Summer, of six weeks standing: pain and tenesmus on hearing or seeing running water.

For several months: offensive mucus from uterus.

For three months: sticking, drawing, squeezing pain in heart.

For seven years: prolapsus uteri.

Tissues—

Affects principally the nervous system.

Great blueness of veins and redness of arteries on wounded arm.

Tearing and shooting as if in bone.

Supraorbital bones feel shattered.

Aching in bones; every bone seems bruised and sore; as if every bone had been broken or violently beaten; never had such pains, had to return to bed and lie there all day.

All his joints cracked on least motion, and pain was quite severe till 10 P.M.

Lost flesh, getting thinner all over.

Quick tendency of body to putrefaction.

Chlorosis.

Touch, Passive Motion Injuries—

He cannot bear to ride in a carriage, feels generally unwell during or after it.

When water (in bath) was least ruffled, so as to touch a fresh surface, convulsions were excited.

Faceache after puncturing a pimple on cheek.

A lacerated wound on right cheek, behind ramus of jaw, one and a half inches, and three lines of abrasion in front of same cheek.

Local sensations of pain in wound or scar continue often after prodromic stage, in an increased degree in higher stage, but are in last scarcely heeded.

Peculiar sensations are frequently experienced at seat of bite, or in adjacent parts; like a sensation of pricking, boring or burning, always proceeding from wound.

Complained of a pain in right arm (bitten part); no inflammation or enlargement of glands of axilla could be discovered.

Tearing pains often proceed from wounded parts, frequently attributed by patients to effects of a cold and to rheumatism thereby induced.

Shooting out from bitten part towards trunk, less frequently extending outward from sensorium, or in some locality other than part injured.

Wound in exceptional cases appears inflamed and swollen; of a reddish or bluish hue.

Sensation of creeping and pain in scar.

Next morning wound red around edges.

Great redness of small bloodvessels around wound.

Soreness in muscles around wound, which is now almost healed.

The wound healed without irritation kindly in course of twelve or fourteen days.

Some are without pain in bitten part.

No pain, swelling or inflammation in lymphatic glands, between bite and thorax.

The wounds heal kindly and are characterized by a striking absence of inflammatory reaction.

The subsequent inflammatory reaction (after caustics) is generally slight, while pain thereby produced is moderated.

Even after application of strong caustics, wounds manifest a strong tendency to skin over without granulating.

Never saw a wound more disposed to heal; he was abroad in five weeks, yet afterwards affected by hydrophobia.

The ready healing of the wound made by the bite of a rabid animal is similar to the rapid healing of wounds in those affected with leprosy.

Touching scar is said to produce peculiar sensations, a shuddering, feeling of anxiety, and sighing.

Sensation of creeping and pain in scar.

| A bite of an angry dog into right thigh had not healed,

turned into malignant ulcers; surrounding bluish red edges, raised and hard, bases badly suppurating and ichorous, with redness and hardness.

| Scars from a bite in nose swollen and red for fifteen months.

| Ulcers remaining after bite of evil disposed dogs.

| Pain on spot bitten became burning, and extended over whole body, and he felt very strangely. Lyssophobia.

Felt a continued pain in spot on right calf where he was bitten, but without a lesion. Lyssophobia.

Wounds from bite of dogs, in sheep.

| A cow bitten by a dog in foot had a large swelling of part, and animal got very restless.

| Two puppies, bitten by their rabid mother, did not get mad after taking Lyssin.

It may be a prophylactic to hydrophobia, but never without at the same time applying radiate heat to the part bitten, and frequent sessions in hot room of Turkish bath; during the attack remedies are to be applied according to symptoms.

Slightest touch: brings on convulsions; along whole vertebrae causes irritability akin to convulsions.

Touch: on head makes it ache; small pustules on frontal eminence; nose very sensitive; pimple on eminence of forehead painful; pain on cheek <.

Pressure: on neck of bladder; causes < pain in neck; causes pain in larynx; muscles of forearm painful; violent pain in right hand.

Disposition to press hand against lower jaw.

Presses head against wall; headache.

Rubbing: headache >; causes ear to pain.

Gentle scratching: headache >.

Scratching: itching in both ears disappears; scurf off pimple, discharge of lymph and blood; sheep's back makes them quiet; < biting and itching in various parts of body; causes small red spots in a circle on inner side of thighs.

Skin—

Quick tendency of the wound to heal (the same in leprosy).

Many underwent smallpox subsequent to reception of bite, and after their recovery died of hydrophobia.

Biting, itching in various parts of body, < by scratching.

Very slight headache and biting itching all over body and legs.

Itching quite severe during night.

Had to scratch frequently, or rather rub.

Through night intolerable itching in lower part of body down to feet.

Itching in right hand, left foot, and in various parts of body.

Bluish discolouration of bitten place (after Laches.).

Itching as soon as he begins to get warm in bed, particularly on inner side of thighs and knees; after scratching there appeared small, red spots in a circle.

When in bed he is compelled to scratch; cannot sleep all night.

| Pustules: on forehead; around inflamed eye; on finger (after bite).

Malignant ulcers from bite of a dog.

| Red scar from bite of a dog.

| Cancerous sores.

Herpes circinatus appeared on left leg, below knee and livid yellow complexion gave way to a healthy colour.

FOOTNOTE

1. An enthusiastic student in Allentown, a Mr. Schmid, made a very good proving; and one of our nearest friends (an experienced prover, a former engraver, Behlert, by name, at that time a paralyzed man) persuaded all his acquaintances, a dozen of women and girls, and some boys, to prove the higher preparations. None of his provers knew anything of the origin of the drug, and they were examined every day with great care, according to the advice of Hahnemann.

MAGNETIS POLI AMBO
(The Magnet)

Symptoms produced by touching either pole of the magnet, indiscriminately, or by laying the whole of the magnetic surface upon the body. The potencies have been prepared by triturating milk sugar which had been saturated when exposed to the emanations of the magnet, a method Hahnemann does not appear to have practiced.

The pathogenesis of the magnet as a whole, and of each pole separately, is from Hahnemann's Materia Medica Pura. It is to the original provings and observations of Hahnemann that we owe these valuable remedies, and no better or more logical introduction perhaps can be given than he has furnished in the Materia Medica Pura:

To the ordinary mechanical, materialistic, and atomistic heads—and there is a vast number of such—it seemed not only paradoxical, but childish and incredible, that, according to the homeopathic medical doctrine, the administration of doses of only very minute fractions of a grain of the more powerful medicines could be of use.

I grant that it may certainly be *more convenient* to regard all diseases as accumulations of gross impurities, and active drugs as rough levers and brooms, or as chemical reagents, consequently as palpable things. This may, I repeat, be *more convenient* than to regard those alterations of the being of living creatures (disease) as pure dynamical affections of the vital force, and medicines as pure, virtual, tone-altering powers, as they are in reality, and to set about curing according to these views.

If we do not adopt these true views, but adhere to those ordinary material ones, the curative powers of medicine must be estimated according to their bulk and the weight of their dose; and hence the scales must determine the efficacy of the dose. But in that case we must first ascertain the weight of the disease, in order to be able to reckon whether a disease weighing so many pounds (it has, indeed, been hitherto not unusual to employ the phrase "*grave* illness") could be pried out, as with a lever, by such a weight of medicine.

I willingly abandon to those colleagues of mine such atomistic views, by which the business of treatment can be carried on very comfortably, even when half asleep; for, as we all know, to us poor mortals nothing is more easy of comprehension than the material, ponderable, palpable, and sensible, because much thinking (and observing), as an Israelitish teacher says, is a weariness to the body. I cannot suppose them capable of regarding disease as immaterial alterations of the vitality, as pure dynamic derangements of our state of health, and medicinal powers as mere virtual, almost spiritual, forces. It is impossible to disabuse them of the idea that for such and such a grave disease a dose of medicine of such and such a weight is required, seeing that they could point to the traditional practice of thousands of years, when palpable quantities of medicine must always be poured into the patient from large bottles, pots, and boxes, in order that any effect should be produced in serious diseases, and *yet even this did not usually succeed.* I can readily believe this; the effect of the ordinary treatment of all times fully corroborates it. But how can they reconcile it with the atomistic, materialistic notions they entertain respecting the action of medicines and their curative powers, that a single *imponderable* spark from a Leyden jar gives a shock to the strongest man, and yet no ascertainable ponderable substance is communicated to his body ? How can they reconcile with their atomistic, materialistic notions the enormous power of mesmerism, when a powerful man with a strong will to do good *approaches* the point of his thumb to the pit of the stomach of a nervous patient? How can they, finally, reconcile with their atomistic, materialistic notions respecting the actions of medicines the fact that a carefully-constructed magnetic steel rod can effect such a powerful derangement of our health, even when it is not in actual contact with the body, but may even be covered with some thick material (such as cloth, bladder, glass, etc.), so that we suffer therefrom violent morbid affections; or what is equally remarkable, that a magnetic rod can quickly and permanently cure the most severe disease for which it is a suitable medicine, when it is brought near the body, for but a short time, even though covered as above described? Atomist! you narrow-minded wiseacre ! tell me what ponderable quantity of the magnet entered the body in order to effect these often enormous changes in its state of health? Is not the centillionth of a grain (a fraction of a grain that has 600 ciphers for its denominator) still infinitely too heavy to represent this absolutely imponderable quantity, the kind of *spirit* that emanated from the magnetic rod into this living body ? Will you now continue to express your amazement at the homeopathic doses of powerful medicines of the sextillionth, octillionth, the decillionth of a grain, which are gross weights compared with this invisible magnetic power?

The subjoined symptoms occurred from various powerful magnets brought in contact with various sensitive individuals, without distinction of the poles. They were observed in experiments conducted for half a year for the purpose of ascertaining the proper and most efficacious mode of stroking the steel with magnets, in which a horse-shoe magnet capable of lifting twelve pounds was held in the hands, which were in contact with both poles for an hour at a time.

Mind and Disposition—

| | While attending to his business in the daytime, he talks aloud to himself, without being aware of it.

He is faint, but excessively solicitous to do his work properly.

Excessive exhaustion of the body, with feeling of heat, and cool sweat in the face with unceasing, and, as it were, hurried and overstrained activity.

Hurried zeal; afterwards a gnawing pain in the arm and in the head of the humerus.

|| Hurried heedlessness and forgetfulness; he says and does something different from what he intends, omitting letters, syllables, and words.

| He endeavors to do things, and actually does things contrary to his own intentions.

Wavering irresoluteness, hurriedness.

He is unable to fix his attention on one object.

The things around him strike him like one who is half dreaming.

Print seems to him very bright, but he has a difficulty to comprehend what he reads.

He inclines to be angry and vehement; and after he has become angry, his head aches as if sore.

He is disposed to feel vexed; this gives him pain, especially a headache, as if a nail were forced into his head.

Sensorium—

Vertigo in the evening after lying down, as if he would fall, or resembling a sudden jerk through the head.

When walking he staggers from time to time, without feeling giddy.

The objects of sight seem to be wavering, this makes him stagger when walking.

Head—

Whizzing in the whole head, occasioned by the imposition of magnetic surfaces on the thighs, legs and chest.

The head feels confused as when one takes opium.

The head feels as if some one were trying to pull it off the trunk.

When endeavoring to think of something and fatiguing his memory, he is attacked with headache.

Transitory headache, one single jerk, composed of darting and tearing sharp pain in the middle of one of the two hemispheres, like the pain that is felt at the moment when one receives a blow.

In the morning on waking, he feels a horrid, digging-up, stupefying headache, going off immediately after flatulence begins to move about in the abdomen.

Headache, as is felt after catching cold.

| | Headache occasioned by the least chagrin, as if a sharp pressure were made on a small spot in the brain.

Pain in the region of the vertex, at a small spot in the brain, as if a blunt nail were pressed into the brain; the spot feels sore to the touch.

Sensation on top of the head, as if the head and the whole body were pressed down.

Face—

Cold hands, with heat in the face and smarting sensation'in the skin of the face.

Intolerable burning prickings in the muscles of the face, in the evening.

| | Sweat in the face without heat, early in the morning.

Eyes—

| Dilated pupils with cheerfulness of the mind and body.

There was no dilatation of the pupils during the spasmodic attacks and the loss of consciousness.

Burning, tearing, and sparkling in the eye.

Burning, drawing, and constant sparks in the affected eye.

Fiery sparks before the eyes, like shooting stars.

Intensely painful stitches through the right eye, disappearing in the jaw, followed by a drawing through the same eye, down the neck, through the chest, abdomen and hips toward the right lower limb.

Sensation in the eye as if the pendulum of a clock were moving in it.

White, luminous, sudden vibrations, like reflections of light, at twilight, on one side of the visual ray, all around.

Smarting in the eyes in the evening after lying down, as from acrid tears.

| Itching of the eyelids and eyeballs in the inner canthus.

Dryness of the eyelids and the inner mouth, in the morning, after waking.

Sensation as if the eyelids were dry.

Twitching of the lower eyelid.

Ears—

The external ear feels hot to him, but is not hot.

Itching or itching burning in the meatus auditorius, early in the morning when in bed.

Fine whistling in the ear, coming and going like the pulse.

Loud strong whizzing in one of the ears, accompanied with headache of the same side, as if a foreign body had lodged in the brain; the pupil of this side is very much enlarged.

Whizzing before the ears.

Noise as of seething water in the ear.

Electric shocks in the ear.

Hard hearing without noise in the ear.

Nose—

Burning pain at a small spot under the wing of the nose.

Illusion of smell: smell of manure before the nose, from time to time he imagines he has a smell before the nose such as usually comes out of a chest full of clothes which had been closed for a long while.

Teeth and Jaws—

Near the vermilion border of the upper lip, not far from the corner, a white pimple, or a red inflamed little tubercle, painful like a sore, in a state of rest, but most painful when moving or touching the parts.

Little ulcer in the centre of the inner surface of the lower lip, painful to the touch.

Painful sensitiveness around the margin of the lips.

Metallic taste on one side of the tongue.

Tearing pain in the periosteum of the upper jaw, coming with a jerk and extending as far as the orbit; the pain consists in a tearing, boring, pricking and burning.

Darting-tearing pain in the facial bones, especially the antrum Highmorianum, in the evening.

When taking a cold drink, the coldness rushes into the teeth.

Drawing pain in the jaws extending as far as the temple, with a crampy sensation in the muscles of mastication.

Looseness of the teeth.

Toothache, excited by stooping.

Beating or jerking pressure, only in single jerks.

Violent grumbling in the teeth, even without any apparent cause.

The gums of a hollow tooth are swollen and painful to the touch.

Aching pain of the hollow, carious teeth.

| Uniform pain in the roots of the lower incisors, as if the teeth were bruised, sore or corroded.

Mouth and Pharynx—

Shocks in the jaws.

Shock in the teeth with burning.

Pain in the velum pendulum palati, as when a large mouthful has been forced down the throat.

Pain of the submaxillary gland as if swollen, early in the morning, in the open air.

Tensive pain in the submaxillary gland.

Single dull prickings in the submaxillary glands, in the evening.

Frequent accumulation of saliva in the mouth, almost like ptyalisrn, with pain of the submaxillary glands..

|| Ptyalism every evening with swollen lips.

| Bad smell from the mouth which he does not perceive himself, also with much mucus in the throat.

Swelling of the throat, redness of the face and increased palpitation of the heart.

| Continual fetid odor from the mouth, without himself perceiving it, as in incipient mercurial ptyalism.

Burning of the tongue, and pain of the same when eating.

Taste and Appetite—

|| Hunger, especially in the evening. He has an appetite, but the food has no taste.

He has a desire for tobacco, milk, beer, and he relishes those things; but he feels satisfied immediately after commencing eating.

Aversion to tobacco, although he relished it.

Want of appetite without any loathing, repletion or bad smell.

Beer tastes like water.

Stomach—

Eructations, tasting and smelling like the dust of sawed or turned horn.

The eructations taste of the ingesta, but as if spoiled.

Frequent attacks of unsuccessful or imperfect eructations.

When stooping, an acid substance rises from the stomach into his mouth.

Pain as from a bandage over the stomach, in both sides.

A sort of rushing through the stomach and the intestines, mingled with stitches.

Pressure in the stomach with cramps in the direction of the upper parts; restlessness which did not permit her to remain at any one place; heaviness of the tongue, paleness of the face, and coldness of the body, the pulse being very small, tight, unequal.

This series of symptoms appeared every day at the same hour, for ten days in succession, in three females, decreasing progressively.

Crackling and cracking in the pit of the stomach, as when a clock is wound up.

Sensation of an agreeable distention in the region of the diaphragm.

Pressure in the epigastrium, as from a stone, especially when reflecting much.

Tensive aching and anxious repletion in the epigastrium.

Abdomen—

The flatulence moves about in the abdomen, with loud rumbling, painless incarceration of flatulence in various small places of the abdomen, causing a sharp aching pain and an audible grunting.

Loud, although painless rumbling, especially in the lesser intestines, extending under the pubic bones and into the groin, as if diarrhea would come on.

Emission of short and broken flatulence, with loud noise and pains in the anus.

| | Loud rumbling in the abdomen, early in the morning when in bed; afterwards colic as if from incarceration of flatulence.

Putrid fermentation in the bowels, the flatulence has a fetid smell and is very hot.

| | Qualmish sensation and painfulness in the intestines, as if one had taken a resinous cathartic or rhubarb, with painful emission of hot, putrid flatulence.

Every emission of flatulence is preceded by pinching in the abdomen.

Tensive and burning pain in the epigastrium and hypogastrium, followed by a drawing and tensive pain in the calves.

Burning and digging-up in the abdomen like a heaving.

Itching of the umbilicus.

Stool—

Frequent but almost unsuccessful urging to diarrhea in the morning, alternating with rumbling of flatulence in the abdomen.

Diarrhea without colic.

Constipation with headache for several days, as if there were something wrong in the brain; the head is uniformly affected, the mind feeling vexed and impatient.

| | Constipation as if the rectum were constricted and contracted.

| | Violent hemorrhoidal pain in the anus after stool, erosive as if sore, and as if the rectum were constricted.

| Burning at the anus when sitting, as in hemorrhoids.

| | Itching hemorrhoids.

| | Blind hemorrhoids after soft stool, as if the varices on the margin of the anus felt sore, both when sitting and walking.

| | Prolapsus recti when going to stool.

Pain on either side of the anus, consisting of itching and soreness, when walking in the open air.

Urinary Organs—

Burning in the bladder, especially in the region of the neck of the bladder, a few minutes after urinating.

Male Genital Organs—

Burning in the urethra, in the region of the caput gallinaginis, during an emission of semen.

| | Early in the morning he feels a burning in the region of the vesiculae seminales.

| | Nightly emissions of semen.

| Violent continuous erections, early in the morning when in bed, without any sexual desire.

| | Want of sexual desire, aversion to an embrace.

| The penis remains in a relaxed condition, in spite of all sexual excitement.

| | The prepuce retreats entirely behind the glans.

Swelling of the epididymis, with simple pain when feeling it or during motion.

Itching smarting of the inner surface of the prepuce.

Burning smarting under the prepuce.

Increased metrorrhagia in a woman advanced in age.

|| Menses had ceased a few days before, returned next day after imposing the magnetic surface and continued ten days.

Larynx—

Frequent fits of nightly cough which does not wake him.

In the evening, after lying down, he has a violent fit of dry cough, sometimes during sleep.

Violent but short-lasting attack of dry cough in the night and at other periods, followed by slight discharge of ordinary mucus from the trachea.

| Convulsive cough.

|| Mucus in the trachea which is easily hawked up, evening and morning.

|| Violent fit of cough, with profuse expectoration of blood.

Chest and Lungs—

Asthma after midnight when waking and reflecting, occasioned by mucus in the chest, diminished by coughing.

Intolerable burning stitches in the muscles of the side of the chest, toward the back.

| Spasmodic cough, with shocks in the chest and anxious breathing, and visible oppression of the chest.

Pricking in the chest, and a cold shuddering burning through the whole body.

A shock in the upper part of the sternum, causing cough and lachrymation.

Violent oppression of the chest, tearing in the stomach and bowels, and beating in the shoulders.

Tearing extending from the right side into the inner parts of the abdomen, mingled with prickings and shocks, as if small pieces of flesh were being torn out, or as if fiery sparks were flying about.

Four burning emanations from the middle of the chest toward either shoulder and side, back, and small of the back, with anxiety, and sensation as if the parts were being dissected.

Burning- emanation from the left shoulder through the chest toward the right side, as if the parts would be severed.

Back—

Painful stiffness of the cervical vertebra in the morning, during motion.

Crackling in the cervical vertebra in the morning during motion.

Pain in the omo-hyoid muscle, as if it would be attacked with cramp.

Pain in the back when standing or sitting quiet.

Burning in the dorsal spine.

Twitching of the muscles of the back, and sensation as if something were alive in them.

||Pain in sacro-lumbar articulation, in the morning when in bed lying on the side, and in daytime when stooping a long time.

Burning emanation from the stomach through the abdomen and back, separating in the small of the back and extending into the lower limbs.

Shock or jerk in the small of the back, almost arresting the breathing.

Upper Limbs—

Pain in the humeral articulation, or in the ligaments, as if the head of the bone were dislocated, not only as if bruised, or sprained and twisted.

Tearing jerkings in the muscles of the arm when staying in a cold place.

Uneasiness in the sound arm.

Drawing pain in the upper part of the lower arm.

In the evening, between the sixth and seventh hours, he feels a tearing and bruised pain in the joints of the arm, more during rest than when bending the arm; the pain returns in twenty-four hours.

Beating in the top of the shoulder with sensation as if torn.

Shocks in the top of the shoulder which caused the arms to recede from the body with a jerk.

Shocks in the arm-joints and head, as if those parts were beaten with a light and small hammer.

Drawing pain in either shoulder, and down the nape of neck, with beating in either arm.

Pulling in the joints and muscles of the arm.

Digging-up around the wrist, elbow, and shoulder-joints.

Pain in the muscles of the arm, as if they would be divided into fine parts.

Burning and cutting in the arms and chest, with cold shuddering.

Burning in the right arm, as from fiery sparks.

Burning pain in the surface of the arm in various parts.

| Prickings in the arm.

The arms are gently elevated, or even crossed as if by spasm; one of the arms is spasmodically tossed, either horizontally or vertically.

| Beating and throbbing in all the joints of the arms and fingers.

| Deep-seated pain in the arm, extending as far as the elbow, the arm going to sleep and trembling spasmodically.

Painless shocks in the elbow.

Burning in the elbow joint, as if torn by hot pincers, with violent burning and sparkling of the eyes.

While removing the magnets from the arms, the fingers, hands and arms become curved and even entirely contracted, in a state of unconsciousness.

| | Drawing from the head down to the tip of the fingers.

The hands are icy cold the whole day, for several days, from touching the centre of the bar.

Pain in the wrist-joint, as if a tendon had become strained, or as if an electric shock were passing through the parts.

Arthritic digging up, and boring pain in a spot of the lower joint of the thumb during rest.

Tearing in the joints of the thumb in the evening when in bed.

Pain as if sprained and bruised, in the morning when in bed, in the lower joint of the thumb, when moving or bending it.

Sudden bending, and sensation as if dislocated in the first and second joints of the thumb.

Prickling and digging-up pain in the tip of the thumb, in the evening after lying down.

Twitching jerking in the muscles of the thumb and in those of the chin.

Continuous burning stitch, accompanied with sore feeling in the thickest part of the muscles of the palm of hand and calf of the leg; afterwards in the lower part of the tibia.

The fingers are liable to be bent and strained.

In the evening the legs and thighs go to sleep.

Lower Limbs—

Sensation in the upper part of the calf, when rising from a seat, as if it were too short.

Attacks of cramp in the calves and toes after waking.

Pain as if bruised in the fleshy part of the leg, on the outer side of the tibia, in the evening when walking.

Pain from the hip down the limb, as if the parts were being divided by a fine instrument.

Drawing from the hips to the feet, leaving a burning along that tract.

Violent shocks of the right lower limb, occasioned by a burning emanation from the chin and neck through the right side.

Fiery burning in the upper and lower limbs; when the right limb touched the left one, it seemed as if the latter were set on fire by the former.

Painful going to sleep of the thighs and legs when sitting, disappearing when walking.

Burning tearing in the left leg, mingled with creeping.

Pricking from the knee to the feet.

Stitches in the leg.

Shocks in the knee, causing the leg to be stretched spasmodically.

Throbbing in the left knee.

In the morning after rising and when attempting to walk, he feels a pain in the tarsal-joint and beyond it, as if sprained.

Stitches in the ball of the heel.

Tearing pain in the heel, setting in with a jerk, passing off immediately, but returning from time to time.

In the evening, prickings with burning in the soft parts on the side of the heel.

Painful sensitiveness and soreness in the region of the root of the nail of the big toe, and in the skin over the root, even when merely touching it.

Sore pain under the nail of the big toe of either foot, as if the shoe had pinched him, and as if the nail would come off by suppuration.

Burning and sore pain of the corn, which is generally painless when commencing to walk.

Pain in the upper part of the tarsal joints, as if the shoe had pinched him, and as if a corn were there.

Sleep—

Coma vigil early in the morning for several hours; after sunrise, sopor or deep sleep set in, full of heavy, passionate dreams, for instance, vexing dreams; the sopor terminates in a headache as if the brain were sore all over, disappearing after rising.

Sleep disturbed by dreams full of oppression and anxiety, resembling nightmare.

| Vivid dreams, as if he saw the thing taking place in his waking state.

| Dreams full of feasting, boasting, and bragging.

|| He wakes at three o'clock in the night; in a few hours he falls into a sopor full of dreams; afterwards, feeling of heat in the limbs without thirst, the limbs requiring to be uncovered at first, but afterwards covered carefully.

He wakes at three o'clock in the morning; at sunrise his eyelids close again, and he lies in a sort of stupor full of heavy dreams.

|| Early in the morning he sleeps on his back, one of his hands lying under the occiput, the other over the region of the stomach, the knees being apart, with moaning inspirations, half-opened mouth, and low muttering, dreaming of amorous things and emissions, although no emission takes place; headache in the occiput after waking, as after an involuntary emission of semen, with asthma, and bruised pain in all the joints, going off after rising and during motion, with copious expulsion of catarrhal mucus.

| Lascivious dreams, even during the siesta, with discharge of the prostatic fluid.

Wakeful drowsiness in the night, toward morning, he hears every noise and has some power of thinking; after sunrise the drowsiness increases to a stupor, during which he hears or feels nothing, except violent pain as after a long journey on foot, and a bruised feeling in all the joints, obliging him to change the position of the limbs constantly, accompanied with loud grumbling in the abdomen, which is interrupted from time to time by emission of flatulence, and a disagreeable feeling of warmth in the body; during which time he generally lies on his back with the mouth open.

The pains in the limbs soon decrease after waking; but in exchange for those pains he is attacked with as painful a headache, increased after rising to a headache such as is felt when a dry coryza is setting in, but disappearing again by sudden sneezing and discharge of mucus from one nostril.

Sweat without heat, early in the morning while asleep, or mild copious exhalation of the whole body, which is not exhausting, and disappears after waking.

When asleep he snores during an inspiration, and wheezes through the nose during an expiration.

Tossing about in bed during sleep.

In the evening before lying down, he is attacked with symptoms of a catarrhal fever; the long bones are painful as if bruised in the middle; accompanied with dull headache causing a cloudiness; he is hoarse, and the chest is lined with tenacious mucus.

In the morning, after waking, the flatulence increases in the abdomen, with loud grumbling; there is emission of flatulence, violent sneezing, copious discharge of mucus from the nose and yawning; all this soon goes off again.

Early in the morning when waking, the mouth is covered with thick, almost dry mucus, and the eyelids are dry; both these symptoms disappear after sneezing and after a discharge of mucus from the nose.

Fever—

Shuddering over the whole body, partly cold, partly burning, and causing an intense pain.

Hot and creeping sensation in the affected part.

Profuse sweat with shuddering.

Slight sweat in the night, especially where the magnet lay.

Sweat in the region of the stomach.

Fever after midnight, no shuddering; disagreeable sensation of heat in the whole body, especially in the palms of the hands and soles of the feet, with dryness in the throat and sweat in the face, nape of the neck or over the whole body.

Dry heat, early in the morning when in bed.

Heat without thirst in the night, requiring one to lie uncovered.

Disagreeable, troublesome warmth in the whole body, with sweat in the face, without thirst.

Imperceptible exhalation of the whole body, having a strong, pungent, though not disagreeable smell, resembling the exhalation which is perceived from a healthy man while sweating.

General sweat after midnight.

Sweat over the whole body, especially in the back, early in the morning while asleep.

Skin—

The recent wound commences to bleed again.

The wound, which is almost healed, commences to pain again like a recent wound.

Boils break out on various parts of the body, passing off soon.

Corrosive pains in various parts, for example, below the ankle.

Itching of the affected parts, the pain is increased by scratching; it is like a sort of burning in a sore place.

Simple, continuous itching of the soft parts, remaining unchanged after scratching.

Burning itching below the joints, after lying down, even for the mere purpose of taking a nap; it cannot be appeased by scratching.

A continuous itching-pricking, here and there, terminating in a burning.

Burning stinging pain in various soft parts of the body, not in the joints; it is more or less continuous.

Single stitches in soft parts, here and there, for instance in the ball of the thumb.

In the evening, after having got warm in bed, he feels single burning stitches here and there, terminating in a smarting sensation.

Pricking, moaning, fluttering sort of a pain at a small place, for instance, in the sole of the feet, as is felt in a limb previous to going to sleep.

Creeping, and sensation as if all the fluids were accumulating in the region where the magnet is applied.

Small pimples on the chest.

Extremely itching eruption where the magnet lay.

The skin under the magnet is painful and corroded, and is surrounded by itch-like pustules.

Red eruption, red spots.

Red eruption in the palms of the hands resembling watery vesicles.

Burning itching where the magnet lay, obliging one to scratch until blood came out; the skin is red, and round about small pimples are visible, passing off soon.

Large pimples around the place where the magnet lay.

Deep, lentil-sized ulcers at the place where the magnet lay.

Wide-spread eruption of pimples and blisters, with drawing and pricking pain; also, red spots here and there.

Secretion of a reddish humor from the wound.

General Symptoms—

Early in the morning, when lying on the side, he feels a continuous, intolerable, simple or bruised pain in all the joints, where the cartilages of the two bones touch one another; the pain abates as soon as one turns on the back, with the head bent backward, and the knees bent and at a distance from one another.

Bruised pain in the joints of that side on which one rests, in the evening when in bed.

Bruised pain of all the joints, or rheumatic pain of the ligaments of the arms and of all the joints of the chest, back, and nape of the neck, during motion and during an expiration.

Paralytic pain in all the joints, especially those of the small of the back, loins and chest, or pain as if the joints were crushed, broken and bruised; worse during motion and when standing, accompanied with a drawing and tearing sensation, especially in the ligaments and tendons, where they are inserted in the bones, particularly early in the morning after rising, and in the evening before lying down; the parts are painless when touched; the pains are relieved by emission of flatulence; an increase of pain obliges one to close the eyes.

The joints are painful when moving the limbs, as if they had been sprained.

Sensation in the limbs during motion, as is felt in the arm when knocking the lunar nerve in the region of the elbow against anything hard.

The limbs go to sleep, especially when standing or walking, after rising from a seat.

In the morning, when lying in bed, and resisting a desire for an embrace, he is attacked with a kind of arthritic pain in the small of the back, knees and all the joints; the pains are bruised or weary pains.

Burning emanation from the head, down the right side; immediately after, the whole body is covered with sweat.

Burning emanations through every part of the body in every direction.

Intolerable burning from the head to the feet, with pain as if the limbs were being torn and divided.

Burning and pricking pains.

During the burning pains there was neither external heat, nor redness of the parts.

Sensation as of flying sparks over the body.

Sensation in every part as if cut up.

Heaviness in all the limbs, and palpitation of the heart from omitting the usual imposition of the magnets.

| Dull, numb pain.

Drawing and pricking pain, mingled with itching.

|| Shuddering movement through whole body.

| The joints are painful when touched.

The places on which the magnets lie, burn as if hot coal were lying near them.

The place where the magnet had been imposed goes to sleep, becomes numb and insensible.

| Jerking shock, causing the trunk to bend violently upward and forward as low down as the hips, with cries.

The trunk, while in a recumbent position, is jerked up spasmodically as it were, the head being jerked forward upon the bed, and then again backward upon the cushion.

The upper part of the body is spasmodically lifted and jerked forward, and then again backward on one side.

Violent shocks causing a general tremor of the body, burning in the chest and through either arm, and sweat all over.

None of the convulsions excited by the magnet after the pulse.

A sort of starting through the body, afterwards sweat on either hand.

Paralysis for ten days, with loss of sensation, the limb having its natural temperature and being moist.

Shocks deprive him of consciousness.

The spasmodic risings and jerkings of the body forward, are followed by a long-lasting loss of consciousness, followed by blowing with the mouth as when one experiences a great heat; after which consciousness and cheerfulness return.

Loss of consciousness with staring eyes, open mouth, almost imperceptible inspirations, and a movement in the chest which is almost like palpitation of the heart, the pulse remaining unchanged and having its ordinary quality.

During the loss of consciousness the fingers are moved one after the other; after the return of consciousness a profuse sweat breaks out.

Languor in all the limbs, accompanied with a swoon, which lasts but a short while and returns several times.

Fits of fainting, palpitation of the heart, and suffocation.

Long-lasting swoons, in which she retained her consciousness.

Swoon, during which she feels her pain, but is unable to complain on account of an inability to speak or move.

Insensibility and deadly sopor.

MAGNETIS POLUS ARCTICUS
(North-pole of the magnet)

MIND AND DISPOSITION.—Out of humor and weary. Weeping mood, with chilliness and a disposition to feel chilly.

Sadness, in the evening; he had to weep, contrary to his will, after which his eyes felt sore.

He felt in the evening as if it were difficult for him to commence the execution of his designs, and it was long before he made a beginning; but as soon as he had commenced, he carried out his designs with great promptness.

| Indolent fancy; he sometimes felt as if he had no fancy at all.

When sitting, he felt as if he had lost all powers of motion, and had grown fast to the chair.

|| Indolent mind.

Anxious, desponding, inconsolable, self-reproaching mood.

Sleep ceased at three o'clock in the morning, and he became anxious; he became solicitous about his health, as if he were dangerously sick; he became gloomy; he grudged every word he was obliged to utter.

Exaggerated, over-scrupulous solicitude.

Irritated and vexed mood; he does not like to be interrupted in his work, and, nevertheless, he does not accomplish anything.

|| While attending to his business, he talks aloud to himself.

| | He makes mistakes easily in writing.

He would like to work a great deal, and does not satisfy himself; he thinks he does things slowly.

He is alternately sad and cheerful.

Acts as if he were frightened and timid (immediately).

Despondency.

Anxious scrupulousness (immediately).

Hasty, bold, quick, firm.

| | Calm, composed mood, devoid of care.

Alternately cheerful and sad, the whole day.

Cheerfulness and feeling of great strength, alternate with want of courage and weakness.

Sensorium—

(Vertigo, sensation as if she would fall in every direction.)

Vertiginous motion in one side of the head.

After having gone up stairs, she feels a motion from the centre of the brain towards either ear like the pendulum of a clock.

Sensation as if his understanding were arrested, and as if something were pressing his brain down, and the eyes out, a sort of fainting turn.

Sensation of intoxication, like a humming in the head.

Dulness of the head with desire for open air.

Weak memory, but he feels cheerful.

Head—

Two days in succession he wakes from his siesta with a violent headache, as if the brain were bruised and obtuse; the headache decreases after he is fully awake, and disappears gradually after rising.

Headache, consisting in a sore and bruised pain in the surface of the brain, in the sinciput and in one of the temples.

The head feels bruised and as if dashed to pieces in one of the hemispheres.

A shock in one side of the head in the morning in bed.

| | Sensation as if the head were pressed down by a load.

Pressure as from something hard in several parts of the brain.

(A good deal of heat in the head.)

Disagreeable, compressive sensation in the head, and as if one part of the brain were pressed in.

The head is concussed by the sound of a hammer.

Headache, especially when raising or moving the eyes.

Tensive sensation in the brain behind the forehead, extending down to the root of the nose.

Stitches in the upper part of the forehead, in the morning after rising, until afternoon.

| Headache, as if the temples were pressed asunder.

| Violent headache the whole afternoon, as if the brain were pressed asunder.

| | Rush of blood to the head, and suffusion of heat in the cheeks.

| Drawing-boring pain in the right temple, accompanied with a spasmodic pain below the right malar bone.

Pressure in the right temple, when walking in the open air, causing a dulness of the head.

| Aching pain over the left temporal region, externally.

Tearing in the head behind the right ear, with sensation as of a shock, gradually moving to the front of the head, when walking in the open air.

| | Pushing tearing in the head behind the left ear when sitting.

Tension of the scalp as if firmly adhering to the skull, causing a dulness of the head (for several hours).

Pressure in the articulation of the condyles of the occiput with the atlas from within outward, obliging him to bend the head forward constantly.

Aching pain in the left side of the forehead.

Aching pain in the outer parts over the right eyebrow.

Tubercles on the hairy scalp, painful when touched.

Smarting itching of the hairy scalp.

Eyes—

Cold movement as of a cold breath in the eyes.

The eyes protrude.

| | Staring look.

Fine prickings in the left eye.

Burning, continuous stitch in the upper eyelid.

Vesicle on the margin of the upper eyelid, pressing on the eye.

Painful sensitiveness of the eyelids when reading.

| | Itching in the inner canthus and in the margin of the eyelids.

| Painful feeling of dryness in the eyelids in the morning on waking.

| | Jerking and drawing in the eyelids.

| | Drawing in the eyelids with lachrymation.

| | Pricking in the eyelids.

Agglutination of the eyelids in the morning.

| Lachrymation early in the morning.

| | Excessive lachrymation; the light of the sun is intolerable.

Dilatation of the pupils; they contract but little in the light (immediately).

Contraction of the pupils during the first hours.

Stinging in the canthus and the left cheek.

Sensation as of sand in the eye.

Itching in the eye.

| | Burning in the weak right eye; it became red and filled with water (the magnet being held in contact with the weak right eye for a quarter of an hour).

| | Coldness in the weak eye for three or four minutes (the magnet being held in contact with that eye for two minutes).

Coldness of the weak eye, as if the eye were a piece of ice;

as the coldness passed off a long-continued pricking was felt in the eye.

Pricking sensation in the eye, resembling the tick of a watch.

| Uneasy motion of the eye, with a good deal of water accumulating in either eye.

|| Sensation as of a cobweb in front of the eyes.

Glare in the eye as of a shooting star.

| Formication between the two eyes.

|| Strong drawing over the eye, in the surface of the cheek, ear, extending into the upper maxillary bone (the magnet being in contact with the eye).

Ears—

Stitch darting from the Eustachian tube to the interior of the ear (when stooping).

| Fine ringing in the opposite ear (immediately).

A few tearings in the interior of the right ear, resembling otalgia.

|| Whizzing and a drawing sensation in the ear.

Tightness of the tympanum.

Crackling in the ear as of burning, dry wood (when holding the magnet in the ear).

Warmth and roaring in the ear, as when water is boiling and bubbling (holding the magnet in the ear).

Ringing in the ear of the same side.

Heat and pecking sensation in the ear (holding the magnet in the ear).

| A kind of deafness, as if a pellicle had been drawn over the right ear, after which heat is felt in the ear.

Nose—

|| Illusion of smell: he imagined the room smelled of fresh whitewash and dust, he imagines the room smells of rotten eggs, or of the contents of a privy.

|| Violent bleeding at the nose, for three afternoons in

succession, increasing every afternoon, and preceded by an aching pain in the forehead.

Sore pain in the nostrils, even without touching or moving them.

|| Redness and heat of the tip of the nose, followed by hot, red, circumscribed spots on the cheeks.

Pimples on the right wing of the nose, with a stinging-itching sensation.

Face—

Intensely-painful tightness in the face, extending as far as the tonsils.

Drawing in the left cheek.

Innumerable prickings in the cheek, with feeling of heat, without any heat being perceptible to others.

Suffusion of heat in the cheeks, with rush of blood to the head.

Tubercle in the face, near the nose, feeling sore when touched; when not touched, a few rare slow stitches are felt in it.

Jaws and Teeth—

Crampy-aching pain in the left submax-illary gland.

Crushing-aching, or pinching pain in the submaxillary glands, without the glands being either touched or moved, as is felt in acute swelling of the throat.

Tearing pain in the cervical muscles, as if too weary.

Painful cramp in the cervical muscles, from one ear to the other.

Drawing in the left jaw and the left cheek.

Tensive pain in the left upper jaw, early in the morning on waking.

Painful drawing in the articulation of the lower jaw when moving it, as if it would be dislocated by force.

| Drawing-aching pain coming from the temple, below the mastoid process, between the sterno-cleido-mastoideus muscle and the ramus of the lower jaw.

Tensive pain in the left submaxillary gland.

Cramp-like toothache in the right lower jaw.

| Toothache as if the tooth would be torn out, worse after a meal, and when sitting or lying down, improving when walking.

|| Toothache in the direction of the eye, a very quick succession of peckings in the hollow tooth, with swollen inflamed gums and a red and burning cheek; the toothache increased very much immediately after a meal, improved when walking in the open air, but aggravated in a smoky room.

| Throbbing in the hollow tooth (immediately), followed by a pressure in the tooth as if something had got into the tooth, with drawing in the temples.

|| Throbbing in the tooth, with burning in the gums, and swollen, red, hot cheeks, with burning pain and heating in the cheeks, in the afternoon.

|| The toothache ceases when walking in the open air, and returns in the room.

Aching in the hollow teeth, with swelling of one side of the face.

Toothache with jerks through the periosteum of the jaw, the pain being a darting-aching, digging-tearing, or burning-stinging pain.

| The toothache is worse after eating and in the warm room.

Numbness and insensibility of the gums of the painful tooth.

Drawing pain in the hollow tooth and fore teeth, increased by anything warm; with redness of the cheek during the pain.

|| Swelling of the gums of a hollow tooth, painful when touched with the tongue.

Toothache, as if the gums were sore or cut, increased by the air entering the mouth.

Mouth—

Sore pain in the left corner of the mouth, when moving it, as if an ulcer would form.

Slow, extremely sharp and painful prickings in the lower lip.

Small pimples on the inner surface of the upper lip.

Itching in the forepart of the tongue, obliging one to rub and scratch.

Accumulation of saliva in the mouth (immediately).

Pain in the left upper incisors, as if something hard were pressing upon them, breaking them.

Pain of the incisors on inspiring air.

Toothache when eating, the teeth feel loose, and as if they would bend over.

| Painful humming in the hollow taeth of the lower jaw, worse on the right side, the toothache ceases during eating.

Appetite and Taste—

Long-continued rancid heart-burn.

He does not even relish the most palatable kind of food, at supper.

When smoking, he feels a scraping sensation in the throat as if he would have heartburn, or had had it.

Sourish taste in the morning, as if one were fasting.

When smoking, he has a bitter taste on the posterior part of the tongue.

Tobacco is disagreeable to him.

She felt so replete at dinner that she was unable to eat.

Greedy appetite at supper.

Chocolate had a flat, disagreeable taste, as if impure water had been added to it.

He relishes his supper, but soon after he has a flat taste in the mouth, and feels a heat in the lobules of the ears.

Stomach—

Eructation, with a sort of painful jerk.

|| Frequent eructations of mere air.

The magnet seems to favor acidity of the stomach.

The tongue is very much coated and covered with mucus; aversion to milk.

Stomach feels as if deranged; food weighs heavily in his stomach.

Sudden griping in the pit of the stomach.

Throbbing in the pit of the stomach (immediately).

Sensation in the epigastric region and in the stomach, as if the walls of the stomach were sensitive to pain.

Drawing in the pit of the stomach, extending into the right chest.

Abdomen—

| She is waked in the night by a pressure in the abdomen as from a stone.

Drawing pain in the abdomen.

Warmth in the umbilical region, causing an anxiety; followed by a sensation as if vomiting would come on.

Coldness in the abdomen (immediately after touching the magnet).

Shocks and jerks proceeding from the abdomen and extending through the chest into the throat (immediately).

A few jerks in the abdomen, like a sort of rumbling, as if something were falling down in the abdomen at intervals (immediately).

A few stitches in the side of the abdomen, and movement in the abdomen as if diarrhea would come on.

Spasmodic contractive sensation in the hypogastrium, externally and internally, early in the morning.

Pinching, especially in the epigastrium, directly after supper.

Violent, continuous pinching, as from incarcerated flatulence, at a small place in the left side of the abdomen.

| Flatulent colic immediately after supper; sharp pressure in every part of the abdomen from within outward, as if the abdomen would burst; relieved when sitting perfectly still.

Flatulent colic early in the morning, immediately after waking; the flatulence was pressed upward toward the hypochondriac region, with tensive pains in the whole abdomen, causing a hard pressure here and there, accompanied with a qualmishness and nausea which proceeded from the abdomen, and was felt both in motion and when at rest.

Continuous aching-pinching pain in the whole hypogastric region, like a sort of colic, but without any perceptible flatulence; it disappears neither by motion nor rest, or eating and drinking, but is excessively increased by reflection and mental exertions, and is in that case accompanied with nausea; the colic is somewhat diminished by strict rest, but it disappears entirely in the space of an hour by touching the zinc.

In the evening and morning he feels a pressure as from flatulence in various parts of the bowels, resembling a pressure on a bruised spot, accompanied with a similar pressure in various parts of the brain; both the headache and colic disappear immediately after the emission of flatulence; the headache and colic return with the return of flatulence, which makes one moreover feel ill-humored; the flatulence has a fetid smell.

(The south pole removed the painful uneasiness in the abdomen, and the headache, within the space of an hour.)

He wakes in the night with a violent colic; it is a sort of continuous, intolerably hard pressure in the pit of the stomach and the hypochondria, continuing to rise in the chest, and increasing in violence up to the pit of the throat, where the breathing threatens to be arrested (this condition was soon relieved by the hands being imposed on the chest with a strong will—a sort of self-mesmerism), the spasm abated, and rest and sleep were restored by a strong but easily emitted flatulence.

Gurgling in the abdomen as if a quantity of flatulence were incarcerated, causing a writhing sensation, which rises up to the pit of the stomach, and causes eructations.

Severe cutting stitches, when walking in the open air, in the middle of the hypogastrium, from below upward.

Stitches in the right lumbar region.

Stitches in the left groin from within outward, in the region of the superior spinous process of the ilium (immediately).

Cutting pain in the left groin, in the region of the abdominal ring, with a feeling of weakness in that region.

| Relaxed condition of the abdominal ring, increasing from day to day; hernia threatens to protrude, especially when coughing.

| Sore pain in the abdominal ring, when walking.

| Boring pain above the left abdominal ring, from within outward, as if hernia would protrude.

|| Inguinal hernia.

Stool–

Drawing, almost dysenteric pain in the hypogas trium, early in the morning, followed by difficult expulsion of the very thick feces.

Blood comes away with stool twice a day.

Sharp pressure in the rectum. Stinging-pinching in the rectum.

Aching-pressing pain in the rectum (not in the anus) after midnight, while slumbering, lasting for hours and disappearing after being wide awake.

Urinary Organs–

Dark urine.

The secretion of urine decreases in the first hours, but increases after the lapse of twenty-four hours.

Copious emissions of urine.

(Relaxed condition of the neck of the bladder from one o'clock at noon until eight o'clock in the evening; the urine dropped out involuntarily.)

Genital Organs–

Continuous smarting pain in the raphe of the prepuce, after urinating.

Itching smarting of the inner surface of the prepuce, obliging one to rub at night when in bed.

Sharp stitches in the left testicle when laying the thighs across one another.

|| Nightly involuntary emission.

Excessive erection, with excessive desire for an embrace and an emission of semen.

Relaxation of the penis and diminished desire for an embrace.

Strangulating pain in the right testicle.

Sharp drawing and cutting in the testicles.

The menses, which ought to have appeared immediately, appeared after the lapse of twenty hours, increased within twenty-four hours beyond the quantity in which they usually appeared, and which was less than ought to have been, until the quantity became normal, without any secondary symptoms (curative effect).

Respiratory Organs—

Dry cough causing a painful rawness in the chest, especially in the night after getting warm in bed, having been chilly first.

Racking and spasmodic cough while falling asleep, hindering sleep.

Suffocative, spasmodic cough about midnight.

The desire to cough is seated in the finest and most remote bronchial ramifications, where nothing can be got loose by the cough; the mucus which is thrown off is secreted in a higher region, the titilation remaining the same, inasmuch as it has its seat lower down; hence the cough is very fatiguing and racking; even the head is concassed, and the whole body becomes warm, after which a general exhalation sets in until morning, when the cough abates.

Unceasing (not titillating) irritation, inducing coughing, in the evening, in bed, immediately after lying down, the cough being short and dry; the irritation is not momentarily diminished by the cough, as is the case in other kinds of cough; this unceasing irritation can only be removed by suppressing the cough, even by a firm, determined will.

He was obliged to breathe spasmodically with deep and

intermittent inspirations, as if his breathing became arrested, at the same time he felt a desire to inspire as much air as possible, and was covered with sweat all over.

Momentary violent turns of cough; three or four.

When walking in the open air the cough becomes much worse, and assumes a suffocative character.

Chest—

Sudden oppression of the chest, with anxiety.

Itching of the nipples.

A few violent beats of the heart.

Burning or sharp stitches in the region of the heart.

Burning stitches, first in the region of the dorsal muscles, afterwards in the side of the chest, and lastly in the fore part of the right chest.

|| Pressure in the region of the heart (immediately).

Sharp stitches in the left muscles of the chest, on moving the arm.

Stitches in the left side of the chest.

Crampy contractive pain through the chest, causing a tremulous anxious breathing, especially the inspirations, when leaning over upon the arms and looking out at the window.

Anxiety and qualmishness about the chest.

When walking in the open air he imagines that heat is entering the chest, passing through the pharynx.

When walking in the open air, he feels a pricking in the left side of the chest.

Continuous stitch in the left side of the chest in the evening.

Back—

Crackling or cracking in the cervical vertebrae, especially in the atlas, during motion.

Pain as if bruised in the middle of the spine, when bending the spine backward.

| Gurgling and creeping sensation between the scapulae.

Twitching in the posterior lumbar muscles.

| Pain as if bruised in the left shoulder-joint both during motion and rest, painless when touching it.

Upper Extremities—

Trembling of the arm, the hand whereof is touched by the magnet.

Cramp-like sensation in the arm, and as if it had gone to sleep.

The left arm is much heavier than the right.

The upper arm which is not touched by the magnet is very heavy.

Itching above the elbow, consisting in a fine stinging and smarting, not diminished by scratching, as if a mosquito had bit him there; the scratching causes a burning.

Jerking in the affected upper arm (the arm and foot seemed to him dead).

Sensation of stiffness in the elbow-joint.

Audible cracking in the elbow-joint during motion (immediately).

Pleasant feeling in the arm-joint, as if it enjoyed rest after great weariness.

Heaviness in the upper limbs, as if the veins contained lead (immediately).

Feeling of heaviness in the arm which touches the magnet.

| Violent coldness in the arm over which the magnet had been moved (in a female in magnetic sleep, after being touched with the north pole magnet).

Prickling pain in the arm as far as the shoulder, especially in the long bones of the forearm.

| Sore pain in the right shoulder when walking in the open air.

Sensation in the arm and hand as if they had gone to sleep (immediately).

Stitches in the forearm near the wrist-joint.

Pressure in the left radius, in the evening, as after a blow.

Pressure and drawing in the wrist-joint, with uneasiness in the forearm, obliging him to bend the arm continually.

Stiffness and rigidity in the right tarsal and carpal joints, at night when in bed.

Trembling of the hand which touches the magnet, and of the foot of the opposite side.

Painful and almost burning itching in the dorsum of the middle phalanx of the little finger, as if the part had been frozen; the place was painful to the touch.

Fine, frequent prickings in the affected spot, and the tip of every finger; worst in the evening after lying down.

Drawing in the fingers from below upwards, with creeping in the fingers immediately; directly after he felt somewhat desponding.

Pain in the finger joints, as if they had been strained by bending them over.

Buzzing in the finger which is in contact with the magnet.

Twitchings in the finger in contact with the magnet, afterwards extending into the arm, with a kind of heaviness in the arm.

Stitches in the muscles of the hollow of the left hand, when walking in the open air.

The fingers go to sleep.

Creeping in the tip of the left index-finger.

Jerking in the thumb which is touched by the magnet, as if there were pulsations in the thumb.

Lower Extremities—

Bruised pain in the hip-joints, aggravated by contact.

Tearing, with pressure and a sensation of strangulation in some parts of the muscles of the thigh when walking or sitting.

Tearing with pressure in the outer side of the knee down to the outer ankle.

Painful sensation in the skin of the calf when walking.

| Burning pulsative stitches in the calf.

Great languor of the lower limbs.

The left leg goes to sleep after sitting, when rising, and especially when standing.

Weariness and numbness of the lower limbs as if they had gone to sleep, without tingling.

| Excessive weakness of the lower limbs, when walking, as if they would break.

Drawing in either knee and in the right lower limb.

Stitch in the anterior muscles of the right thigh, from above downwards.

| Voluptuous itching of the left thigh, on the anterior and internal surface, but more on the former.

Stitches in the tendons of the left thigh, toward the bend of the knee.

| Rigid tension in the hamstrings, when rising from a seat, as if too short.

Painless buzzing in the left leg, with sensation of heaviness, as if the leg had gone to sleep.

Pain in the upper part of the toes, as if they had become sore by walking.

| Sore pressure in the corns, which had been painless heretofore, when pressing the feet ever so little.

Sore pain in the heel.

Occasional pain in the heel, like pressure.

Violent pressing around the ankle of the ulcerated foot.

| Sudden lancinations in the heels, big toe and calf when sitting.

Painful crawling in the toes of the right foot.

Voluptuous itching under the toes of the left foot.

Sleep—

Excessive spasmodic yawning with pain in the articulation of the left jaw, as if it were on the point of being dislocated.

Sopor: several times he was attacked with a sudden sensation as if he ought to shut his eyes, and as if he were going to fall into a pleasant sleep; an irresistible sensation which threatened to deprive him suddenly of consciousness.

In the evening he fell into a deep sleep; all his limbs felt paralyzed or bruised.

| Constant drowsiness in the day-time.

Deep sleep toward morning.

Slept on his back in the night.

She sings in the evening during sleep, wakes by her singing, recollects that she ought not to sing, falls to sleep again, sings a second time and is again waked by her singing.

Vivid, but innocent and impassionate dreams about events; he is unable to recollect them on waking.

| Lascivious dreams the whole night.

She dreams about midnight that she is falling from a height; this startled her and caused her to tremble all over.

About midnight she dreams of murder, which causes her to weep and cry.

| She saw a person in a dream, and next day she saw that person in reality for the first time.

He has vivid dreams the whole night about objects which are not disagreeable but have no connection with one another; on waking he is unable to recollect any of them.

He is unable to go to sleep before a couple of hours in the night.

| At two o'clock in the morning he is half awake, his internal consciousness being very intense, his memory very vivid and his mind filled with ideas; he composes in the very best style in a foreign language which he neither spoke nor wrote fluently, as if he had been in a magnetic sleep; but is unable, when waking, to recollect distinctly what he had thought.

He suddenly wakes in the evening after going to sleep, with a violent jerk in the muscles of the head and neck, as if the head had been pushed back.

He wakes about midnight from a violent pressure across

the abdomen, directly over the umbilicus, and remaining unchanged either by motion, or rest, or by changing one's position.

Violent pain in the pharynx in the evening when in bed, as when one has swallowed too large a morsel; the pain went off when turning to the left side.

He tosses about in his bed in the night, half waking.

He wakes in the night with a good deal of troublesome heat of the whole body, and has to uncover himself from time to time; his mouth being dry, without any thirst.

|| Restless sleep; he tosses about and his bed feels too warm.

Warmth in the night as if sweat would break out.

Very vapory night-sweat, without heat.

He waked in the night, feeling very warm; he felt still warmer after drinking a glass of cold water.

Frequent shudderings in the night while in bed, and jerks in the arms causing them to start.

Frequent waking as if in affright.

He frequently wakes in the night with a burning heat of the whole body, and is sometimes obliged to uncover himself.

Fever—

Chilliness with yawning, early in the morning.

(Chilliness the whole day, over the whole body, but especially along the back.)

| Sensation of coldness or coolness over the whole body, as if she were dressed too lightly, or as if she had taken cold, without shuddering; immediately after she had a small loose stool which was succeeded by pressing.

| Shuddering all over at the moment when the north pole was touched by the tip of the tongue.

Sensation of coldness in the tip of the finger which was in contact with the magnet, accompanied with drops of sweat on the fingers of this hand and the dorsum of the hand (immediately).

Sweat in the palms of the hands, the hands being cool.

| Cool sweat all over.

Towards morning he is covered all over with a strongly, but not disagreeably smelling, vapory, slight sweat.

Sweat about two o'clock in the morning, all over, even in the face, mostly on the chest, except the hair on the head and those parts of the hairy scalp on which he was resting; only while asleep; the sweat disappeared entirely on waking, and was not accompanied with thirst.

Heat in the face.

In the evening the blood rushes to the head and the face feels hot, accompanied with chilliness of the lower limbs, especially the feet.

| Heat in one of the cheeks, accompanied with a feeling of internal heat, irritable disposition and talkativeness.

Sensation of warmth in the feet.

Feeling of heat over the whole body, with quick and strong pulse, without any external warmth; even the hands are cold, although they feel hot to him, without thirst.

Fiery redness of the face, oppression, stronger pulse.

Heat over the whole body in the evening, with anxiety driving him to and fro.

Heat, especially down the back and over the whole body, with an anxious, unsteady appearance.

(Fever: chilliness in the small of the back, along the back, from noon till evening without any perceptible coldness and great thirst; at nine o'clock in the evening, he has a good deal of heat in the face, without thirst; after midnight she is covered with a profuse fetid sweat, lasting until morning and disappearing on waking.)

Fever: frequent flushes of heat in the afternoon, only in the head, with a red, hot face (for two or three minutes); accompanied with some drawing in the head.

Fever: at three o'clock in the afternoon there came on a small burning spot on the foot for one minute, disappearing suddenly, and succeeded by a sudden heat in the head, with redness of the cheeks and sweat in the face, for some minutes.

Fever: frequent shudderings in the back lasting a few minutes, followed by an equally short heat spreading from the back over the head, the veins of the hands becoming distended, without sweat.

Flush of humid warmth over the whole body (immediately).

Skin—

Stitching in a steatoma.

| Crawling over the skin.

Burning pain in the existing herpes.

Crawling itching, as of a fly or flea, terminating in a sensation of soreness, first in the inner, then in the outer side of the limbs, in the evening when in bed, and in the morning after waking.

General Symptoms—

Continuous digging-up stitches in various parts, becoming sharper and more painful, in proportion as they penetrate more deeply into the flesh.

Darting jerks in the part touched by the magnet (immediately).

Tremulous, vibrating, numb sensation.

Sensation as if the blood were rushing to the place touched by the magnet, as if the blood would come out there.

Twitching in the adjoining parts.

Twitching and beating near the part touched by the magnet.

Tensive sensation in the adjoining parts.

| Bruised pain in the adjoining parts, and as if one had carried a heavy burden.

Creeping in the adjoining parts as if they were going to sleep.

|| Tremulousness through the whole body, especially in the feet.

|| Tremor in the part touched by the magnet (immediately).

Nervousness with trembling, uneasiness in the limbs, great distension of the abdomen, anxiety, solicitude, and great nervous weakness.

|| Sensation of coldness in the part which was touched by the magnet.

Warm sensation in the adjoining parts.

Drawing in the periosteum of all the bones, as is felt at the commencement of an intermittent fever (but without chilliness or heat).

In the right side of the tongue, in the neck and across the foot he feels a sudden drawing, or a movement to and fro, and jerks resembling stitches.

Heaviness in single limbs (with a sensation as if their strength had increased).

Sensation of dryness and tightness in the body, with want of strength.

He is very faint, had to rest himself while walking in the open air, and was melancholy and desponding.

The faintness, the bruised and painful sensation in the limbs were worse in the open air.

In the morning there was a general faintness with a sweat as of anguish; want of appetite at dinner; he had to lie down; afterwards diarrhea.

In the morning she felt so languid that she was scarcely able to drag herself along, as if oppressed by a sultry atmosphere.

MAGNETIS POLUS AUSTRALIS
(South Pole of the Magnet)

Mind and Disposition—

After walking in the open air he feels quarrelsome and peevish.

After an evening nap he feels exceedingly peevish and ill-humored.

He is liable to start when touched.

Want of cheerfulness; he is low-spirited, as if he were alone, or as if he had experienced some sad event, for three hours.

Weeping immediately.

Despondency (the first hours).

Great discouragement, dissatisfaction with himself.

Want of disposition to work, and vexed mood.

Taciturn, he is not disposed to talk.

He wants to be alone, company is disagreeable to him.

Cheerful faces are disagreeable to him.

Violent anger excited by a slight cause; he becomes trembling and hurried, and used violent language.

Wild, vehement, rude, both in language and action (he does not perceive it himself); he asserts with violence, reviling others, with distorted countenance.

Feeling of warmth, gradually increasing to heat (in a woman in the magnetic sleep, after touching the south pole of the magnet).

Great quickness of fancy.

Sensorium—

Unsteadiness of the mind; he is unable to fix his, ideas; things seem to flit to and fro before his senses; his opinions and resolutions are wavering, which occasions a kind of anxious and uneasy condition of the mind.

This mental disturbance is removed by touching the metallic zinc.

| Vertigo as if intoxicated, as if he were obliged to stagger, some vertigo even while sitting.

Head—

Rush of blood to the head, without heat.

| Heaviness of the head, with a sort of creeping or fine digging in the head.

| Fine crawling in the brain as of a number of insects, accompanied with heaviness of the head.

Creeping in the vertex, as if something were running about there, and a sort of tearing.

Shocks in either temple.

Pain in the right side of the forehead, composed of tearing and beating.

A few beatings over the forehead, accompanied with a tearing pain.

Tearing at a small spot on the left temple.

| Drawing-tearing pain in the left brain, resembling a slow, burning stitch.

| Pressure in the occiput, in alternate places.

Headache, pressure on the top of the head, or in either temple, an intense violent pain, as is felt in a catarrh, being violent when sitting straight, more so when shaking the head or when reflecting, diminishing when walking, and disappearing almost entirely when bending the head forward or backward (in the first hours).

Headache in the occiput, most violent in the room, but disappearing in the open air (in the first hours).

Creeping, mixed with prickings, in the anterior and middle part of the forehead, in the evening.

Sharp, pointed, aching pain in the left side of the head, with pressure from within outward; continuous stitch accompanied with pressure (relieved by the north pole).

Simple and tensive pain over the whole brain, commencing while walking in the open air, and speedily going off in the room.

Pulsative beating in the right side of the head, when lying down.

Jerkings in the head.

Spasmodic contractive headache in the region between the eyebrows.

A certain spot in the hairy scalp is painful as if bruised, still more so when touched.

A glandular tubercle in the nape of the neck becomes suddenly inflamed, the skin all around was painful as if sore, and the least touch was unpleasant to it.

The skin on the forehead feels as if dried fast to the skull.

Face—

Sensation in the face (and in the rest of the body) as if cold air were blowing upon it.

Blunt stitches in the cheek.

Eyes—

Slow, burning stitch in the margin of the eyelid.

|| Watery eyes from time to time.

Erosive pain, morning and evening, especially in the outer canthus, and when touching the eyelids, as if a hair had lodged in the eye, a sort of inflammation of the margin of the eyelids.

|| Painful, smarting dryness of the eyelids, especially perceptible when moving them, mostly in the evening and morning.

Swelling of the Meibomian glands of the lower eyelid, in the morning, as if a stye would form, but the pain was merely aching.

Smarting in the inner canthus (in the morning).

Pressure and dull sticking in the left eye.

Spasmodic contraction of one of the eyes, in the morning.

The skin around the eyes is sore.

When holding the magnet to the eye, he feels a little coldness in the eye for a short time, but a severe itching in the eyelids.

The eyes feel agglutinated in the morning.

Beating and itching in the eye.

| Deficient sight: things looked dim, also double, when touching the nape of the neck.

Faintish sort of cloudiness, with disposition to sit down; the objects seem veiled; afterwards they become much more distinct and much brighter than before, accompanied with an ecstatic mood.

In the commencement the dilatation of the pupils is easier, and their contraction more difficult.

Ears—

An almost painless drawing behind the ear from below upwards, and extending into the head, almost continuous.

| Tearing pains in the cartilages of the outer and inner ear, extending very nearly as far as the inner cavities.

| Roaring in the ears, which he felt more in the upper part of the head.

| Noise in the ears, like the motion of a wing.

| Sensation as of the whizzing of the wind in the ears, early in the morning; he feels it as far as the forehead.

| Inflammation of the outer ear, the grooves of that portion of the ear assuming the appearance of sore rhagades.

| Occasional stitches and ringing in the ear.

Painful jerk in the ear as if its parts would be pressed asunder: a sort of otalgia.

Sensation as if a cold wind were blowing upon the ears.

Sensation as of warm breathing upon the outer ear.

Two painful vesicles on the right side of the neck below the ear.

Jaes and Teeth—

Pain of the submaxillary gland, as if swollen.

The skin under the chin is painful, as if sore.

Toothache, aggravated by warm drink.

| Tearing jerking in the upper jaw towards the eye, in the evening.

Dull pain with intensely painful stitches in hollow teeth.

Mouth—

Single stitches in the left margin of the tongue.

Sensation of swelling in the tongue, and heat in the organs of speech.

Throat—

Sore feeling in the throat during and between the acts of deglutition.

Putrid smell from the throat, early in the morning (the mouth being clean), not perceptible to himself.

| Burning in the pharynx, a sort of strangulation from below upwards, with a feeling of heat.

Heat in the organs of speech, with difficulty of speech; sensation as if the tongue were swollen.

Accumulation of a quantity of watery saliva from the mouth, flowing out of the mouth when stooping.

Appetite and Taste—

Slight appetite, without loathing or abnormal taste, the general health being good.

Indifference to eating, drinking or smoking; he relishes the food, but he has no desire for it, and is satiated before beginning to eat.

| Indifference to milk, bordering on aversion, early in the morning.

Food and coffee taste bitter to him.

Food has no bad, but too little taste.

Metallic taste, partly sweetish, partly sourish, now in the upper, then in the lower part of the tongue, with a feeling of coldness, as from saltpetre.

He loses his taste while eating warm food; the taste returns after eating.

White wine has an acrid taste to him; after taking a swallow he feels a violent aversion to it.

Canine hunger, in the midst of his feverish chilliness.

Canine hunger, noon and evening.

Want of hunger, immediately.

Nausea and Vomiting—

Inclination to vomit, early in the morning after waking.

Inclination to vomit, shortly after dinneright

Fits of nausea when stooping forward, apparently in the stomach.

Eructations of mere air.

Emission of flatulence after dinner.

Stomach—

Pain in the stomach, as when one presses upon a bruised spot; after eating, this pain gradually passes into the intestines.

A kind of violent aching pain in the pit of the stomach, occasioned by a continued exertion of the mind.

Abdomen—

A kind of griping, directly over the umbilicus.

| Loud rumbling in the abdomen.

Flatulent colic, early in the morning when in bed.

Pinching in the abdomen, brought on by a draft of air.

The flatulence is pressed upwards, below the short ribs; flatulent colic in the hypochondria, in the evening.

Colic after supper: sharp pressure here and there throughout the bowels; during motion the colic becomes intolerable, and passes off suddenly while at rest without emission of flatulence.

| Flatulent colic at night: portions of flatulence seem to

spring from one place to another, which is painful, and causes a disagreeable grumbling sensation, or a sore pinching pressure from within outward in many places, depriving him of sleep; short flatus goes off now and then with pain, but affords no relief.

Flatulent colic early in the morning after rising; the flatulence is pressed toward the diaphragm, causing intensely painful dull stitches.

| Drawing pain in the right side of the abdomen, scarcely permitting him to walk.

| Tearing colic occasioned by (reading?) and walking, and appeased by sitting, especially in the epigastrium (early in the morning).

| Distended abdomen in the evening immediately before going to bed, with colicky pains.

Feeling of repletion in the abdomen, while affected with shortness of breathing.

|| Emission of a quantity of flatulence.

A few stitches in the left side of the abdomen.

Continuous stitch in the abdomen, toward the cecum, not going off till one turns to the opposite side.

Sensation as if the left abdominal ring were enlarged, and as if hernia protruded; every turn of the cough causes a painful dilation of the ring.

Stool—

Frequent desire for stool, causing nausea; but she is unable to accomplish anything.

Sudden desire for stool, which nevertheless is expelled with difficulty.

Cutting in the abdomen, with chilliness, followed by diarrhea.

Involuntary discharge of thin stool.

Continual contraction and constriction of the rectum and anus, permitting scarcely the least flatulence to be emitted.

The tough stool is mixed with mucous filaments.

Itching of a hemorrhoidal tumor at the anus.

Itching creeping at the anus, while walking.

A few long stitches in the "region of the right kidney (immediately).

Urinary Organs—

Stitch in the fold near the genital organs.

Ahing pain in the fold near the genital organs.

Relaxation of the sphincter vesicse (immediately).

|| Incontinence of urine.

| Smarting pain in the forepart of the urethra, during the emission of urine, as if the urine were acrid or sour.

Male Sexual Organs—

| Drawing in the spermatic cord, early in the morning when the testicle is hanging down, as if pulled or distended; the testicle is even painful to the touch.

| Jerking in the spermatic cord.

| Slow, fine, painful drawing in the spermatic cord.

Tearing in the spermatic cord.

| Spasmodic drawing up of the testicles, in the night.

Tearing, strangulating jerks in the testicles; they swell.

Fine itching in the scrotum.

Pain in the penis, as if several fleshy fibres were torn or pulled backwards.

| Red spot, like a pimple, on the corona glandis and on the internal surface of the prepuce, without sensation.

| The glans is red and inflamed, with itching and tension.

Blood dropped from the sycotic condyloma.

The temperature of the genital organs increases in the night.

Creeping and tickling of the glans; semen seemed to be emitted without the person being aware of it.

| Nocturnal emission (in a person affected with hemiplegia); it had not taken place for years past. (Note by Hahnemann. —After this emission the paralysis became worse; the sick limb seemed dead to him.)

Emissions two nights in succession, with much talking during sleep.

During the first two days, the genital organs were greatly excited.

Violent excitement of the sexual desire after dinner.

Impotence: embrace with the proper sensations and erection; but at the moment when the semen is about to be emitted, the voluptuous sensation is suddenly arrested, the semen is not emitted, and the penis becomes relaxed.

Females Sexual Organs—

| The menses, which had already lasted the usual time, continue to flow for six days longer, only during motion, not when at rest; every discharge of blood is accompanied with a cutting pain in the abdomen. (Note by Hahnemann---This woman held the south pole, touching at the same time the middle of the bar. The south pole appears to excite hemorrhage, and especially from the uterus, as its primary effect; the north pole seems to act in the contrary manner.)

The menses, which were to appear in a few days, appeared four hours after the south pole had been touched, but the blood was light-coloured and watery.

Heat and burning in the pudendum, with fine stitches.

Respiratory Organs—

Coryza, and cough with expectoration of green mucus, and short breath.

Several turns of fetid cough, at night when asleep, not occasioning a complete waking.

Oppression of breathing, along the lower rib.

Deep inspiration, resembling a kind of sobbing, and accompanied with involuntary deglutition (as is generally the case when sobbing).

| Shortness of breath in the pit of the stomach.

In the evening after getting into bed, he is scarcely able to recover from the shortness of breathing.

Oppression of the chest, as if the breathing were tremulous, and as if the breath which he inspires were cooling (immediately).

Pain in both sides of the sternum, consisting in pressure and drawing, accompanied with an anguish which does not permit him to remain anywhere, as if he had done something wrong.

Chest—

Pressure in the lower region of the lower end of the sternum, with anxiousness and arrest of thought (immediately).

|| Palpitation of the heart.

Sharp stitches in the right chest, arresting the breathing.

Pressure in the left chest, making her feel nauseated.

Aching pain in the chest, afternoon and evening.

Dull pressure in the left chest, during motion and rest.

Itching stinging in both nipples at the same time.

A few sudden stitches in the surface of the scapula.

Below the scapula she feels a fine, not entirely pointed stitch (immediately).

Back—

Heat commencing in the cervical vertebrae and extending through the whole of the spinal column.

Pinching in the muscles of the back.

Gnawing and smarting in the back.

Shuddering from the nape of the neck down the back.

Aching, and at the same time burning pain in the small of the back, during rest and motion.

Dull stitches in the small of the back.

Pain, as if sprained, in the sacro-iliac articulation, afterwards pain as if bruised in that part.

After rising from his seat he feels stiff in the small of the back, hips and knees.

Violent smarting and stinging over the os sacrum and between the lumbar vertebrae, arresting the breathing when stooping.

Upper Extremities—

Intolerable pain, as if bruised, at night when in bed, in

the biceps muscle of the upper arm, upon which he does not rest, especially when lifting the arm upward and backward, going off immediately when turning on the affected side.

| Crawling in the left arm, from above downward, resembling small snakes.

|Sense, as of rumbling and gurgling, down the left arm (immediately).

Rumbling up and down in the veins of both arms, for several hours.

|| Quick, painful jerking, in the arms, from above downward.

Stinging itching in the upper arm (between the joints), in the evening before and after lying down.

Sense of fullness and puffiness in the arm, as if the arteries in the arm were beating.

Painful stiffness in the elbow-joint of the arm which is touched by the magnet.

Feeling of coldness in the left arm, as if ice were lying upon it, the arm had its natural temperature.

Drawing-paralytic pain, early in the morning; first in the left arm when lifting it, then in the small of the back when bending forward, afterwards in the left hip, and in the muscles of the left thigh and leg when stretching the knee.

Great languor in the right arm in the evening.

Sense of heaviness in the forearm, or as if one had worked too much.

Pain in the arms, as if the blood in the arms had been arrested; now in one, then in another place.

Stiffness of the elbow-joints (immediately).

The left arm is much heavier than the right, accompanied with creeping in the tips of the fingers.

Sensation in the arm as if it had been asleep.

Sensation as if the hand had gone to sleep, with swelling of the veins and quicker pulse (immediately).

Sensation as of a cold breath touching the hands.

Sensation of coldness in the hands, which, nevertheless, felt warm to others.

Painful drawing in the fingers and finger-joints.

| Jerking in the fingers which are touched by the magnet.

Pain of the lower joint of the thumb, as if sprained.

Jerk in the right index-finger, occasioning a visible twitching.

The tip of the finger which touched the magnet, became numb and insensible.

Creeping in the tips of fingers.

| Sense of heat and jerking in the finger touching the magnet.

Beating in the finger in contact with the magnet.

Beating in the tip of the thumb (immediately).

Ulcerative, beating stinging pain in the root of the nails.

Lower Extremities—

Paralytic and bruised pain in the hip-joints, when lying on the affected side.

The thigh and leg go to sleep easily in the morning, when sitting, not soon going off when rising.

| Drawing, with pressure, in the muscles of the thighs, worse during motion.

Paralytic drawing in the evening, from the middle of the thighs down to the feet.

Stinging itching in the thigh, in the evening, also when in bed.

Stinging jerking in the muscles of the thigh next the perineum.

| Sense of coldness in the right thigh.

Drawing pain in the outer side of the bend of the knee.

Dull, bruised pain in the tendons of the bend of knee; beating and jerking, the limbs being convulsively contracted; most violent during motion.

Violent drawing jerking in the hamstrings, accompanied with a bruised pain; the legs were evidently contracted by the pain, especially during motion.

When walking she felt a sticking in the knee.

| Tearing with pressure in the patella (worse during motion), and aggravated by feeling the part.

The knees gave way in walking.

| Cracking of the knee-joint during motion.

Very painful drawing in the hamstrings, sometimes accompanied with painful jerkings in the calves.

Dull pain in the knee after dinner, aching and tearing, aggravated by touching the part.

Cramp-pain, extending from the left tarsal joint to beyond the knee; stretching did not relieve the pain.

Beating in the muscles of the legs on sitting down after walking.

Drawing or tearing with pressure, in the tibia.

Cramp-like drawing pain in the calves.

Intolerably-painful jerking in the calves, accompanied with painful drawing in the hamstrings.

His legs ache when hanging down while sitting; beating in the legs all over.

| Itching-burning, slow stitch in the side of the calf.

Drawing or tearing with pressure, in both tarsal joints and ankles.

Sticking below the ankles, followed by drawing in the hamstrings and painful jerkings in the calves.

The tarsal joint is liable to become strained on making a wrong step.

Pain as if sprained in the tarsal joint, when making a wrong step.

Cramp of the sole of the foot, when bending the foot backwards.

Stitches in the soles of the feet, especially during motion.

Stinging in the dorsa of the toes, and in the sides of the feet (in the evening), as if they had been frozen.

| | | Soreness of the inner side of the nail of the big toe in the flesh, as if the nail had grown into the flesh on one side; very painful, even when slightly touched.

| | Pinching occasioned by the shoes on top and on the sides of the toes, and near the nail of the big toe when walking, as from corns.

Drawing from before backwards, in the middle three toes, only when walking (in the open air).

Miss ———, Nov. 8th, 1878. For three weeks, *aching* in middle front of left *lozver* leg (where she had varicose veins for eight months), when standing, or *when leg is hanging down,* removed by placing it horizontally; frequent feeling of hot water running down'affected part, but only *when leg is down,* at times throbbing there, *when leg hangs down. Magnetis Australis,* c. m., one dose.

1879, June llth. Reports that the hot water feeling never returned, and the pain quite ceased in two days.—*Berridge.*

Mr. C. suffered two years from an inverted toe-nail; had tried three of the best physicians and an endless variety of remedies without any relief. About a year ago he submitted to the painful operation of having his nail pulled out by the root, but in three months it grew in and troubled him more than before. He took *Magnetis Australis* 1m, and in about five weeks was entirely cured.—*Swan.*

Mrs. D., nervo-sanguine temperament, has suffered for five years from an ingrowing toe-nail, outer side of left great toe. During most of this time she has not been able to wear a shoe on this foot—and never without greatly increasing the pain— or even bear the weight of the body on it. Any misstep would be followed by a discharge of blood and pus. The outer side of toe was very much inflamed and swollen, so that nearly half the nail was hidden. No treatment, even cutting out half the nail, gave more than temporary relief. One drop of *Magnetis*

Australis 1m was given. Relief soon followed. The toe looked better, was less sensitive to pressure, and she could wear her boot without causing much pain. The swelling had nearly disappeared at the root of the nail, giving the appearance of a piece having been cut out. Gave three doses of the same remedy, one every night, and in a few days the toe was perfectly well.—*Ballard.*

Mrs. C. S., aged 31, blonde, complains of a pain in left lower jaw as if out of joint; worse in morning and on moving it, sensation as if the head of the bone were squeezed and crowded into the socket. *Magnetis Arcticus* 1m, three doses, one every night, removed all the symptoms.—*Conaut.*

A young married lady rapidly gained flesh and weight after her confinement; this, with the unnatural pressure on the ball of the foot, induced by high-heeled shoes, caused the flesh on inner side of left great toe to grow over the corner of nail. Through neglect and injudicious local medication, ulceration and large unhealthy granulations followed. The attendant pain was so great as to prevent the use of the foot. *Magnetis Australis* 1m every night for a week. In ten days the toe was well, and has remained so.—*Ostrom.*

Sleep—

Frequent yawning (with chilliness).

| Sleepless and wakeful before midnight, and no disposition to go to sleep.

Great desire to sleep at day-break, without feeling able to sleep.

| Restless, frequently turns from side to side, in the night when in bed.

Frequent loud talking during sleep, with a number of confused dreams.

He starts in a dream; this wakes him.

|| Dreams about fires.

He dreams that a horse is biting him in the upper arm, and is giving him a kick on the chest; on waking he felt a pain on the outer side of the chest.

| He quarrels and fights in a dream.

He dreams about the same subject for a long time uninterruptedly, exerting his mind.

Vexed dreams.

Slow, whizzing expiration during sleep, before midnight.

Slow, loud whizzing inspirations after midnight.

Quick shaking of the arms and hands during the siesta.

Unusual beating in the region of the heart.

Fever—

Disagreeable feeling in the periosteum of the long bones as is felt at the commencement of an attack of fever and ague.

Seems to predispose one for colds.

Short shuddering in the afternoon.

In the afternoon he is frequently attacked with a short shuddering all over; when walking in the open air, her sight was obscured, and when standing still, she had a shaking and tossing of the muscles of the limbs, being unable to hold them still, for several minutes, without feeling chilly; on sitting down he was attacked with heat in the head and face.

| Chills in the room the whole day, especially after an evening nap.

| Chilliness of the legs up to the knee, with ascension of heat and blood to the head.

Shaking chilliness, with feeling of coldness, for two hours, without being either thirsty or cold; followed by great warmth, even while walking in the open air, with thirst, and sweat on the forehead and chest, especially in the pit of the stomach (immediately).

Feeling of coldness on the left arm, as if ice were lying on it.

Feeling of coldness in the region of the knees (immediately).

Shuddering in the calves when drinking.

Sensation of coldness in both arms and the left side.

A good deal of itching of the back, during chilliness.

Sensation as of a breeze blowing into the ear, during the chilliness.

| Feeling of coldness all over, in the evening (without shuddering), without thirst (except at the commencement of the chilliness), and without being actually cold; at the same time he feels out of humor, everything was disagreeable to him, even the meal; two hours after he was covered with heat and sweat all over, without thirst.

Internal coldness in the affected part.

The left hand seems to him much colder, but has the same temperature as usual, or it is even increased (immediately).

Internal dry warmth, a few hours after the sensation of coldness, during a walk.

Increase of coldness of the thighs, with feeling of coldness to the prover, and heat of the genital organs.

|| During the chilliness, or the feeling of coldness, he was quite warm, but he was obliged to lie down, and to cover himself well; his mouth was very dry; afterwards he was covered with a profuse sweat all over, without feeling hot; on the contrary, he felt a constant shuddering over the perspiring parts, as if they were covered with goose-skin; accompanied with a sensation as of a breeze blowing into the ears.

Wakes in the morning with a violent headache, heat and alternate chilliness, and was unable to leave the bed.

Increase of internal warmth, without thirst.

Heat in the face after a meal.

Warm sensation in the region where the magnet was applied.

Hot hands after midnight, while in bed.

| Warmth all over, especially in the back.

Sweat during sleep, two mornings in succession.

General sweat in the night.

Thirst for two days, without heat.

Great aversion to the open air; even when not cold, it penetrates bone and marrow, accompanied with a weeping mood and ill-humor.

Sensation as if cool water were poured over the head as far as the chest (immediately).

Small, scarcely perceptible pulse.

Uncomfortable, unusual warmth, accompanied with a peevish mood.

Flush of heat from one part of the body to the other, at different times, for instance, from the thigh down to the tibia.

Sensation as if the blood were jumping in the veins, when lying down, in the evening when in bed.

Skin—

| Corrosive itching in the evening, when in bed, on the back and other parts of the body.

| Itching-stinging, tearing, here or there, in the evening, when in bed.

Fine itching, here and there, in the evening, when in bed, and on waking, easily going off by scratching.

Itching here and there (also in the nates), in the evening, when in bed, and soreness after slight scratching.

During slight coldness of the air, his nose, ears, hands and feet feel chilly and benumbed; in a warm room they feel hot, with creeping and itching in the parts (with pricking).

General Symptoms—

Creeping sensation in the left side and the left arm (immediately).

A sort of anxiety in the limbs (immediately).

Pinching in the flesh here and there.

Pinching in many outer parts of the body, in the afternoon.

Pinching and squeezing in various parts of the body in the afternoon.

Pain in the limbs, as is felt when growing too rapidly.

| Darting pains here and there, disappearing again immediately.

Jerking sensation in every part of the body, as when one has been running fast, and feels moreover anxious and fidgety.

Stinging-burning pains here and there, in the body, especially in the tips of the fingers.

Bruised pain in all the limbs, so that he imagined he was lying on stones, on whatsoever side of the body he lay.

Bruised pain in all the joints early in the morning, when inbed, and on rising, even in the articulations of the pelvis, with a feeling of weakness in both abdominal rings, as if hernia would protrude.

| Stiffness of the joints.

| Cracking of the joints during motion.

Speedy increase of mobility of all the muscles, and quickness in all the movements; the mind being calm.

| Lightness of the whole body.

Weakness of the feet, on going up stairs.

When walking in the open air the legs feel bruised, and he is suddenly attacked with sleep.

He becomes faint while taking a walk, and the faintness increased while sitting.

| Laziness and heaviness of the whole body, accompanied with a feeling of anxiety, as if he were threatened with paralysis, and as if he would fall, accompanied with a feeling of heat in the face and the whole body, mingled with shuddering.

He was unable to lie still in any position.

Great rush of blood to the brain, early in the morning, in bed.

MALANDRINUM
(The Grease of Horses)

The crusts vary in form and character, and the appearance differs as much in animals as many skin diseases of the same family do in the human. Dr. W. P. Wesselhoeft reports a case in which: "The crust assumed a conical form; a thick layer of crusts, if allowed to remain without removal, heaped up one-half an inch. They were fragile, moist, yellow, about the consistency of honey-comb. When removed a raw surface remained with deep fissures and thick crusts reformed into their original size in 48 hours. There was evidently no itching, but some soreness after removal of the scabs."

These crusts resemble some forms of eczema and rupia.

From Jenner we have it that the origin of cowpox is infection of the udders of cows by contact with grass, on which a horse infected with grease has trodden; while the other historical origin from a similar source of infection, also from Jenner, is that it was from the unwashed hands of the stable neys who milked the cows after grooming the horses infected with grease. These assertions are to some extent confirmed by the clinical experience of many homeopaths, who have successfully used Malandrinum against infection with smallpox, and for the bad effects of vaccination.

John H. Clarke says: "It has been used on inferential grounds with great success in bad effects of vaccination. I have cured with it cases of unhealthy dry, rough skin remaining for years after vaccination; in small-pox, measles and impetigo."

Burnett cured with it a case of knock-knee in a child who was constantly handling his penis. His indications are: "Lower half of body affected, greasy skin and greasy eruption. Slow pustulation never ending, as one heals another appears."

For the bad effects from vaccination: The late Dright Fellger, of Philadelphia, probably had a more extensive experience in treating variola and the effects of vaccination than any other man of his time. He had given much thought and many years of study to the subject and came to rely almost wholly upon Malandrinum as a prophylactic for variola, and as the therapeutic remedy in acute cases. He used Malandrinum for confluent small-pox with great success. Where the skin has an unnatural colour between the pustules, and small-pox takes on the confluent form, it is always serious and often dangerous. When the eyeball becomes congested and red, it enables the physician to prognose danger.

Dright Boskowitz, of Brooklyn, was the first to introduce and use Malandrinum. He made the first potencies up to the 30th from the crusts of the "grease of the horse." To the observations of Dright Boskowitz in the use of this remedy, both as a prophylactic and therapeutic remedy against small-pox and the bad effects of vaccination, are added those of Drs. Raue, Carleton Smith, Wm. Jefferson Guernsey, Selfridge, Wesselhoeft, Burnett and Clarke. The potencies of Boericke and Tafel were obtained from Dr. Raue; those of Fincke, Swan and Smith, of New York, came direct from Dr. Boskowitz. It is needless to add that these original preparations were hand-made, but we believe all are reliable. The remedy has had an extensive proving by W. P. Wesselhoeft, H. C. Alien, Steere, Holcombe and students of Hering College, in 1900 and 1901 The provings were made with potencies ranging from the 30th and 35th to the 200th. No prover knew what was being taken.

We consider it a deep long acting remedy, to be repeated not oftener than once a fortnight.

Impetigo, ecthyma; fat, greasy looking pustular eruptions

are especially affected by this remedy. A. L. Marcy, H. R. Vol. XIV, p. 530, relates a singular experience with Malandrinum 30. During a small-pox epidemic he vaccinated himself, taking at the same time Malandrinum 30 night and morning. The vaccination did not take. It was twice repeated and still did not take; nor was small-pox contracted. Called to vaccinate four children in a family whose parents had small-pox, he vaccinated all and gave Malandrinum 30 to three of them at the same time; the remaining child was the only one whose vaccination "took." This was so severe that Malandrinum had to be given to modify its intensity, which it did effectually. The other three were re-vaccinated but none "took." Of five children from six to seventeen years of age, only the eldest had been vaccinated, and he had a good scaright All except the eldest were given Malandrinum, and were vaccinated and none of the four "took." The eldest took small-pox. Malandrinum was then given, and in a few days he was convalescent. In another case of small-pox Malandrinum was given, and the disease only lasted a few days, the eruption drying up.

The only previous attempt at proving was made by Straube with the 30th potency, published in the H. R. Vol. XV, p. 145, and the H. W. Vol. XXXV, p. 504. These symptoms are included.

Mind—

Confusion and lassitude of the mental faculties with a dread of any mental exertion and a lack of concentration, an entirely new and unusual experience which continued several weeks after stopping the remedy.

|| Comprehension difficult.

|| Memory weakened and impaired; great difficulty in remembering what was read.

Confused feeling in head with severe pain in left temporal region, finally located in left eye and felt as if a saw was being drawn up and down vertically through globe, < by light and reading.

Sharp darting pain first in left temple then in right. Confusion and lassitude of mental faculties; lack of concentration and a dread of any mental exertion.

Melancholy with general fatigue.

Head External—

Pustular eruption on scalp. Sensation of weariness at junction of atlas with cranium, every morning on rising.

Itching on scalp, especially in the evening.

Excessive oily dandruff (an entirely new experience) the fourth week after pustules dried up.

Prover contracted a digital chancre, from surgical infection in May, 1891; was treated homeopathically. Ever since a tendency to crusty pimples on the scalp, chiefly on vertex; discrete, scattered, entirely free from itching, neither painful nor sore, small at the base but considerably elevated in form of a dry crust. Condition had existed eleven years. Malandrinum 30, three times a day, caused the eruption to disappear entirely for three months, after which it gradually re-appeared.

Impetigo covering head from crown to neck and extending behind ears.

Thick, greenish crusts with pale, reddish scabs, itching < in the evening.

Impetigo, covering back of head, extending over back to buttocks, labia and even into vagina.

Head—

Frontal and occipital headache, backache, weariness and chilliness, lasting one day.

Frontal headache, no appetite, bilious vomiting and weariness.

Dizziness.

Terrible headache and backache.

Splitting headache in the forehead, chilliness, salty taste in mouth.

Frontal headache, backache and weariness.

Temporal headache, dizziness, backache.

Terrible headache, bone pains, vomiting (bilious), chilliness, diarrhea, malaise.

Pain in forehead, left after Malandrinum.

Heaviness in the head.

Pains all over head.

Pain in back of head, no appetite, inability to sleep.

Headache and backache, stiffness of neck, loss of appetite, constipation, and great weakness (following vaccination).

Headache, worse in forehead, with pain in back and abdomen, attended with general debility (following varioloid).

Eruption on forehead, crusty with intense itching.

Eyes—

Red stripes under eyes. Severe pain in left eye as if a saw was drawn up and down vertically through eye ball.

Nose—

Dry rawness in floor of left nares, more marked on left side.

Face—

Skin of face and neck chaps and smarts after shaving; must shave on warm moist days.

Eczema facialis; intense burning, much edema, oozing viscid fluid.

A yellowish honey-comb crust on upper lip.

Ears—

Profuse purulent, greenish yellow discharge, mixed with blood.

Left ear painful on waking.

Mouth—

Tongue, coated yellow; with red streak through middle, cracked and ulcerating down middle; swollen.

Horribly offensive breath.

Canker on left border of tongue, which spreads in all directions; tongue sore, unable to speak.

In one case in which I was using Malandrinum 30 as a

prophylactic of variola, it cured a very stubborn case of aphthae.—*H. S. Taylor.*

Throat—

Sore and swollen < left side. Left tonsil swollen; yellow ulcer with clear cut, well defined edges persistent for several days; rough scraping sensation like a corn husk or a foreign body, which must be removed mechanically; painless swallowing.

January 24 commenced taking Malandrinum 200.

Thursday, Feb. 6th, awakened with first sore throat of my life.

Left tonsil swollen and inflamed.

Left ear ached and gums on left side of mouth inflamed and swollen; marked salivation.

These symptoms continued and severely < until March 5th, when they became so severe that he was compelled to seek antidote (Meright s. cm.).

Throat symptoms and pains in throat begin on left side, and extend to right.

Ulcerative patches, grayish in colour, on tonsils and fauces, with a tickling sensation on swallowing.

Ulcerated sore throat had tendency to extend downward, invading the larynx.

Severe ulcerated sore throat beginning on third day, worse on left side.

Appetite; Throat—

Thirstless; water nauseates.

Entire absence of thirst.

Teeth and Gums—

Teeth covered with viscid mucus; must clean them with cotton several times daily.

Gums swollen, ulcerated, receding from teeth; bleed easily when touched; unable to brush the teeth from sore and bleeding gums.

A dark, brown, tenacious mucus mixed with blood and pus exudes from ulcerated gums.

Sordes on the teeth.

Stomach—

Nausea after eating; vomiting of bilious matter.

Very hungry.

Empty, faint, "all gone" sensation, with faintness and trembling, not > by eating, though desire for food is very marked.

Abdomen—

Pains around umbilicus.

Stool—

|| Diarrhea: yellow, bloody, slimy; very changeable, worse in the morning; acrid, excoriating; child had a dried-up mummyfied appearance; sleepless and has not nursed for 24 hours.

| Dark, thin, cadaverous-smelling stool.

|| Diarrhea: acrid, yellow, offensive, followed by burning in anus and rectum.

|| Dark brown, foul-smelling, almost involuntary diarrhea; pains in abdomen.

|| Dark brown, painless diarrhea.

| Black, foul-smelling diarrhea; weariness, nausea, dizziness.

| Yellow, foul-smelling, almost involuntary diarrhea, and great weariness.

||Black, foul-smelling diarrhea, malaise and weariness.

Bowels inactive, no desire; move after enema, but leave sore bruised sensation in rectum for hours; dreads stool.

Urine—

Great sensitiveness of bladder on walking; bladder irritable, frequent desire to urinate.

Male Sexual Organs—

(Child constantly handles the penis.)

Violent erections the seventh and eighth nights.

Painful erections the seventh and eighth nights.

Painful erections second night with great sensitiveness of bladder.

Females Sexual Organs—

Vagina closed with thick impeti-ginous crusts; yellowish, greenish, brown in colour.

Back—

|| Intense pain across small of back.

|| Pain along back as if beaten.

| Backache was intense in the sacral region; in the dorsal region, under the shoulder blades, chiefly the left side; it was almost unbearable. (Dr. B. from three doses of the 200th.)

Upper Limbs—

Impetiginous crusts on extensor sides of forearms. Rhagades in palms and fingers.

Had a case of varioloid to treat; I took four doses of Malandrinum 30, one dose a day, and had a sharp proving in the form of a severe backache for several days.

Lower Limbs—

Pains especially in left tibia, with petechia-like patches on anterior aspect of left leg from knee to ankle.

Petechia on both thighs < on left.

Knock-knee.

Weak ankles, easily turn on making a false step.

A sore spot in right quadriceps extensor femoris as eruption disappeared, later it changed to muscles of left leg with increased pain and tenderness.

Dull pain in crest of left tibia for several days before sore throat and headache began.

Left foot drenched with sweat; right foot dry. Four days later (after dancing 2½ hours) both feet drenched with perspiration.

Toes felt as if scalded and itched terribly underneath; was compelled to change hose twice a day, and bathed with cold water morning, noon and night, which gave relief.

Intense itching < by rubbing or scratching.

Skin underneath toes cracked and bled.

Profuse foot-sweat with carrion-like odor; toes so sore unable to walk; only > was when feet were bared and elevated.

The itching or sweating would return on covering or letting the feet hang down.

|| Soles of feet bathed in sweat, scald and burn when covered or warm.

Large blisters on soles of both feet—no change of shoes—skin exfoliated on both feet.

| Feet 'go to sleep' upon least provocation, a sensation never before observed.

Cold perspiration on soles of feet; sensation of a draft of air blowing on feet at night, must get up and tuck in the bed clothes which relieves.

|| Deep rhagades, sore and bleeding, on soles of feet > in cold weather and after bathing.

Aching in the limbs for several weeks, much worse when weary (during small-pox epidemic).

Sore in all limbs and joints.

'Run arounds' on all nails of hands and feet.

On Oct. 22, 1901, a man, 56, had three doses of Malandrinum 30, to be taken 24 hours apart.

On Nov. 11 complained of burning, stinging itching of face and scalp < at night. In a few days there was a well developed eczema which continued four or five weeks despite antidotal treatment.

SKIN.—On the 6th day a pustular eruption covering chest and shoulders with hard nodules and intense itching; eruption began to crust with little or no discharge from pustules.

Two ladies had taken the 200th, one dose, daily; on the third day with one and on the fourth day with the other, a slight pustular eruption appeared on the face and chest. The eruptions were similar in character and ran their course in a week.

A few small pustules appeared on the left arm near the

site of infantile vaccination, some days after a dose of Malandrinum 200. — *Geo. H. Clark.*

A sensation of rawness of the skin over chest and shoulders, after bathing, as if the skin had been scraped with burning acid, smarting by covering parts.

A nodular eruption over chest and shoulders, extended down the arm to elbows, with slight vesication, disappeared, leaving thin crusts.

A burning itching sensation beneath the skin in the palm of the hand, appeared upon contact; after the eruption had disappeared, continued for several weeks.

Eczema of face and scalp, with burning, stinging itching.

Impetigo on extensors of forearms.

Small dusky red spots on legs, not disappearing on pressure.

Dry, rough, unhealthy skin remaining for years after vaccination.

Skin rough, dry, harsh.

Palms and soles thick; deep rhagades < in cold weather, < from washing with any kind of soap.

Skin greasy; oily eruption, and'hair excessively oily.

Pustules slow to develop but never ending; as one healed another appeared.

Eruption in hollow of arms and knees, red, scaly with intense itching < when becoming warm.

Sleep—

Restless sleep; dreams of trouble, of quarrels.

Malandrinum 30, while being used as a prophylactic of variola, cured a stubborn case of aphthae, which had resisted many well selected remedies.

Malandrinum 30, one dose daily for four days, produced a severe backache for a week or more.

For the bad effects of vaccination has been used with best results.

Each member, in a family of six, had been vaccinated; three receiving Malandrinum, and their arms were only slightly affected by the vaccination and ran a short course of a few days; the other three, who did not receive Malandrinum, were very ill, arms sore for weeks and required treatment.

Bad effects of vaccination: A lady, with an ulcer as large as a silver dollar and three-fourths of an inch deep, which continued to suppurate and would not heal; but under the curative effect of Malandrinum, recovered promptly.

When used as a prophylactic for variola has proved protective in many cases, and also prevented vaccination from "taking."

Skin symptoms produced in nearly all who took Malandrinum as a prophylactic; itching rash on various parts of body and face, plainly visible under cuticle, with a few scattered eruptions on surface.

Malandrinum was given to nearly 600 persons, many of whom had been exposed by personal contact with various patients, before and after taking the medicine; only one case of so-called varioloid occurred, and this may have been a proving of Malandrinum.

Malandrinum 30 given to many persons during smallpox epidemic as a prophylactic produced in a number of cases marked premonitory symptoms; headache, backache, general soreness, malaise, thickly coated tongue, loss of appetite, and more or less fever.

Blood boils. Malignant pustules. Vaccinal ulcers.

"The crust assumed a conical form; a thick layer of crusts, if allowed to remain without removal, heaped up one-half inch. They were fragile, moist, yellow, about the consistency of honey-comb. When removed a raw surface remained with deep fissures and thick crusts reformed into their original size in 48 hours. There was evidently no itching, but soreness after removal of the scabs."—*Wesselhoeft.*

Malandrinum 30: produced burning, stinging, itching of the face scalp, worse in the night; a few days later a well developed eczema.

Malandrinum 200: produced a number of small pustules on the left arm, near the site of infantile vaccination.

Mr. H——, aged 42, American, youngest of ten children; father died at 45, of pneumonia; a brother died at 20, of pneumonia; mother died in old age. Two sisters complain of rheumatism.

Brunette, black hair, dark blue eyes, healthy and athletic, until 21 years old. Never used tea, coffee, alcoholics or tobacco; lived a chaste life; father and brothers the same.

From birth his skin has been rough, dry, harsh; one brother has the same. Skin of palms and soles thick, cracks in cold weather; deep rhagades, sore at bottom; < dry cold weather; < when using soap or any alkali; skin of face and neck chaps and smarts after shaving. Must choose moist warm days for shaving.

At 21 had malaria, and was given very large doses of Quinine. Never had another chill; but has been constipated ever since, and sciatic rheumatism then set in, < in cold weather, <^ before storms.

Was nearly crippled from it for ten years.

Had sphincter dilated; papillee removed at two different times, but with no permanent benefit.

Bowels inactive, no desire for stool. Move after an enema, but leave a sore bruised feeling in rectum; dread of stool. *Thirstless;* water nauseates.

Was vaccinated Feb. 1901 A slight "take."

Lower half of body affected; greasy skin; greasy eruption. Slow pustulation, never ending, as one healed another appeared. —*Burnett.*

Bad effects of vaccination; has cured cases of unhealthy, dry, rough skin, remaining for years after vaccination in small-pox, measles and impetigo.—*Clarke.*

Eczema facialis; oozing of a viscid fluid; intense burning;-much edema; small scales, exfoliated < from bathing at night; > in cold air.—*Thompson.*

In a family of eight persons, none of whom had been vaccinated, the oldest boy took small-pox. One of his brothers.slept with him and broke out all over; the mother expecting to be confined in a few days, we sent him away, and I at once put the rest of the family on Malandrinum 200, with the result that none of them took small-pox. The boy that slept with his brother had a light fever the twelfth day, but that passed off without any further trouble.—*Bryant.*

A yellowish honey-comb crust on upper lip; would crumble off, leaving moist surface, which would soon reform.

Sharp, stabbing pain through upper lip with occasional burning.

Small pimples on chest and back, with intense itching extending to other parts of body and limbs < by cold air, when undressing.

A large crust of a light yellowish-gray colour on right side of forehead extending to the temple and borders of the hair.

Eruption in the popliteal space and hollow of elbows; scaly, crusty, moisture under the crusts and intense itching.

"Malandrinum in small-pox:" The following symptoms are reported cured with Malandrinum:

Aching in limbs; headache; pains in left side of head with great debility; pains in back, head and abdomen; pain in head and back, fatigue, chilliness and vomiting; stiff neck; constipation; inability to go up stairs from weakness; lazy, weak feeling; terrible itching after an attack of small-pox; foul smelling diarrhea, chilliness, weak, tired feeling; great pain around the navel, sore aching in bones, sleeplessness during an attack of smallpox. Crying and ill temper of children during small-pox; pain in back extending to heels, soreness of abdomen, every bone in body aches. There was no smell from the eruption after Malandrinum was given.—*Straube.*

"Malandrinum has been given to numbers of unvaccinated children who were directly exposed to the contagion of variola, and they have invariably escaped the disease. I have given it to many persons (one dose each), directly after vaccination and been unable to make that or a re-vaccination 'take' with virus which had proven effectual with others who had not had the medicine. One girl who suffered terribly from pain and an enormously swollen and inflamed arm and forearm, following vaccination, I entirely relieved of the pain in a few hours by two doses of Malandrinum, and with an almost complete disappearance of the objective symptoms in twelve hours."—*Guernsey.* As therein stated, one or two doses are given, 24 hours apart, and not repeated until a succeeding epidemic or 'scare'— at all events it is believed to be sufficient for at least a year.

Impetigo covering back of head, extending over whole back to buttocks and even into vagina, covering labia and extensors of forearms.

Boils.

Malignant pustules.

Bad effects of vaccination.

Small dusky red spots on legs, not disappearing on pressure.

Proving—

Miss A. W. C.; a large brunette; unusually well and strong; aged 50, a nurse.

Wednesday, Dec. 6. Took twenty pellets of Malandrinurn, the 35th, at 5:30 P.M.

Thursday evening, Dec. 7. Toothache in right upper eye-tooth beginning about 8 P.M. and lasting for two hours until bed time.

Friday evening, Dec. 8. Peculiar feeling of snuffles in the nose without discharge, with an unusual feeling of apprehension.

Saturday, Dec. 9., 9 A.M. A peculiar dull ache in my left chest near the heart lasting about two hours.

In the afternoon about 2 P. M. a severe dull pain in ball of foot, under big toe; worse when stepping on it. This lasted all the rest of the afternoon.

Sunday, Dec. 10. Felt very well today and with the exception of the above sensations have felt an unusual exhilaration and have had an especially good appetite during the last four days.

No more symptoms until December 19th, when I took ten pellets of the two hundredth in the morning before breakfast.

Had a dull, uncomfortable headache which passed off after sundown.

December 21 Back of head aches from early morning all day, after a sleepless night with a patient.

December 22. Have had unusually vivid dreams and very unpleasant ones.

December 23. Dreams again vivid, but not as unpleasant (I very rarely dream).

Felt very well otherwise except an unusual apprehension about patient, for no reason that I can account for.

December 25. Unusually vivid dreams.

December 26. All night quarrelsome dreams. Woke in the morning with left arm very lame and a peculiar restlessness in the arm, which was exceedingly uncomfortable.

Sudden pains in my right hand which come and go quickly and have continued during the whole afternoon.

Mrs. G. F. S., widow, aged 58. Blonde, well developed, inclined to obesity. Remarkably healthy woman, whose appearance and vivacity would place her at the age of 40.

Dec. 6, 1905. Took fifteen pellets of the 35th potency at 10 P.M.

Before eleven o'clock began to feel a creepy sensation in my skin, particularly in the face, like the crawling of ants over it, accompanied by itching.

It was red, and I had to resist a desire to jerk my fingers and twist my hands; this continued and increased even after I had taken my warm bath.

Went to bed about twelve very sleepy, but could not get to sleep because I could not lie still on account of creepy sensation which spread over my arms, shoulders and upper part of my body, with jerking of the limbs.

I turned from one side to the other, but could not be quiet long enough to get to sleep. Accompanying this was a ringing in my head, as it once had when years ago I had taken quinine, but it was not of long duration.

At half-past one I got up and wrote this. My lower limbs did not seem to be affected by any of these sensations, but I kept scratching my arms and face, head and shoulders, and my hands and fingers felt particularly restless and nervous. Had no internal disturbance other than my head. Finally fell asleep at half-past two and slept soundly until six.

Dec. 7. Awoke with all the symptoms of the night before gone, but had a sharp headache, and a bad taste in my mouth. Byseven o'clock these too were gone, and I arose feeling all right.

While I was out walking I was taken with a severe pain in the back, or, rather, at the left side of the sacrum low down, with stitching pains in rectum. It lasted about an hour.

At two o'clock began to have a bad headache over eyes, and with a sense of fulness in my head.

My feet were somewhat swollen when I put on my boots in the early morning, but by twelve o'clock after walking (not without some pain) the swelling left. By half-past three in the afternoon my headache was entirely gone (it lasted only one and a-half hours), also the sense of fulness in the head. Have felt perfectly well ever since until Friday morning.

Dec. 8. About eleven o'clock when I suddenly had another attack of headache, and I find that I am liable to a return of these attacks, with the sense of fulness, at odd times, apparently without any reason.

Friday had three attacks, but they did not last long; from half an hour to an hour and a-half, not longer, also since Wednesday evening, when I took the pills, until Friday night, Dec. 8th, I have not had any discharge from my bowels.

Dec. 9. When I went to bed last night, after lying down, my head had a sharp pain for perhaps ten minutes. This morning when I woke I had that disagreeable taste in my mouth, but felt all right until about 9 o'clock, when I went out, and I did not have any vitality, and found it hard work to lift my legs. I thought it might come from not taking coffee (which you have asked me not to do during the proving), as I have done for so long a time, so I went and had some rolls and omelet and drank a cup of weak tea, but did not feel any betteright My movements seemed to be uncertain. I was afraid of falling, or tripping. It was difficult work getting in and out of the cars. I had occasion to go up two flights of stairs, very old, narrow and rickety, and was afraid that I should fall on my way down.

I have had all day, not a headache, but a feeling that made me scowl, and keep closing my eyes. I felt as if I must get home as soon as possible.

For two days, several times, I have been troubled by feeling very hot in the face; never cold. Sometimes when the face felt burning hot I would perspire on the face and head.

This morning I had a movement of the bowels, the first since Wednesday, Dec. 6th.

I have been troubled a great deal with rheumatism in my hand, the right one, and thigh and hip, although the pain was not constant, but since taking the pellets on Wednesday last, I have not had any pain of this kind anywhere. I have had a slight eruption on my cheeks and sometimes a place larger than a dollar would be burning red and shining on my right cheek at the side of my nose.

Sunday, Dec. 10. No symptoms today until now, 7 P.M., both cheeks are burning and have the inflamed shiny look. Perhaps it is also another symptom that I have been very irritable all day.

Dec. 11. The rheumatism has returned in right hand and hip. After I have been walking a very short distance, my legs pain me and get so heavy and my back and hips drag so that I have to sit down, and when I sit down, all these feelings go away. Two or three times today my right eyelid has kept twitching.

Tuesday, Dec. 12. Twitching in left eye only. Same trouble in my hips and legs and back, when walking. My stomach and abdomen have been much swollen for two days.

Wednesday, Dec. 13. Nothing more.

Thursday, Dec. 14. Nothing.

Dec. 17. Took two hundredth potency in solution at eleven o'clock P.M. A. tablespoonful of twenty pellets dissolved in four tablespoonfuls of water.

At 12:30 A.M., my skin began to itch and my legs were very fidgety, also all my body was very restless. Arms and shoulders were not affected as before, however, with itching and restlessness. It seemed to be the lower part of my body this time, although my face felt some of the irritation, but in a much less degree.

Monday, Dec. 18, 7:30 A.M. Slept soundly from 12:30 to 7:30 this morning, with all the symptoms of the night before one gon awaking.

At 4 P.M. began to have excruciating pain in my forehead over the left eye, which continued until about midnight. Once it ran down behind my left ear for a short while. It left me as suddenhy as it came. Took the last tablespoonful that night. Slept well without disturbance.

Dec. 19. That day was without pain or other disturbances,

except I felt in a state of collapse nearly all day. Had no strength in my arms or legs, and every little while was obliged to lie down wherever I happened to be. Would almost fall asleep and my breathing was very deep and heavy, like puffing. My body felt heavy, and I had difficulty in lifting my legs and walking. Frequently low sighs would come. This was all much better by 6 P.M.

While taking the medicine this time, I have had no operation of the bowels, and the last day there was more or less of an eruption on my cheeks and at the side of the nose, but not the red shiny look I had when taking the remedy the first time in pills (the 35th).

Each time I took the medicine (the first time in pellets and this time in solution) I had a slight return of the breaking out round my waist which I had when afflicted with shingles years ago. I was not rheumatically affected this time as I seemed to be when I first took the pills. Ever since I began taking the pills, from the first day until now, I have found that when I started out walking, however well I felt, after a short time I gave out all over, and especially in my bowels, thighs and legs, also the toes of my left foot, except the bigtoe, were affected in a way I never before felt, not like cramp or gout; and whereas I am always light on my feet and move quickly and easily, during these days it has been hard for me to get about and I have felt heavy and moved heavily, also a great deal of headache, a thing unusual for me; also often a shortness of breath with an inclination to wheeze.

Dec. 20th, 7 A.M. Woke with a bad headache (the bad taste which I had in my mouth when waking while I was taking the medicine in pellets (35th) I have not had at all this time). Since December 20th I have had no more symptoms.

Mrs. J. F. C., aged 62; a large well developed woman, gray hair, former blonde, born in England, and has lived for twenty years in Munich, Germany.

May 8, 1900. Has always been remarkably well until eight years ago when an eruption appeared on the upper lip, which formed a yellowish, honeycombed crust. Portions would crumble off and leave a moist surface, which again would form a similar crust; occasionally a burning and, at long intervals, sharp stabbing pains through the upper lip.

Had received all kinds of external treatments by German specialists, without effect. Once after cautery, it remained absent for six months. Then Dr. Jochner, of Munich, advised surgical interference, which was not acceded to. On her return to America, further local experiments were tried without success.

I could not elicit any symptoms of a constitutional characteright Neither could I establish any connection with vaccination, or revaccination, as she told me she had never been revaccinated since childhood, which is a remarkable record for a life in Germany of twenty years.

The appearance was so unsightly that she had excluded herself largely from contact with society and was consequently mentally much depressed and anxious. From May 8th until February, 1901, she received at long intervals of at least three weeks single doses of Sulphur, Arsenic and Kali carb. The latter remedy was given June 20th, 1900, and some improvement was noticed until February, 1901, during which time she was under placebo, when she reappeared with the condition as bad as ever.

The character of the eruption reminding me so strongly in appearance of the 'scratches' of horses, led me to give her one dose of Malandrinum 24m., on February 5th, 1901.

April 1st. There was on the whole a decided change in the diameter and elevation of the crust, but still there existed the sticky moisture under it. Repeated Malandrinum 24m., and placebo, with slight improvement. On April 27 she received Malandrinum cm., with gradual improvement during May and June.

July 15. The crust had decreased one-half, but still mois, ture underneath it, Malandrinum cm.

October 26th. She reappeared with an entirely clear lip- which has remained so to this date, Dec. 11, 1906.

Miss M. N. H., aged 19, medium brunette. Student.

Dec. 27, 1904. Eruptions first appeared three years ago on chest and back.Small pimples with intense itching, extending to other parts of the body and limbs; < when exposed to air and on undressing.

For the last two months a different form of eruption has appeared on face, a very unsightly crust of a light yellowish gray colour, on right side of forehead extending to the temple and under the hair on that side. Has used external medicinal applications more or less for the last three years without benefit. There is some irritation and itching of the eruption on the forehead, but less intense than that on the body.

Complains of faint, gone sensations in stomach without real hungeright This is especially evident since the previous July, and is not > by eating. All functions normal.

Was vaccinated repeatedly before her twelfth yearight In that year the vaccination 'took' followed by a tedious suppuration at the point of vaccination.

Sulphur cm. in water to be taken during forty-eight hours, a tablespoonful morning and evening.

Jan. 21, 1905. Has more eruption and more intense itching. No faintness. Appetite rather abnormal, craves hearty food.

Psorinum cm. in water, morning and evening for two days.

Feb. 18. Itching continues intense. Eruption has appeared in popliteal space and hollow of elbows. Thinks there is less moisture after scratching. Placebo.

March 15. No improvement whateveright All symptoms remain the same, except the faintness at the stomach disappeared. Malandrinum 24m., one dose dry.

April 15. Eruption on forehead appears to be less thick, but itching remains intense. Malandrinum 24m., one dose dry.

May 13. Decidedly less itching; less moisture, both on face and body. Chief discomfort on forehead. Crust less thick. Malandrinum 24m., one dose dry.

June 12. Decidedly better. Placebo.

July 10. Most marked improvement. Forehead entirely free from the crust, and all eruption. Skin normal, where the large crust was located. Eruption on body also much improved; no itching. Hollows of elbows and knees clear of eruption.

Dec. 9. Has been free from eruption all summeright Since the cold weather slight reappearance on forehead and neck, but no crust. Small pimples with some itching. Says her hair is falling out. Malandrinum 24m., one dose dry.

March 10. No eruption anywhere. Skin of body normal. No itching. No falling of hair.

In November, 1906, received letter from a relative, who reports her as perfectly well, and the happiest girl in her town.

Miss G. W., aged 40, light blonde, full habit, very healthy.

Dec. 6th. Ten pellets, 38th potency, at 12 M. Wednesday.

While sitting at lunch at 2 o'clock momentary light-headedness lasting perhaps two minutes.

Friday, 8th. Woke at 4 A.M., attack of sinking weakness; rose and walked about the room a few minutes; was chilly for half an hour after returning to bed.

Monday, llth. All day nausea, > after eating, uncertain, shaky feeling in stomach.

Tuesday, 12th." Same nausea continued <afternoon, with *dull headache in forehead.*

After dinner at 7 o'clock nausea with eructations tasting of food.

Wednesday, 13th. Slept from 11 till 4 A.M., then an attack of eructation of gas tasting of food; no nausea to-day; took cup of coffee this morning, which relieved nausea.

Feels week and exhausted all over.

Has felt so ill that she declines to take more of the medicine, and begged me, with tears in her eyes, not to give her any more, as she knew she would have "nervous exhaustion," which she had during a whole year, four years ago.

Sleep—

Restless sleep; dreams of trouble, of quarrels.

DAY BOOKS OF PROVING.

By W. P. Wesselhoeft, M. D.

Miss E. M. B., a strong brunette inclined to obesity, age 50, no menses for 18 months.

Dec. 6th. Took ten pellets at 1 P.M., 35th potency.

Wednesday night, Dec. 6th. Did not sleep well, woke frequently, mind unpleasantly active, darting from one idea to another.

Thursday, 7th, A.M. Feeling of fulness in head, ache in back of neck (joint at top of spine, running down into arms and up behind ears).

Friday evening, 8th. Slight soreness and swelled feeling around palate and between nose and throat.

Saturday, 9th. Little blisters *with crust* at left angle of lips; larger one on lower lip came two days before.

Saturday night wakeful.

Sunday, 10th, A.M. Soreness and rawness between throat and nose continue, more prominent on left side.

Seven P.M. Shifting pains in lower abdomen. Sudden urgent movement of bowels gives relief (twice during the evening), fulness and heaviness in lower abdomen with dull ache, but not very marked.

Monday, 11th, A.M. Mouth dry on waking, very thirsty all day. Sensation of large tongue, dryness succeeds soreness between nose and throat (left).

7 P.M. Return of sensations in abdomen described yesterday.

Tuesday, 12th. Dry mouth in morning. Thirst and large tongue continue.

Wednesday, 13th. Dry mouth, large tongue continue. Feeling of soreness and lameness under jaw and chin when mouth is opened very wide. Soreness under jaw (almost half way back from point of chin) felt when pressed deeply on outside, both sides.

Dec. 18, 1905, 8 A.M. Took first dose of remedy in wateright 10 P.M., took second dose.

Dec. 19th, 9 A.M. Third dose. Four or five small red pimples on left forearm. No itching about them.

10 P.M. Fourth dose. *Itching* on back, neck and shoulders, more marked on left side. Very troublesome for more than an hour on undressing, and after going to bed.

Dec. 20th, 10 A.M. More than an hour after breakfast. Intense discomfort in head, hard to describe.

Feeling of lightness, yet of pressure on top of head; sensations confined to region above ears.

Sensation of motion in the eyes. Vision not clear or steady.

Quick pulse, conscious of its beat in ears and neck; quick, short breathing.

Feeling of weakness in hands and wrists.

Tingling sensation in arms and hands.

Throbbing in top of head; hissing sound in ears, with rhythm of pulse.

Exhausted feeling was present all day.

Dec. 21st, 11 A.M. Return of yesterday's symptoms, not quite so severe.

10 P.M. Great discomfort on lying down in bed, from heart beating very quickly with occasional skipping of a beat; hissing in ears, weak feeling in arms.

More comfortable with head propped high.

Heartbeat quickened by slightest movement.

Foregoing symptoms continued for an hour or more.

Waked suddenly at 12 (by noise); first sensation a quivering or vibration inside of or back of eyes.

Sensation of *great heaviness of body,* bed seemed insufficient support.

Dec. 22d. Did not sleep after 4 A.M.

11 A.M. *Slight* return of symptoms of previous days at same hour.

Depressed, worried, anxious.

Slept somewhat better.

Dec. 23. Depression continued through forenoon, began to wear off towards evening.

Dec. 28, 10-11 A.M. *Itching* or *prickling* on back, arms and legs; less marked elsewhere on body; relieved by warmth rather than by scratching.

This has recurred at irregular intervals of one to four days up to to-day (Jan. 10).

Dec. 31st. Feeling of swelling and soreness in throat or between nose and throat, back of palate; pain running up into ears, left side. Thirst.

Chilly feeling on changing clothes at night (the same on dressing next morning); *headache.*

Jan. 1st. Symptoms return at evening with sneezing, dryness in throat, left side.

Jan. 2. Some mucus cleaned from nose and throat afforded relief, and the trouble gradually disappeared, though the dryness of nose and throat on left side continues (Jan. 10).

MALARIA OFF

We are indebted to the late G. W. Bowen, Fort Wayne, Ind., for this valuable remedy.

Hahnemann had an extensive experience in Malarial Fevers in the valleys of the Danube, and the fevers of the Pontine marshes on the Tiber are historical.

Dr. Bowen lived on the Wabash River at that time, a noted malarial region, and for many years he was called upon to treat hundreds of patients suffering from all forms of malarial affections.

Malarial affections have been attributed to marsh, exhalations in summer and autumn when the water has been evaporated by heat. These poison vapors of decaying vegetation Dr. Bowen had to contend with, Malarial fevers and their resultant diseases, intermittent, remittent, continued, typhoid, etc., for years, not only in their acute, but in their suppressed forms, in which he found all forms of chronic diseases, very frequently, could be traced to maltreatment of the acute manifestation. He conceived the practicability of testing the effects of artificial toxin prepared from peat, or decayed vegetable matter, taken from a marsh during the dry season, when the malaria toxin was most active. This vegetable matter was placed in glass jars, filled with water and allowed to decompose, which were numbered I, II, and III, according to the time, one, two or three weeks' of decomposition.

At the end of each period, or stage, provings were made by inhaling the gases given off, just as the patient would naturally inhale the marsh miasm. Provers were paid so much per day to inhale the gas in its different stages of decomposition, and a careful record of its effects was made. This constituted the provings of the crude gases.

For medicinal purposes a tincture was prepared by putting ten drops of No. II, in which the matter had been decomposed for two weeks, into 90 drops of alcohol; this formed the 1st dec. potency, and all Bowen's reported cures were treated with this.

Boericke and Tafel made a 30th from this tincture, which Yingling inhaled, and resulted in his involuntary proving. Later Boericke & Tafel made a 30th potency of No. III, which was run up into the higher potencies by Gorton, and used by Yingling in his clinical experiences.

The paid provers of No. II, which was not very offensive, obtained the following uniform results in from one to three hours after inhalation: "Headache, nausea, distressed stomach, white-coated tongue." These symptoms passed off in two or three days.

Provers of No. II obtained results in from twelve to twenty-four hours, which were much more severe and long lasting. They were: "Fearful headache, nausea, vomiting in some cases, aversion to food, distress in stomach, hypochondria, first in the spleen, then the liver and stomach, and on the third day pronounced chills, which were so severe that they had to be antidoted."

No. III, which was "fetid to a fearful degree," produced little result except nausea within three or four days, but then symptoms began to appear; first, extreme lassitude, chills and fever, pains and aches, impeding locomotion.

When taken internally the results were much more severe:

No. I caused bilious colic, nausea, cramps, headache.

No. II, the stomach, liver, spleen and kidneys became in volved, with quartan or tertian intermittent fevers.

No. III setting up a more profound type even, a genuinetyphoid or semi-paralytic state, which compelled the provers to take to bed.

On the day I received from Boericke and Tafel Malaria off. 30 I was foolishly led to try Hahnemann's inhalation. The thought just occurred to me on the spur of the moment, and without stopping to think I took three strong inhalations, with both sorrow and a proving resulting. None of the symptoms were distressing, yet marked and clear cut. The remedy commenced its work promptly and in the order following:

Aching in both elbows.

A kind of slight concentration of feeling in root of nose, and just above, as though I have a severe cold, similar to that complained of by hay-fever patients.

Aching in wrists.

A tired ache in hands.

A tired ache in knees, and for a distance above and below.

A feeling as though I should become dizzy.

Pain in top of left instep.

A tired feeling in wrists.

Aching in an old (cured) bunion on left foot.

sensation on point of tongue as though a few specks of spice or pepper were there.

Itching on right cheek over malar bone; > by slight rubbing or scratching.

When leaning face on left hand, elbow on the table, perceptible feeling of the heart beats through upper, body and neck.

Slight itching on various parts of the face and extremities; > by slight rubbing.

Sense of heat in abdomen.

Chilly sensation in left forearm. Soon followed by chilly feeling in hands and fingers; feet are cold with sensation as if chilliness was about to creep up the legs. A few moments later knees feel cold. A sense of coldness ascending over body from the legs.

Arms feel tired.

Belching several times, easy; no taste.

A drawing pain in right external ear.

Lumbar back feels tired as though it would ache.

Neck feels tired, with slight cracking in upper part on moving the head.

Shallow breathing which seems from languor, with a desire to take a deep inspiration occasionally.

A kind of tired feeling through abdomen and chest.

A general sense of weariness.

A feeling about head as though I would become dizzy.

Pain in upper left teeth.

A sensation as though I would have a very loose stool (passed away without stool).

Feeling rather stupid and sleepy.

A sensation in the spleen as though it would ache.

Saliva more profuse than usual; keeps me swallowing often.

Pain in abdomen to right of navel.

Dull aching through forehead.

Face feels warm, as if flushed, also head; becomes general over body, as if feverish.

Aching across upper sacral region.

Legs very weary from short walk.

Pain at upper part of right ilium.

General sense of weariness from a very short walk, especially through pelvis, sacral region and upper thighs: I feel strongly inclined to lie down and rest.

Qualmishness of stomach, as though I should become nauseated.

General sense of malaise and weariness becoming quite marked.

Aching above inner angle of right eye.

A kind of simmering all through the body.

Felt impelled to lie down, and on falling to sleep a sense of waving dizziness passes all over me, preventing sleep.

At times I feel as though I should become cold or have a chill, then I feel as though I should become feverish or hot, though neither is very marked.

Eyes feel heavy and sleepy.

Uneasiness in lower abdomen.

Gaping, yawning and desire to stretch.

Legs are restless; feel like stretching and moving them.

I feel very much as I did one time before having the ague, twenty-five years ago.

Odor from cooking is pleasing, but I have no desire for dinneright Yet when I sit down I eat a good dinner with relish.

Dizziness on rising from a reclining position.

Feel generally better after eating dinner.

Aching in occiput.

During the afternoon leg weary.

Unusual hearty appetite for supper (the good appetite keeps with me for some days).

A good night's rest following, and have felt much brighter and generally better ever since the first day. (Healing.)

"I know several localities in South America, Africa and Spain where the marsh miasma has unquestionably arrested and cured that fatal scourge of the human race, phthisis pulmonalis, without any other treatment or restriction in food or drink. And why should not the climate of the fen lands of Lincolnshire, in the neighbourhood of Spalding, prove as curative an agent for this disease as the climate of so many foreign regions where patients go and die, deprived of all the comforts of home? Penzance, among the British localities, is reported to be superior to nine-tenths of the places to which patients are sent. Penzance, then, and Spalding should be particularly studied by medical men and recommended to consumptive individuals who wish to enjoy the benefits and advantages of a national place of relief, if not of cure."

C. F., aet. 28, a. Kansas volunteer, after a week or ten days of rainy and chilling weather in camp, came home sick. Had a chill, followed by feveright Aching all over body; nausea continuous, vomiting bile and retching. Wants cold drinks. Can't eat anything; vomits everything, except once he could eat raw tomatoes. Craves sour. Tongue white and thickly coated. Lips parched dry. Urine highly coloured, like strong tea. Retching and gagging from hawking mucus. Ipecac cm.

Nausea some betteright Vomited twice since yesterday. Thirsty, would like much cold water, but is fearful to drink, yet it does not sicken. Slight dizziness, especially on rising up or on raising head. No appetite; aversion to food, thoughts of it sicken. Costive. Feels very weak and languid. Mouth very dry; saliva pasty. Skin dry all over; no sweat at all. Bry., 9m.

No nausea; sight of food does not nauseate now, but the thought of his army life gags him. Mouth very dry, subjectively, but really moist. Thirsty, but desires less quantity.

Very weak and tottering. Great uneasiness through abdomen, a sense of heaviness. Has eaten nothing, but drinks some cherry juice. Throat dry and sense of slight drawing. Face, eyes and skin very yellow. Constipation; vomited bile; skin very dry. Aside from nausea seems betteright Malaria off., 1m.

Feeling better generally. No nausea. Has eaten twice for the first time. Bowels sluggish; no sweat; skin dry and yellow; feels weak; mouth less dry. Sac. lac.

Much betteright Less thirst. Has eaten with relish. Mouth less dry. Slept all night. No sweat, but skin some better in colouright Sac. lac.

Generally improving. Had a good dinner yesterday and breakfast this morning with much relish. Feels like getting up. No nausea. Less yellow.

Doing well. Weak and totters yet. Appetite improved; eats

with relish. Tongue cleaneright Bowels moved normally. Mouth dry, at times with plenty of saliva. Skin yellow and dry; no sweat. Malaria off. 1m.

Doing finely. Walked a mile to the office. Yellowness of eyes and skin fading. Rapid restoration to better than usual health.

R. A., aet. 22, another soldier boy, with similar symptoms to the above, was promptly cured by Malaria off.; no other remedy given.

Mrs. S. A. H., aet. 63, sick for some days. Shooting pains all over in the muscles; bones ache. High fever during the night. Restless tossing about. Thirsty for lemonade; not so much for wateright Diarrhea; five or six stools this morning; no pain; weakness in bowels; tenderness in right iliac region; stools watery, thin, yellowish, somewhat foul. Bitter taste; mouth parched; tongue white. Ravenous appetite for some days past; none now. Dizziness on rising. Head feels badly, as though it would ache. Pulse 98. Skin hot and dry. Restlessness most marked in the arms, tossing them about. Very stretchy and gaping. Malaria off., 1m. Relieved and up and about next day.

M. H., aet. 16. 'Dumb ague' a year ago. Last four days has been very tired and languid. Backache in lumbar region, shoots up the back; worse when first lying down, then gets better; worse after walking; better lying on the abdomen. Bowels loose yesterday, but no stool to-day. Aching through forehead and temples. Feels well on rising in the morning, < after being about for awhile; < towards evening. Last fall had slight chills and fever; no sweat. Yawning. 'Malarious feeling.' Poor appetite. Thirsty all the time. Malaria off., 6m. Improvement at once, and in a few days said she felt no further need of medicine.

M. H., aet. 12, sister of above. Peevish for a few days. Last night had severe frontal headache. Restless, tossing all night. Pain in chest and upper abdomen; worse breathing; may be from indigestion. Fever during the night and also this morning. Pulse 112, soft and yielding. Tongue white, with brown streak down the middle. Malaria off., 6m. Prompt cure.

M. B., aet. 13, each evening, about dark, getting earlier

each day, he will be chilly with flushes of heat, great desire for fresh air and cannot breathe on account of pain in the liver; worse lying down, must jump up; better from hard pressure on region of liver; during the day has no trouble and no tenderness. Seems entirely well, except that he is getting weakeright Slight fever for a couple of hours in the evening; raves, sings and talks all night; restless. Appetite variable; craves potatoes, apples and beefsteak. Tongue about clean. Malaria off., 1m. The next morning ate breakfast with the family, the first time in several weeks; much better in every way, and had no trouble with the liver the next evening following the remedy. Cure rapid and remains.

G. C., aet. 28, ague every other day, icy cold from hips down, chilly all over; < about the trunk, and general sweat, but slight. Begins about noon. Used to have ague often and long at a time when living in Missouri, and had it very hard on the Pacific coast, and is now run down. Feels languid, weak and drowsy between attacks; unable to be up. Pulse weak. Very poor appetite. Foul breath. Flashes of heat all the time. Very thirsty. Has taken much quinine. Dizzy when up, with nausea. Has taken salts for constipation. Stool hard, bleeding after stool, at times. Intense headache, as though it would burst. Malaria-off., 1m.

No chill next day, except the soles of feet felt cold, almost numb. No fever, except very slight on back for a few moments. Sweat over body. Dizzy when up, with some nausea.

"Feels wonderfully better; did not think one could feel so much better so soon." Head is heavy and aches some. Thinks it is from the quinine he took. Bowels have moved twice, thin, watery, foul odoright Urine smells very strong and is very red some days. Short, hacking cough for some days; better today; not so languid and weak. Is sitting up, which he could not do before. Missed two or three chill days, and made general improvement, so as to be able to go home, hence went from under my supervision.

F. B., aet. 80, very active. Three times, one week apart,

has had 'dumb ague,' feeling bad all over, head feels thick and mean, bones ache some, no chill but profuse sweating. Sweats very easily and profusely on least exertion. Right knee weak and painful, worse when bending down to work and raising up; must help himself up. Dizzy when getting up in the morning and on rising up. "Thirst like a horse." Sleepy, falls asleep reading. Has had chills and fever several times. Malaria off., 6m. Prompt relief.

Three months after he came for help. "Feels bilious," as though he was "going to pieces," Feels tired, uncomfortable. No pain, but very languid; don't want to move, listless. "Feels malarious." No chill, no fever. *Dizzy* when getting up, must steady himself before starting to walk. Sleepy and drowsy when reading or sitting quietly. Malaria off., 6m. Prompt relief and no return in eight months.

L. H., aet. 50, for three weeks has had pain in the right side of back, about the floating ribs (posterior aspect of liver), hurting through the right side; aching, worse sitting, lying a long time, possibly in the evening; better from walking a little. Had something similar four years ago, and was sick for a long time. Feels weak and languid. Good appetite; eats a good deal without inconvenience. No trouble with the urine or bladder. Constipation. Drawing or puckering feeling in the region of the liver, a kind of cramping. Tongue coated slightly yellowish-white. Had malaria and ague badly years ago; took lots of quinine. Had "dumb ague" badly; took ironwood tea. Has used much Mercury and physic. Malaria off., 6m. Reports himself a great deal better, "The drawing feeling let go within three hours and has not returned." Pain in posterior aspect of liver much better.

Could hardly walk to office before, but now "feels as if he could walk all over town." A month later, after hard work and picking up potatoes, he felt some trouble in the liver, which was relieved by the same remedy.

Mrs. H. H., aet. 36, is feeling 'malarious,' feels depressed and languid. Is sleepy all the time; can go to sleep standing.

Had a 'dumb chill' eight days ago, and again in one week. Occasionally has a sudden cold spell at night. Back seems as though it would break; pain goes into the hips. Limbs get numb and cold. Frequent spells of headache, forepart of head. Malaria off., 6m. Soon feeling much better and over the trouble.

Mrs. J. E. G., aet. 25, for four days, about 11:30 A.M., she has great aching all over, commencing in small of back; then hot fever, short of breath; headache all the time, day and night; each day the trouble gets later. During the morning feels weak, head whirls, sense as if the head made the stomach sick; eyes feel heavy. When in the open air she feels cold and 'shakes inside' till she 'fairly cramps.' Dull and stupid. Aching under right scapula; cramping, and very sore and sensitive in the region of the liver; worse from pressure, and at times has sharp pains; sleepy and drowsy, but sleep does not rest her; wakes up tired and feeling bad all overight No appetite; no thirst; breath seems very short; eyes burn like coals of fire. Must urinate often; urine high coloured, very strong odor, scanty; feels like a burden, she wants to urinate, but cannot. In the morning feels as if getting over a long spell of sickness. Dizziness; feels that she does not have any sense; worse walking or turning around, rising up, stooping. Cannot have the house closed up, for it aggravates the head and stomach, but fresh, cool air chills her. Very bad taste, bitter, nasty. Tongue about clean; headache in forehead and down cheek bones. Malaria off., 6m. Reported a very prompt relief.

H. F., aet. 35, a farmer; rumbling and burning in stomach and abdomen; burning of stomach, feels very weak and nervous; frontal headache, going all over the head; face feels stiff; dryness at root of tongue; draws up like from green persimmons; feels drowsy and sleepy; aching all over body, in arms and legs; chilly feeling, then breaks out in a slight sweat for a while, both come and go. Sighing, takes a deep breath; restless and nervous. Hands seem to be useless, but can use them by force of will. Malaria off., 6m. Reports every symptom markedly and promptly relieved.

G. E., aet. 15, chill every second day at 6 P.M. Thirst variable. Slight hot stage after chill. Sweats during the night, profuse; wakes up chilly and gets cold from the sweat drying up. Feels pretty well between times. Sleepy during day of the chill. Lips dry and parched. A constant hacking cough, half minute guns, when talking and when turning over in bed. Malaria off., 6m. Reports a prompt cure.

E. W. E., aet. 56, pain in right side in region of liver; steady, dull ache, better after urinating. Throbbing in scrobiculum, lower part of stomach, worse lying down. Very cold hands during the day, and both hands and feet are cold at night. Skin yellowish. Piles for many years, external, bleeding some, not painful, but unpleasant. Worse using tobacco. Bowels inactive. Malaria off., 30m. Reports all symptoms greatly better, with continuous improvement.

Dr. B. reports that he has been feeling tired and weak for several days. No time of aggravation. Weakness as though he had been sick with loss of appetite. No other symptoms. Malaria off., 6m. Improvement set in in less than an hour after the one dose. At the end of four days he was in usual health.

Mrs. B., wife of the above, chilliness, followed by feveright Pain in upper left chest through to scapula. Burning in left chest. Bodily aching. Malaria off., 6m. Better two months. For the past six days has burning of external chest. Darting in left chest during fever. Burning begins about 10 A.M., lasting during the heat of the day. Occipital pain begins with fever, worse at night, lying on back, lying on left side. Throbbing all overight Malaria off., 50m. All symptoms > for nearly five months, when she received a dose of the 5cm., with amelioration. Soon after this the patient had la grippe.

Stools—

For the past four days cramping in lower abdomen, with urging, which comes on after rising in the morning. Four or five actions daily of thin mucus with bloody spots, a teaspoonful; no fecal matter. Urging and tenesmus each half hour until bedtime. Muscular stinging over body while straining at stool when mucus passes. Desire for stool returns as soon as he sits down. Walking > pain and the desire for stool. Stinging sensation all over at times, if he gets too warm from exercise. Desire to be near the fire.

Stomach—

Faint, empty feeling in stomach at times, day and night; sensation as though he had not had food.

Abdomen—

Pains are > from walking about.

Back—

Pain in small of back, as though strained; > when sitting; < walking or lifting.

Neck—

Pain in back of neck, as though head was being pulled forward.

Limbs—

Pain in legs, better from motion. Feet go to sleep while sitting.

Mouth—

Bitter taste. Dryness.

Appetite—

None. Thirst for a little every hour, caused by dryness in the mouth.

General—

Weakness as though from a spell of sickness. No desire to lie down during day. Desire to walk about. Rhus tox., 50m., was given two days ago, with no >, excepting pains in legs. All other symptoms unchanged. Malaria off., 6m.

In less than a half hour after taking the dose the bad taste in mouth, urging to stool and weak sensation were betteright Improvement uninterrupted, no more trouble with stool until the fourth day; he had some urging to stool while moving about, but the stool was normal. Another dose of same cleared up the case fully.

Mrs. R., aged 45, weighing 245 pounds, could scarcely walk or get into a buggy for two years from the effects of rheumatism in her back and limbs. Malaria lx three or four times a day. In one week she could walk as well as ever and has no rheumatism or lameness since.

Mright S., foreman of a large saw mill, has been afflicted with rheumatism for years, stiff neck and right arm and shoulder helpless and painful. He wished to keep it from his chest and heart. Malaria lx every two hours, when better every three hours. In three days he was better and could turn his neck and use his arm fairly well. One week later gave him two drams more of Malaria, to be taken six hours apart. He has not had any rheumatic troubles since that time.

Mr. C., proprietor of two large saw mills, one in Arkansas, where he passes part of his time (and frequently gets wet), has been afflicted with so-called gout. I found it was of a rheumatic nature (caused by malaria) and made < by Quinine and external applications, I gave him Malaria 1x. In three days he was better and did not have half as many pains or aches. He took only four drachms, from three to six hours apart, and has not had any rheumatic or gouty pains since.

Mr. I. S., aged 55, a veteran and pensioner of the civil war, emaciated, bronzed in colour; had not been able to walk for years. After repairing his heart, chest, stomach, curing his piles and regulating his bowels he was content, yet he could not walk. His back had been injured in the army, and his limbs would not move at will and he could not walk alone or get out of a chairight I gave him for a week Ruta graveolens and Rhus. tox,, of each the first cent., three hours apart. This > for a time. Concluding his trouble was due to rheumatism, caused by malaria, gave him lx three or four times a day. In one week he rode to my house and came up and down steps alone. I gave him two drachms more and in five days he came to my office, having walked nearly three miles that morning alone. I need not say I was surprised, could hardly believe it was all due to Malaria. But it certainly was, as nothing else was taken or applied; has gained flesh and seems at least ten years younger.

Mind—

Feels stupid and sleep.

(Very thoughtful.)

Head—

Feeling as though he would become dizzy.

Waving dizziness on falling asleep.

Dizziness on rising from reclining position.

Dull aching through forehead and temples.

(Dull headache, dizzy and drowsy.)

Intense headache, as though head would burst.

Vertigo on rising in the morning and on rising from stooping; must steady himself before starting to walk.

Frequent attacks of headache, especially in the forehead.

Pain in occiput, begins with fever, worse at night, < lying on back or on left side.

Throbbing pain all over head.

Vertigo; confused sensation; worse by walking, turning around, rising or stooping.

Headache in forehead and down cheek bones.

Headache beginning in forehead, extending all over head.

Eyes—

Aching above inner angle of right eye.

Eyes feel heavy and sleepy.

(Eyes weak, blurring, reading difficult.)

Eyes burn like coals of fire.

Ears—

Drawing pain in right external ear.

Nose—

A kind of concentration of feeling at root of nose and just above, as though I should have a severe cold like hay-fever.

Catarrh; hard, yellow lumps from posterior nares; nose stopped up at times; bloody discharge from nose mornings.

Face.—Itching on right cheek over malar bone (and various parts of face and limbs); > by slight rubbing or scratching.

Face becomes warm as if flushed; and spreads over body.

Mouth.—Pain in upper left teeth.

Sensation on point of tongue as if a few specks of pepper were there.

Saliva more profuse than usual, keeps him swallowing often.

Had a good night's rest and felt better and brighter from that time (curative).

Tongue coated slightly yellowish-white.

(Bitter taste, parched mouth; tongue white.)

Tongue white, with brown streak down the middle.

Tongue white and thickly coated.

Throat dry and sense of slight drawing.

Lips parched and dry.

Mouth very dry, subjectively, but really moist.

Mouth very dry; saliva pasty.

Appetite—

Wants cold drinks.

Can't eat anything; vomits everything.

Craves sour.

Thirsty; craves cold water.

No appetite; aversion to food, thoughts of it sicken.

Thirsty for lemonade; not so much for water.

Variable; craves potatoes, apples, beefsteak.

Bitter, nauseating, bad taste in the mouth.

Dryness at root of tongue; buccal cavity seems constricted and contracted.

Stomach—

Unusually hearty appetite (for supper).

Odor from cooking is pleasing, but no desire for dinner; on sitting down eats a good dinner with relish.

Feels better after eating dinner.

Easy belching, several times, no taste.

Qualmish.

Nausea.

Retching and gagging from hawking mucus.

Nausea continuous, vomiting bile and retching.

Throbbing in scrobiculurn.

Rumbling and burning in stomach and abdomen.

Abdomen—

Sense of heat in abdomen.

Tired feeling through abdomen and chest.

Sensation as though he would have a very loose stool (it passed off without).

Sensation in spleen as though it would ache.

Pain in abdomen to right of navel.

Uneasiness in lower abdomen.

Liver, spleen and kidneys affected.

(Cannot breathe on account of pain in liver, < lying down, > hard pressure.)

(Drawing or pricking in liver.)

(Cramping in liver; pain under right scapula.)

Great uneasiness through abdomen, a sense of heaviness.

Constipation.

Diarrhea; no pain; weakness in bowels.

Pain in upper abdomen and chest; worse breathing.

Drawing or contracting feeling in liver, a kind of cramp.

Steady, dull pains in region of liver > after urinating.

Aching under right scapula; cramp with soreness and sensitiveness in region of liver; from pressure < by lying down.

Stool and Anus—

Diarrhea.

Diarrhea in morning, stools thin, yellow, foul.

Urinary Organs—

Urine highly coloured, like strong tea.

Urine high coloured, with strong urinal odor; ammoniacal.

Frequent urination; urine high colour, scanty, very strong odor; feels oppressed; desires to urinate but cannot.

Respiratory Organs—

Shallow breathing, which seems from languor, desire to breathe deep, occasionally.

Residence in malarial districts is said to cure phthisis.

A consumptive constitution is protected against malaria.

(Singing causes some irritation in the throat.)

Chest—

Tired feeling through chest and abdomen.

Constant hacking cough, half minute guns, when talking and turning over in bed.

Pawn in upper left chest through to scapula; burning in left chest.

Burning in chest begins about 10 A.M., continuing through the heat of the day.

Frequent sighing, takes a deep inspiration; restless and nervous.

Heart—

When leaning face on left hand, elbow on table, perceptible feeling of heart-beats through upper body and neck.

Neck and Back—

Neck feels tired, with slight aching in upper part on moving the head.

Lumbar region tired as though it would ache.

(Rheumatism of back and limbs, with lameness.)

(Stiff neck, and right arm and shoulders painful and helpless.)

(Aching under right scapula; cramping in liver.)

Backache in lumbar region, shoots up back; worse when first lying down; worse after walking; better lying on the abdomen.

Pain in right side of back, over the region of the posterior aspect of the liver and through the right hypochondrium; the aching is worse while sitting, > from walking slowly.

Back seems as though it would break. Pain goes into the hips.

Backache commencing in small of back about 11:30 A.M. for four days; then fever with shortness of breath; headache all the time day and night; paroxysm postponing every day.

Upper Limbs—

Chilly sensation in left forearm; soon followed by chilly feeling in hands and fingers; feet are cold with sensation as if chilliness were about to creep up the legs; a few moments later knees feel cold.

A sense of coldness ascending from body from the legs. Gout.

Limbs get numb and cold.

Aching in both elbows.

Aching and tired feeling in wrists; tired ache in the hands.

Arms tired.

Hands seem to be semi-paralyzed, useless, but can use them by force of will.

Very cold hands during the day; hands and feet very cold at night.

Lower Limbs—

Pain, upper part of right ilium.

Tired ache in knees and for some distance above and below.

Pain top of left instep.

Aching in an old (cured) bunion on left foot.

Legs weary from a short walk.

Legs restless, feel like stretching and moving them.

Soles of the feet cold, almost numb.

Right knee weak and painful worse when bending, and raising up.

Generalities—

General sense of weariness; from a very short walk; especially through pelvis, sacral region, and upper thighs; strong desire to lie down.

A kind of simmering all through the body.

Typhoidal, semi-paralytic condition (No. III).

Rheumatism.

Rheumatic paralysis and emaciation.

Feels very weak and languid; restless; does not want to move.

Great weakness as though he had had a long illness, with loss of appetite.

Great exhaustion.

Must have doors and windows open; a close room < head and stomach, and fresh, cool air chills her.

Skin—

(Skin, eyes, and face very yellow.)

Skin dry all over; no sweat at all.

Sleep—

Impelled to lie down, and on falling asleep a sense of waving dizziness passes all over, preventing sleep.

Gaping, yawning, and desire to stretch.

Sleepy, falls asleep while reading.

Sleep all the time; can go to sleep while standing.

Sleepy and drowsy, but sleep does not relieve; wakes up weary and unrefreshed.

Fever—

(When in open air seems cold and shakes inside till she fairly cramps.)

Coldness ascending over body from legs.

Face feels warm as if flushed, also head; spreads over body as if feverish.

A feeling as if he would have a chill, then as if he would become feverish, though neither is very marked.

Intermittent: quotidian; tertian (No. II).

Chills for one hour followed by fever for six hours (No. II given to a consumptive patient, whom it cured).

(Ague every other day, weak and drowsy between attacks.)

(Dumb chills.)

Shooting pains all over in the muscles; bones ache.

High fever during night; also in the morning.

Pulse 98; skin hot and dry; restlessness most marked in arms, tossing them about. Very stretchy and yawning.

Chilly, with flushes of heat, and great desire for fresh air; unable to breathe on account of pain in liver < lying down; > from hard pressure over region of liver.

Slight fever for several hours in the evening; raves, sings, and talks all night; restless.

Chill begins about noon, every other day. Icy cold from hips down; chilly all over; fever worse about the trunk, and slight general sweat.

Feels languid, weak and drowsy during apyrexia; unable to be up.

Flashes of heat all the time; offensive breath.

Sweats very easily and profuse on least exertion.

Feels malarious, depressed and languid.

Dumb ague, chills every week.

Weakness in the morning, vertigo and nausea. Eyes feel heavy.

Coldness and internal chilliness in the open air.

Aching all over body, especially in arms and legs; chilly sensation, then breaks out in slight perspiration; frequent recurring attacks.

Chilly every second day followed by heat; profuse sweat during the night; wakes up chilly and takes cold as perspiration ceases.

Stool—

Hemorrhoids for many years; external bleeding; no pain but very unpleasant.

For past four years cramping in lower abdomen < after riding in the morning.

Diarrhea; four or five motions daily of thin, bloody, streaked mucus; no fecal matter.

Limbs in General—

Sensation of fatigue in upper extremities first; later extending to lower extremities and entire system.

Dull pain in the muscles of the back, lumbar region; uneasy; tired.

Burning sensation, apparently nervous, which is associated with intense fatigue in the extremities.

Dull, aching pain in left sciatic nerve, and on outer surface of left hip.

Sensation of burning flush, rising from knees to throat, but without sweat; relieved by lying down.

Dull pain in right hip with soreness and tenderness on pres sure in the sheaths of the muscles about the hip and tendons of muscles of the thigh.

Waking at midnight, feet extremely hot with burning palms and soles; this was followed by profuse sweat on lower part of body, more marked on flexor surfaces and on the back.

Drawing, shooting pain on left hypochondrium, extending down left leg.

Arms feel heavy.

Burning of hands and feet; aching of hands and arms.

Nerves—

Great restlessness all night, worse towards morning. Could not find a position in which he could rest.

Hypochondria—

Dull, throbbing pain in hepatic region for three days, relieved by pressure of corset and by lying on the painful side.

MEDORRHINUM

Potencies made from the gonorrheal virus. There are two preparations; the acute and chronic. From the virus of the acute stage to the chronic, or gleet stage, both of which are supposed to contain the gonococcus.

Introduced by Swan.

Provings by Swan, Ren Dell, C. H. Alien, Finch, Norton, Frost, Farrington, Cleveland, Laura Morgan, Berridge, Wilder, Higgins, Ostrom, Nichols, Peace, Sawyer, Carr, Bigler.

Macdonald, in Great Britain, and Noegerath and Lydston, in America, have published fatal cases, and the effects of the poison. The symptoms produced by the virus in acute cases have been included in the pathogenesis, just as the toxic symptoms of Arsenic, Mercurius, Opium and Plumbum are included in the pathogenesis. The potentizing of the virus has developed latent dynamic forces, which is just as effective in homeopathic practice, prescribed strictly on its symptomatological basis as any other remedy. If the symptoms of the patient call for this remedy it should be prescribed with the same confidence as any other in the Materia Medica, entirely irrespective of the sycotic history in the case. Like every other nosode, it should be prescribed according to its strict indications, just as we prescribe Arsenic, Opium or Sulphur, irrespective of its origin or the diagnosis.

We append the following graphic description on the effects of:

Mind—

| Great weakness of memory.

|| Dulness of memory and desire to procrastinate, be-

cause business seemed so lasting, or as if it never could be accomplished.

Entirely forgot what she had read, even previous line.

| Forgetfulness of names, later of words and initial letters.

| Cannot remember names; has to ask name of her most intimate friend; forgets her own.

Cannot spell right; wonders how the word 'how' is spelled.

Reads a letter and thinks the words look queer and are spelled wrong.

|| Time moves too slowly.

| Dazed feeling; a far off sensation, as though things done today occurred a week ago.

Momentary loss of thought, caused by sensation of tightness in brain.

Loses constantly the thread of her talk.

|| In conversation he would occasionally stop, and on resuming make remark that he could not think what word he wanted to use.

Seems to herself to make wrong statements, because she does not know what to say next, begins all right but does not know how to finish; weight on vertex, which seems to affect mind.

| Great difficulty in stating her symptoms, loses herself and has to be asked over again.

Difficulty in concentrating his thoughts or mind on abstract subjects.

Could not read or use mind at all from pain in head.

Thinks some one is behind her, hears whispering; sees faces that peer at her from behind bed and furniture.

Persons come in, look at her, whisper, and say 'come.'

| One night saw large people in room; large rats running; felt a delicate hand smoothing her head from front to back.

|| Fears he is going to die.

Is sure that she is worse, knows she is not going to live, cannot see any improvement, even when it is pointed out; has no fear of death, speaks calmly about it; and gives directions as to the dispositon of her affairs.

| Sensation as if all life was unreal, like a dream.

| Wild and desperate feeling, as of incipient insanity.

I Cannot speak without crying.

Tendency to suicide, gets up in night and takes his pistol, but his wife prevents him.

|| Is in a great hurry; when doing anything is in such a hurry that she gets fatigued.

Strange exhilaration of spirits.

Alternation of happiness and gloominess.

Spirits in the depths, weighed down with heavy, solid gloom > by torrents of tears.

| Is always anticipating; feels most matters sensitively before they occur and generally correctly.

| Anticipates death.

Dread of saying the wrong thing when she has headache.

| Everything startles her, news coming to her seems to touch her heart before she hears it.

Woke at an early hour with a frightened sensation, as if something dreadful had happened; heavy weight and great heat in head; could not rest in bed; felt as if she must do something to rid her mind of this torture.

Fear of the dark.

Feeling as if he had committed the unpardonable sin and was going to hell.

A word or look of seeming harshness puts her in despondency for hours.

Indisposed to work or make mental effort; desire for rest and dread of change; noise, confusion, disorderliness of surroundings distressing; depression and much anxiety, especially after sleep; irritable if the room is not light enough to make everything distinct; craving for stimulants, but cannot endure the effects, for they cause a wild, crazy feeling in brain after the first sleep; same effect from using eyes.

Usually depressed; easily tired; disinclined to any exertion, and yet often unable to keep still; forgetful; unable to think connectedly; mind wanders from subject, even in reading; cannot think at all if hurried.

Always wakens tired in the morning; hates to do anything that must be done, even nice things; gets nervous and excited about riding and driving as soon as the time is fixed.

Constant state of anguish. Always a feeling of impending danger, but knows not what. There is no cause for such feelings, as she is not obliged to do anything when disinclined; is so situated that nothing need cause her trouble.

Inability to think continuously, to talk or to listen to talking when weary; vacant feeling in head.

Forgetful, cannot remember the least thing any length of time; writes everything down of any importance; cannot trust herself to remember it; great irritability and disgust with life.

The impatience, excitement, wild feelings; the unreal, dazed condition; the gloom and fear in the dark; the difficulty of speaking without tears, are marked evidence of functional derangement of the nervous system.

Medorrhinum is forgetful of names, words, etc., but instead of forgetting *occurrences,* during certain periods of time, like Syphilinum, it forgets what it is reading, even to the last line read; it cannot concentrate its attention; thinks words spelled wrong and have no meaning, etc.

Medorrhinum develops a peculiar sensitivity especially in relation to occurrences affecting itself.

It feels the evil coming to it, and the bad news before it arrives, of course it is selfish, and it is easily hurt by a harsh word.

It is also introspective, self-accusative, remorseful. Time moves slowly to it, therefore it is hurried.

We find a dazed condition from the loss of the thread of thought, which annoys and causes a dread of saying the wrong thing, and a difficulty in stating symptoms.

It is always anticipating, fearing evil will happen, loss of reason or suicide.

It fears it has committed the unpardonable sin, and cares little for the result, because of the seething, restless, uneasy, unbalanced nerves.

Feeling of desperation; did not care if he went to heaven or hell.

Cross through day, exhilarated at night, wants to play. Irritated at little things.

Nerve trembling, with worry.

| Very impatient.

Reading and writing make her nervous and enrage her.

Great selfishness.

Time moves so slowly that things done an hour ago appear to have occurred a year since; asked the time of day, and in five minutes insisted that half an hour had elapsed and could not believe it had not till she had seen the watch.

Head—

Vertigo: when stooping; several times during day sudden attacks, seemingly in vertex, with danger of falling; things did not seem to go round, but there was a sensation and fear of falling, only slightly > lying down; < on movement; always woke with it; as if intoxicated; walks *zigzag;* in occiput extending to vertex, with sensation of enlargement of occiput.

Head light, not exactly *dizzy.*

Sensation of tightening in head, causing intense vertigo.

Tensive pains in head, with a wild sensation as if she would go crazy, with a sensation as if she would do something desperate in spite of herself; afraid to be alone.

| Intense itching of scalp.

Great quantities of dandruff.

Hair lustreless, dry and crispy.

Dryness and electrical condition of hair; it will not remain brushed.

Great deal of fugitive itching in scalp.

Sharp itching of scalp, whiskers and eyebrows.

Severe pain at the base of the brain, running to the vertex, in two cases suffering from retroflexion.

Frontal headache; with nausea; feeling of a tight band across forehead, < leaning head forward; as if front half of brain would come through forehead; as if skin was drawn tight; with fluent coryza, with pressure back of eyes, as if they would be forced out; extending over brain to neck.

Brain seems weary; slightest sound annoys and fatigues her.

Neuralgia first in left temple and parietal bone, then in right, next day in left eye.

Wakes with headache over eyes and in temples; < from sunlight.

Headache in right temple; a good deal of aching over left eye. Nocturnal enuresis.

Neuralgic headache in left temple and around middle part of cranium, at times terribly severe, with sensation of great weight and pressure in vertex; has lasted twenty-four hours and is gradually increasing in violence.

Pain in centre of brain; in evening sharp pain through temples; pains commence and cease suddenly.

Heat and throbbing in temporal region both sides.

Brain exceedingly tender and all mental work irksome.

Pain in left parietal bone when the wind blows on it.

Pain circling through head and around crown.

Terrible pains all through head in every direction, with continuous and violent vomiting, followed by aching in sacrum and down back of legs to feet.

Constant headache, < while coughing; light (through the eyes) seems to hurt it.

Intense headache for three days, with inflammation of eye.

Headache and diarrhea from motion of ears.

Headache with menses.

Dull headache in a broad ring around head.

Intense cerebral suffering, causing continual rubbing of head in pillow, rolling from side to side.

Dull pain in cerebellum.

Intense burning pain in head, < in cerebellum.

Tensive pain in left side of head as far back as parietal eminence and to middle of crown.

Tensive pains in head as if she would go crazy; could not read or use mind.

Sensation as of three points of tension in head, in centre of each hemisphere and cerebellum; as if large cords were drawn to each from every part of lobes and cerebellum; extremely painful, caused a disposition to run wildly through streets tearing hair; seemed as if tensive pains would break, when suddenly they relaxed and a bubbling sensation passed from centres to circumferences; when reached, the tensive pains began again.

Sensation of tightness and contraction, extending from eyes and meeting in brain; extends down whole length of spine.

Aching in occiput and medulla; pain sharp on motion; drowsy.

Aching and exhausted feeling in cerebellum and medulla, with a subjective tenderness of spine from cerebellum to kidneys.

Aching pain in base of brain, with swelling of cords of neck.

Burning glow in cerebellum and down spine.

Head feels heavy and is drawn backwards.

Severe pain in back of head as though it had been struck; pain spread over to front, with severe neuralgic pain in left eye; headache lasted all night; eye bloodshot.

Pain in back of head and in right eye.

Simmering in head, does not know whether it is heard or felt.

Sensation as if occipital protuberances were enlarged.

Hair lustreless, dry and crispy.

Dryness and electrical condition of hair; it will not remain brushed.

Intense itching of scalp; quantities of dandruff.

Eyes and Sight—

When eyes were shut, felt as if pulling out of head to one side or other; when open all things seemed to flicker.

A blur over things; numberless black, sometimes brown spots dancing over her book; sees objects double; things look very small; sees imaginary objects.

| Feeling as if she stared at everything, as if eyes protruded.

| Aching in eyeballs, pressure and heat in vertex, a tendency to shut eyes.

I Neuralgic pain in eyeballs; when pressing eyelids together; < when rolling them.

|| Continuous watering of eyes, great heat and sensation of sand under lids.

| Feeling of pain and irritation, and sensation of sticks in eyes, lids and especially inner canthi, redness and dryness of lids, congestion of sclerotic and sensation of a cool wind blowing in eyes, especially inner canthi.

Ptosis of outer end of both upper lids, particularly left, requiring exertion to open them.

| Swelling of upper lids; soreness and smarting of edges.

| Decided tendency to irritation of edges of lids.

Pulling pain in left lower lid from outer canthus; could see lid twitch between these points.

Hardness of upper lid as if it had a cartilage in it.

Eyebrows itch; brows and lashes fall off.

Swelling under eyes.

Sometimes cannot raise lid of right eye after being asleep; cough when tired or nervous.

Miss X., 23, had chronic blepharitis since eleven. Her suffering was intense. Light, especially gas-light, was intolerable, and this prevented her from going into society. She could not read in the evening, and in the morning the lids would be closed, and she suffered much on getting them separated. There was much discharge. Before coming under me she had been under strict homeopathic treatment all the time. I remembered treating her father for gonorrhea before his marriage, and I suspected the taint had reappeared in this form. Medorrhinum was given in high potency, single doses repeated as the effect of each wore off, and she was entirely cured.—*Deschere.*

Ears and Hearing—

Nearly total deafness of both ears, with very little noise; had to use a trumpet.

Partial or transient deafness; pulsation in ears.

|| Child hard of hearing for six days.

Singular sensation of deafness from one ear to the other, as if a tube went through head, while yet there was an over acuteness of hearing.

Is sure he hears people in conversation, but on carefully watching, finds that sounds have reference to arterial pulsation, but where he cannot discover.

When whistling, the sound in ears is double, with peculiar vibration as when two persons whistle thirds.

Noises seemingly in mastoid cells, frying and hissing.

Pain passes up Eustachian tube and out of both ears with a tickling sensation.

After sleeping feels as though parchment was drawn over ear, on which she was lying.

Sensation of a worm about an inch long crawling in right ear, and as if it commenced boring in anterior wall of auditory canal.

Itching, aching, or boring pain in left ear.

Aching in cartilage of ear when lying on it at night.

Soreness to touch of right concha.

Quick, darting pains in right ear, from without inward, pains followed each other in close succession.

Ringhole in left ear sore and almost gathered.

Nose and Smell—

Intense itching in nose, internally near point, had to rub all the time.

Very great burning in both nostrils when breathing through them.

Coldness of end of nose.

Entire loss of smell for several days.

Soreness of outer wing (inside) of left nostril.

Nose constantly running.

Nasal catarrh, with continual running down throat.

Sensation of action in bones; obstruction at root of nose as if mucous membrane was hypertrophied.

Nose goes to sleep.

|| Epistaxis.

Nose inflamed, swollen.

Catarrh of posterior nares.

Posterior nares obstructed, > by hawking thick, greyish mucus, followed by bloody mucus.

Heavy fluent coryza, with hard headache all day in frontal region, < 10:30 A.M.

Soreness and crawling feeling as of a centipede in left nostril in morning.

Nose stopped up, cannot breathe through it in the morning; snuffles in children not relieved by other remedies.

Face—

|| Great pallor; yellowness of face, particularly around eyes, as if occurring from a bruise (greenish yellow); yellow band across forehead close to hair.

Greenish, shining appearance of skin.

Blotches on face.

Flushes of heat in face and neck.

Fever blisters near corner of right upper lip, small but very sore.

Enormous fever sore on lower lip near left commissure.

Sweat of face; on upper lip.

| | Neuralgia of right upper and lower jaws, extending to temple.

Swelling in region of left submaxillary gland, the size of a goose egg; whiskers over tumor came out; softened in centre, at times sharp, shooting pains; on being opened discharged a large quantity of thin, bloody pus; was opened several times, finally the aperture formed raised embankment-like edges; the pus burrowed until arrested by clavicle, where it formed an enormous swelling (> after Thuja 3m.); the tumors left fistulous openings which were a long time in healing.

Face covered with acne; dry herpes; freckles.

| | Tendency to stiffness in jaws and tongue.

| | Rigidity of muscles of face, especially of lower lip, drawing it up tight to teeth; jaws stiff, unable to open them; deglutition nearly impossible; throat filled with saliva.

Swelling of submaxillary glands.

Sensation of constriction and aching in throat and jaws when weary.

Teeth and Gums—

| | Teeth have serrated edges, or are chalky and easily decay (Syphilinum; teeth are cupped, decay at edges of gums and break off).

Sore teeth, particularly eyeteeth; feel sore and soft.

Yellowness of teeth.

| | Hard swelling on right upper jaw, as if in socket of a tooth gone since four years; intense neuralgic pains extending to whole head, causing sleeplessness; severe pains all over head, with external heat.

| | Pale gums.

Taste and Tongue—

Taste: coppery on rising; disagreeable; bad in morning.

Tongue coated: brown and thick; thickly in morning, with bad taste; white at base, the rest red; white, with papillae showing through.

Tongue blistered.

Small sores, pustules (canker sores) on edge, tip and under tongue, very painful; also inside lips and in throat.

Mouth—

Foul breath in morning.

Dryness of mouth; feels burnt.

| | Very sore mouth, ulcers on tongue and in buccal cavity, like blisters.

| | Blisters on inner surface of lips and cheeks, skin peeling off in patches.

Excitement of submaxillary glands, pouring out saliva profusely.

Stringy mucus comes out of mouth during sleep.

Throat—

Irritation in throat as if scraped.

Pharynx inflamed and feels very stiff and sore; swallowing painful.

Great dryness of throat, with swollen glands.

Back part of throat constantly illing with mucus from pos terior nares.

Sore throat and cold in head > by salt water bathing.

Soreness of throat, hurts to swallow; sensation of lump in larynx; deglutition painful; raw, irritated, as if scraped.

Expectoration greenish yellow, catarrhal cold of the head with burning of septum of the nose to bronchi, complete loss of taste and smell—cannot taste tobacco.

Appetite, Thirst, Desires, Aversions—

Appetite in creased; ravenous hunger immediately after eating.

Absolute loss of appetite; thirst.

Enormously thirsty; even dreams that she is drinking.

Insatiate craving for liquor, when before she hated it.

|| Great craving for salt.

Craving for sweets; hard, green fruit; ice; sour things oranges; ale.

Appetite poor. Can digest but a limited amount of food.

Belching, hiccough, nausea and vomiting. Hiccough.

Nausea; with frontal headache; after drinking water; after dinner; always after eating; before eating.

Vomiting of thick mucus and bile, without nausea.

|| Violent retching and vomiting for forty-eight hours; first glairy mucus, then frothy and watery, and lastly coffee grounds; accompanied by intense headache, with great despondency and sensation of impending death; during paroxysm was continually praying.

Vomiting black bile without nausea, tasting bitter and sour with considerable mucus; no odor.

Scrobiculum and Stomach—

|| Sensation in pit of stomach as of a paper of pins that seemed to force themselves through flesh, causing her to rise and double up and scream; pins seem to come from each side. Abscess of liver.

A sick or gnawing feeling, not relieved by eating or drinking.

Trembling at pit of stomach.

Sometimes a burning (like a flame) in pit of stomach, as if heart palpitated there.

Dull pain in epigastric region, deep in.

Feeling of a lump in stomach after eating.

Throbbing in sides of stomach.

Clawing in stomach, < drawing up knees.

|| Cramps in stomach as from wind.

|| Intense pain in stomach and upper abdomen, with a sensation of tightness.

Sensation of sinking and agonizing sickness at stomach, with a desire to tear something away.

Sensation of nausea from using eyes or when weary.

After a hearty meal, sensation as though stomach pressed upon a sore spot at left side.

Hypochondria. Terrible pains in liver, thought she would die, they were so acute.

| | Bilious colic with frequent vomiting and nausea; diarrheic stools, chilliness and perspiration on face and neck.

| | Congestion of liver.

| Grasping pain in liver and spleen.

| | Burning heat around the back, like a coal of fire. Abscess of liver.

| | Severe pain from abscess extending to right shoulder and down elbow.

| | Throbbing and thumping in region of suprarenal capsule, seeming to come from abscess or sore spot just below fifth rib, right side; creeping chills in region of right kidney, throbbing, contracting, drawing and relaxing as if caused by icy cold insects with claws.

Abdomen—

| Intense agonizing pain in solar plexus; surface cold; eructations tasting of sulphuretted hydrogen and, after eating, of ingesta; applied right hand to pit of stomach and left to lumbar region.

Pressure in lower abdomen as of a heavy weight.

A feeling as of a tumor in right side of abdomen.

Tensive pain in right side of abdomen, as of a hard, biconvex body; with heat and gnawing aching pain, continued a short time; it was between spine of ilium and recti muscles.

Darting pain from centre of right ovarian region to lower edge of liver.

| | Ascites; abdomen greatly distended; palpitation showed water; urine very scanty and high coloured.

Beating as of a pulse in abdomen vertically.

Left inguinal glands sensitive and slightly swollen.

Cutting in right lower abdomen running into right spermatic cord; right testis very tender.

Bearing-down sensation in abdomen and pelvis upon standing or walking, and after movement of bowels.

Sensation of want of power in rectum. Accumulation of fecal matter at times which seems impossible to pass.

Stool and Rectum—

Bilious diarrhea, verging on dysentery, with mucous stools.

Pains of most intense kind (threatening cramps) in upper abdomen (darting and tearing pains) coming on at stool; stool diarrheic, thin and hot, but not copious; after stool, profound weakness and mild cramp in left calf.

Profuse bloody discharges from rectum, sometimes in large clotted masses, followed by shivering.

|| Black stool.

|| White diarrhea.

Stools tenacious, claylike, sluggish, cannot be forced, from a sensation of prolapsus of rectum.

|| Can only pass stool by leaning very far back; very painful, as if there was a lump on posterior surface of sphincter; so painful as to cause tears.

| Constriction and inertia of bowels with ball-like stools.

|| Child, act. 15 months, brought on a pillow to clinic, apparently dead; eyes glassy, set; could not find pulse, but felt heart beat; running from anus greenish yellow, thin, horribly offensive stool.

|| Baby, aet. 7 months, after summer complaint, great emaciation, diarrhea green, watery, slimy, yellow, curdled, like boiled potatoes chopped up with greens, thin, cream coloured, watery, smelling like rotten eggs; stools pass involuntarily; apparently lifeless, except that it rotates head on pillow.

|| Cholera infantum with opisthotonos, vomiting and watery diarrhea; profuse discharge of blood and pus.

Sharp, needlelike pains in rectum.

|| Painful attacks of piles, not bleeding, hot swelling of left side of anus; pin worms.

Oozing of moisture from anus, fetid like fish brine.

Sycosis of the rectum, seven cases, three in women and four in men, thin ichorous discharge from rectum, producing very intense itching and burning, which prevents sleep, worse the first part of the night, one case in a man had to use Opium suppositories in order to sleep. The rectal discharge in one case produced blisters on healthy flesh where it touched; there is also a full, stuffed feeling in the rectum.

Patient suffering with infantile diarrhea which persistently relapsed despite most careful prescribing. Remembering the father's history whom he had treated for gonorrhea a year and a half before the patient was born, Medorrhinum was given with a perfect cure.

Urinary Organs—

Intense renal colic; severe pain in ureters, with sensation as of passage of calculus; during kidney attack, great craving for ice.

Dull pinching pain in region of suprarenal capsules at 11 A.M.; fingers cold at same time; great pressure in bladder, greater than amount of urine warrants; urine scanty and high coloured.

|| Pain in renal region, profuse urination relieves.

|| Very distinct bubbling sensation in right kidney; sensation of three bubbles in right renal region, moving like bubbling in water, causing faintness; deathly feeling in kidneys, with great depression of spirits, similar to effect of cold settling in renal region; prostration after urination.

| Urine high coloured.

A child, severe attack of cystitis, with light coloured urine filled with mucus; extreme pain in urethra on urinating; end of penis inflamed; analysis gave albumen, phosphates and triple phosphates.

Urine watery, colourless.

After urinating, great coldness and shivering.

Burning on urination, like incipient gonorrhea.

| Strong smelling urine.

|| Urine covered with a thick greasy pellicle.

|| Nocturnal urination entirely ceased, the chamber empty in morning, a thing unknown for years.

|| Painful tenesmus of bladder and bowels when urinating.

|| Passes an enormous quantity of high coloured, strong smelling urine in bed every night; thinks it is in afterpart of night, as he is always wet in the morning; overwork and too much heat, or being in cold, aggravates this condition.

Debility after prolonged or complete urination.

Syncope after urination.

Intensely yellow urine.

In urinating very slow stream, with sharp, cutting pains transversely across root of penis; once flow intermitted; no burning; pains come on just as last drops are voided.

||Diabetic condition; profuse and frequent urination.

Almost constant desire to urinate; if there be any delay, an intensely nervous sensation, with sometimes burning and sometimes chilliness all over body. Urine dark and scanty.

Frequent urination with slight burning at the meatus; dull heavy ache in the region of the prostate, marked in two cases; very sore in perineum extending to rectum; frenum red and swollen in three cases. Red vesicles on the glans penis that have a burning itching sensation, very irritable.

Urinates every half hour; urgent, can't wait a moment; worse at or during the menstrual period.

Sycotic warts cured by one dose, after nine months careful treatment had failed. He contracted sycotic gonorrhea December, 1886; was nearly cured. In May, 1887, another sycotic attack, with chancroids. The ulcers were all over prepuce, and as they improved the warts began to grow all over glans, back of corona, inside of prepuce and frenum; enormous seed warts; the head of penis was two or three times natural size; the warts were very moist, and secreted a yellowish, stinking fluid, and bled very easily, and the odor was very perceptible in a room with him; but his general health was much improved. From May 26th he had Merc, sol., Nit. ac., Sulph., Corallium, Cinnab., Silic., Thuj., Phos. acid, Sabin., Staphis.—all in high potencies, but got no better. March 7th, 1888, Dr. W. P. Wesselhoeft advised Medorrhinum, gave cm. In a week he was better, discharge and odor gone. In two weeks warts were about one-third their size on March 7, and in six weeks were entirely gone.

Male Sexual Organs—

Nocturnal emissions, followed by great weakness and miserable feeling all day.

Emissions during sleep: watery, causing no stiffness of linen; transparent, consistence of gum arabic mucilage, too thick to pour, and voided with difficulty; thick, with threads of white, opaque substance.

|| Impotence.

||Gonorrheal flow thin, transparent, mixed with opaque, whitish mucus, stains linen yellow.

|| Intense and frequent erections day and night.

|| Pains along urethra while urinating, drawing burning.

|| Gonorrhea for ten months; during eight months mostly suppressed by drugs and injections; for past two months flow persists, watery, transparent, but acrid and abundant, mixed with creamy liquid, stains linen yellow brown; pain at end of penis during urination; since third month of infection had heavy, drawing, wandering pains in right arm, right hip and left calf, < damp weather.

| | Gleety, gonorrheal discharge for twenty years; urine stains clothes a dirty brown, discharges extremely slow, sometimes it takes half an hour to empty bladder, leaving him in a weak condition; during urination, painful rectal tenesmus; chilliness when bladder is too full, > by urination; if he urinates after getting warm in bed, has to urinate every hour rest of night; faint, indefinite sense of chilliness, followed by frequent calls to urinate, urine being hot, copious and followed by spinal chill and incontinence of urine on getting cold.

| | Burning in meatus during urination, and a feeling of soreness through whole urethra; also after urinating, a feeling as if something more remained in urethra.

| | Scanty, yellowish, gleety discharge, of many months' standing, showing most plainly in morning, gumming up orifice.

| | Profuse, yellow, purulent discharge from urethra, most copious in morning.

| | Cannot retain urine more than an hour, after 5 or 6 P.M.

| | Cannot retain urine through night.

Chancrelike ulcer on prepuce (never had syphilis or gonorrhea); six months later there came for several months successive crops of vesicles on prepuce, very sore to touch, which soon opened at the tip, and left a little ulcerlike sore lasting a few days; a round, clean cut, sharp edged elevation with depression, however not filled with pus as in genuine chancre. Soreness, swelling and dragging of testes.

Females Sexual Organs—

| |Great sexual desire after menses, in a single woman.

A great deal of pain in left ovary, with a sensation as if a sac was distended and if pressed would burst; sensation as if something was pulling it down, causing it to be sore; pain when walking passed to left groin, as if leg pushed something, with a great amount of heat.

Left ovary seemed enlarged, with intense heat and severe

aching pain; could not bear pressure, though it seemed as if she must press it; with a burning heat.

Tense pains passing diagonally in right ovary, followed by a bubbling sensation.

Intense, excruciating, neuralgic pains in whole pelvic region, extending downwards through ovarian region to uterus; cutting like knives, forcing tears and groans.

||Ulceration of neck of uterus, which looked ragged and torn, inflamed and covered with stringy pus; had gonorrhea.

Distinct soreness and nervous pain in one spot in lower part of uterus on left side, < walking or moving left leg.

Pulling and pain in sacrum and pubic region, as if menses were coming on.

Profuse menses; dark clotted, also bright blood, with faintness and some pain.

|| Menses very dark; stains difficult to wash out.

Intense menstrual colic, causing drawing up to knees, with terrible, bearing down, laborlike pains, with pressing of feet against support, as in labor.

A burning pain in lower part of back and hips during menses.

|| After very profuse menses, neuralgia in paroxysms in head, with twitching and drawing in limbs and cords of neck, which were like wires; pain in lower abdomen, with profuse, yellowish leucorrhea.

Itching of vagina and labia, thinking of it makes it worse.

Small chancres on edge of right labia (had no sexual intercourse for three years, never had venereal disease).

Short, shooting pains, passing outwards, chiefly in breasts.

Breasts cold as ice to touch, especially nipples (during menses), rest of body warm.

Large but not painful swelling of left breast.

Nipples sore, sensitive and inflamed.

Breasts and nipples very tender to touch, also inflamed.

Soreness of nipples, a gummy secretion drying on orifice; when picked off nipple bleeds freely.

Soreness of breasts, very sensitive to touch, at nonmenstrual periods.

Peculiar tenderness of breasts.

A patient had convulsions at every menstrual period; coming on in the early morning.

Ulceration and inflammation of os uteri, and chronic intrauterine inflammation.

Leucorrhea: albuminous, white-of-egg-like consistency.

Painful hypertrophy of uterus.

A burning, drawing sensation in uterus after driving, standing on feet or when weary.

Dull, aching pain in pelvis from leaning over or if back is not supported.

Membranous Dysmenorrhea: Menstruation was accompanied by terrible pains of a grinding character. Flow scanty, and on the second day there was a passage of a firmly organized membrane. The mental symptom was a constant feeling as if something was behind heright She could not get away from that sensation. It was of nothing definite, simply something terrible behind her, peering over her shoulder, causing her to look around anxiously. Under Medorrhinum I found many of her symptoms, including the peculiar mental symptom, and gave it to heright The next period was without pain and without membrane. Repeated the remedy and the third period was painless again.—*Close.*

Sharp shooting pains like knives, much soreness and tenderness to pressure—the slightest pressure causes her to suffer pains for hours, bearing-down sensation, especially in the left ovary, relieved by pressing upon abdomen; pains run from left ovary to uterus.

Uterus: subinvoluted, sensitive to slightest pressure, a sensitive spot above and to the right of the cervix.

Leucorrhea: thin, acrid, producing severe pruritus, itching intolerable, worse by rubbing, also better by bathing frequently with tepid water; it has odor of decayed fish; sharp pains run from uterus to rectum.

Leucorrhea in a pure young girl, act. 13; thick, yellow, profuse, running down the clothes to the feet, stiffening the linen. Sycotic.

Voice and Larynx, Trachea and Bronchia—

Hoarseness, especially while reading, with occasional loss of voice.

Slight hoarseness with hawking up of mucus.

|| Choking caused by a weakness or spasm of epiglottis, could not tell which; *larynx stopped so that no air could enter, only > by lying on face and protruding tongue.* (Acet. ac.) (Asthma: Dright Miller, Glasgow.)

At night dryness, soreness and choking very severe; thrusting tongue in cheek brought on coughing and choking as if epiglottis was closed; a tearing sensation as if lining of larynx and pharynx had been torn off.

Dryness of glottis, very annoying, with pain during deglutition; great hoarseness.

During day hoarseness, soreness and elongation of palate.

Soreness in larynx as if ulcerated.

Larynx feels sore when coughing.

Tenacious mucus in larynx.

Sensation of a lump in larynx; severe pain on deglutition.

|| Bronchial catarrh spreading into larynx, swelling of tonsils and glands of throat extended also into ears, causing transient deafness.

Constricted and frequent swallowing, painful deglutition with dyspnea as if caused by something foreign in larynx.

Cough: harsh, whistling, barking, croupy.

Respiration—

Desire to breathe deep; wakes gasping for breath.

Difficulty in breathing, with momentary faintness; very marked stuffed feeling in chest made her grasp for breath.

Great oppression of breathing every afternoon about 5 P.M.; sense of constriction.

Has to till lungs, but no power to eject air.

Faint suffocative sensation when sitting up in bed, as if throax was full.

Spasm of glottis, with clucking in throat, air expelled with difficulty, but inhaled with ease.

Breath hot, feels so even when breathing through nose.

After a deep inspiration singular piping and croaking in bronchia.

Cough—

Cough from tickling under upper part of sternum.

Inscessant dry cough, < at night; wakes just as she is falling asleep; < from sweet things.

Hacking cough, causing darting pains through scapulae.

Dry, hacking cough, with a weak, sinking sensation under sternum.

Severe dry cough, < at night; sensation of a lump; dryness and excoriated sensation in glottis, with great hoarseness (relieved by Ipec.).

Terrible, painful cough, as if larynx would be torn to pieces, and as if mucous membrane was torn off, with profuse discharge of viscid, greyish mucus, mixed with blood.

Cough deep and hollow, like coughing in a barrel; bronichal tubes appear to be very much enlarged and cough spasm causes a flabby feeling, as if lining membrane was a loose fold of tissue.

Great rattling of mucus, which appears to be low down in chest, while cough does no seen to reach there, but only to throat pit, consequently hard cough does not reach phlegm unless he lies on his face. When cough brings up a greyish yellow, or a pale greenish yellow, gelatinous mucus without taste.

When lying on back or either side when coughing, rattling, wheezing or whistling.

Cough: with aching across kidneys; causes painful shock at base of each ling; with a peculiar shrill, barking sound, some expectoration; on a entering a warm room; after eating.

|| Cough, < on lying down, > lying on stomach.

|| Cough, < at night, causing retching.

Hawking of tenacious mucus.

Expectoration: yellow white, albuminous, or little green, bitter balls; ropy, difficult to raise; as if flecked with infinitesimal dark spots.

A young French Canadian of delicate constitution, after working in a factory all winter, began coughing in spring and running down in health. He returned home and came under my care in May. The cough persisted and prostration increased, in spite of carefully selected remedies, and the patient took to his bed. It was then observed by me that the cough and general condition was > *from lying on the face*. This, coupled with a knowledge of their being a syphilitic taint in the boy's parentage, suggested Medorrhinum, which was given. The next day a profuse gonorrheal discharge appeared, and the cough and all threatening symptoms promptly disappeared. Exposure to contagion had occurred several weeks before, but from lack of vitality the disease could not find its usual expression and was endangering the patient's life.—*D. C. McLaren.*

Girl of twenty years of age had a violent cough for many months, that nobody could (or did) cure, until I learned that her father had had gonorrhea a year before her birth; then a few doses of Medorrhinum worked like magic.

Inner Chest and Lungs—

Oppression of chest: < left side; with difficult breathing and a tendency to take a long breath; wakes gasping for breath.

Hoarseness seems to be in chest; feels like an accumulation in chest; as if it was painfully contracted.

Sharp pain in bottom of left lung.

Darting pain through lung, which makes her start.

Chest sore to touch, at times burning extends over chest; cold seems to increase it; a piece of ice cools it for an instant, then it is hotter; lung feels as if beaten or bruised.

Feels as if her breath was fanning a blistered sore in lung.

Singular sensation through chest; bounded by a line drawn across lower end of sternum and another about middle; as if there was a cavity extending from side to side, filled with burning air, which dilated in puffs in all directions and could be felt impinging on walls of cavity.

Heat like a furnace in chest, with itching of ears.

Pain in upper part of right lung when moving arm.

|| Pain in right shoulder as though it came from left, straight through.

Chest feels sore throughout.

Darting pain from centre of right lung to lower edge of liver.

Cold pain in right lung and liver with coughing.

Very sharp stitching pain in bottom of right lung; also over surface of both lungs.

Aching in back part of left lung.

An old sore spot in top of left lung aroused.

Fatigue of left lung after talking, as if collapsed or paralyzed.

Walking in sun, left lung becomes excessively, hot, right lung cold.

Pain in left upper chest through to shoulders; cough arising from chest; incessant, dry cough, < at night.

Aching in left lung under scapula, indescribable aching as if it was drawn up in hand and then let loose, < after walking; at same time aching in base of brain.

Sharp pain along right edge of sternum, changing to left edge, and afterwards into left lung.

Left lung very painful, feels drawn towards right side;

left side of chest from top of lung to waist hot as fire; heart beat very fast and felt hot, too; heat spread over right side, but was very mild, only a warm feeling, while left side was consuming; face pale grey, nose pinched and deathlike.

Bottom of left lung sore to pressure (slight urging to cough from lower bronchia); afterwards slight pain in bottom of right lung.

|| Constricted sensation at bottom of both lungs; finally dull, heavy pain at top of left lung.

Intense boring pain in chest, but most below left scapula, a place, the size of a dollar, on outer edge extremely sensitive to touch; pain from upper lung to this spot.

Coughing gives great pain in chest, as if it was painfully contracted.

Sore spot size of silver dollar begins at top of left lung and like a red hot bolt extends through to lower part of back; chest sometimes feels as if something had grown to sore spot in front and was drawing back the chest; she feels for a cavity.

Pain in heart and lungs, especially at night.

|| Awful pains, in phthisis, in middle lobes.

|| Incipient consumption.

Takes cold at the slightest exposure, begins in the head and goes down on the lungs; severe burning in the base of the tongue extending down the bronchi as if he had inhaled hot steam; worse in the morning, a raw feeling extending from throat to lungs as if the mucous membrane was scraped with a knife; aggravated by breathing cold air, sensation as if the lungs were stuffed with cotton.

Deep, hollow, rattling > by lying on the abdomen and face.

During a maneuvre in the army in 1885, Dr. V. got wet by a heavy rain coming into the tent during a whole night. From this he got a hacking cough, on rising in the morning and in the open airight It sounded as if he would call some one, and people would turn and look at him with angry eyes. His throat was thoroughly examined by a specialist, but nothing was found. In 1901, after 16 years of coughing, he consulted Dr. Ide, one of our greatest homeopathic physicians. He ordered the doctor to take Medorrhinum one dose, and await the result. On reaching home he took the dose, and next morning had no cough, nor did he cough afterwards, even in the open airight As an officer he had had a gonorrhea, of which he could not get rid. From this he always had an unpleasant feeling and burning pain. All this vanished like magic.

Heart Pulse and Circulation—

Difficulty of breathing through oppression of heart.

Fluttering about heart.

Palpitation after slight exertion.

Heavy heart throbbings.

With heat in chest, heart felt very hot, beat very fast and felt large, accompanied by a bursting sensation.

Soreness in heart in morning after having slept on left side.

| | *Feeling of a cavity where heart ought to be.*

Pain in heart: acute, sharp, quick; dull, quick.

Sharp pains around heart, passing thence to head; preceded by nausea.

Sharp pain at apex of heart; < on movement.

Intense pain in heart, seemed to radiate in different parts of left side of chest; < from least movement.

Pain from sore spot below left scapula to heart, with violent palpitation.

Dull pain in heart, with pain in left arm and sensation as if hand was swollen.

Burning in heart, went through to back and down left arm.

Dull pain in left side of heart, with pain in left arm and a sensation as if the hand were swollen.

Great pain in cardiac plexus, extending to left arm and throat; pulse 64; next day no pain, pulse 100.

Outer Chest—

Pain and soreness through chest and mammae.

Sensation of an abscess on left chest between pectoralis major and minor where they form anterior boundary of axillary space, hard and sensitive to touch, drawing pains in every direction, < motion of arm; great heat extending about three inches from spot and through to back of shoulder, no redness and very slight swelling.

Great soreness to pressure of muscles of lower left chest front and back, soreness when moving of 1 shoulder-blade.

Neck and Back—

Drawing in cords of neck, causing desire to throw head back.

Swelling of cords of neck, with aching pain in base of brain.

Spasms of neck muscles, notably sterno-mastoid, drawing chin firmly down to breast.

Sensation of an enlarged gland in right side of neck under upper part of sterno-cleido-mastoid muscle, painful when moving head.

Pain in nape and between scapulas, running to either side, shoulder and down to lumbar region.

Contractive pain from superior angles of scapula, passing to Seventh dorsal vertebra and extending straight down spine to ninth vertebra, drawing shoulders back tight as if bones would be crushed; < moving shoulders, neck or arms.

Pain in back between scapulae.

Intense burning heat, commencing in back of neck and extending gradually down spine, with a contractive stiffness extending into head and seeming to thicken the scalp.

Pain under right scapulae.

| Pain straight through from left to right shoulder.

Burning glow in cerebellum and down spine.

Weak, stiff, aching back.

| Heat in medulla and spine for a whole week.

Whole length of backbone sore to touch, also ribs of left side.

Tenderness of spinal column when stretching.

Aching across and in kidneys.

Occasional creeping sensation in region of left kidney.

When she stoops cannot rise again without violent pain region of kidneys.

Pain in region of left kidney, darting over left hip, especially when spine is pressed upon.

|| Throbbing and thumping in region of right suprarenal a sule seeming to come from abscess or sore spot just bellow fifth rib, right side, under breast; creeping chills in region of right kidney, throbbing, contracting, drawing and relaxing; as if caused by icy cold insects with claws. Abscess of liver.

Lumbar vertebrae sensitive to touch.

|| Pain in lumbar portion of spine; myalgic; induration testes.

Sensation of water dropping out of a bottle in lumbar region (opposite third lumbar vertebra), between posterior and superior spine of ilium and vertebra.

|| Lumbago caused by straining in lifting.

Pain in back of hips, running around and down limbs.

Pain in sacrum and coccyx.

Upper Limbs—

Rheumatic pain in top of left shoulder, from motion; occasional little darts of pain if kept still.

|| Rheumatic pain in right shoulder and arm.

Rheumatic pains in shoulders, notably left, also in hanc with pains on closing them.

Brown, itching eruption on left shoulder.

|| Severe pain from abscess, extending to right shoulder and down to elbow.

|| Pain commencing under left scapula, running down left arm to little finger, which pricked as if asleep.

Cold numbness on outer side of arms, just below elbow.

Itching and irritation inside of elbow joints.

Sharp pain in elbow when moving it.

Cracking of joints, especially elbows.

Left forearm and hand numb, unable to hold anything with force; any attempt to raise arm caused a sense of discomfort and irritability.

Pain in left arm and sensation in head as if swollen; connected with heart; numbness down left arm.

Aching in bones of arm after headache.

Numb pain in left arm; cannot even hold a paper any length of time; the veins become enlarged; it is very painful to raise arm.

Trembling of arms and hands.

Right arm cold.

Crampy pain in first and second fingers of right hand.

In night, sensation of a boil coming on back of hand, just above metacarpal phalangeal joint of left index finger; sore to touch, with drawing pains from every direction; expected to find a boil there in morning, but found only a red spot, not elevated.

Burning of hands, wants them fanned and uncovered; always cold hands.

Intense burning in palms; burning and itching of hands, first left, then right.

Itching of hands at roots of and between fingers, as in itch.

Palms and sometimes feet burning hot. Right hand is cold, then left.

Cold hands, with coldness extending all over body.

Sharp rheumatic pains across middle knuckles of left hand, also rheumatism of arms and legs.

Hot numbness of back of hands.

Back of hands rough.

Small yellow spots on hands.

Middle finger of left hand swollen and cannot be bent without pain; cannot touch palm with it; top of this finger painfully sensitive, numb and dead, she cannot grasp anything with it, can hardly touch anything.

Hardness at base of ball of little finger.

Transverse depression on nails as if they were bent.

|| Consumptive incurvation of nails.

Acute lancinating pain of right arm at the level of the deltoid attachment, deep down near the bone.

Aching in right shoulder and arm; dull, sore pain, and soreness and stiffness of arm when moved. Hurts most to move it back or straight out from side. Worse at night or from any pressure on back of shoulder that pushes shoulder forward. Weight of bedclothes on arm hurts it. Aching at times extends to fingers, and the fingers swell when used.

Nails dry and brittle.

Rheumatism: of the wrists and ankles with complete loss of power in the part affected. If in the ankle, was unable to walk; if in the wrist, it had to be carried in a sling.

Lower Limbs—

Woke with a sharp pain over left hip, preventing stooping, makes walking difficult; it is like a stiff neck, but more aching.

Slight aching pains to hip joints and knees.

Pains in both legs, at times from hips down to knees, at other times in left; only when walking.

Sensation of heaviness, or want of power to move limbs, in walking.

Heaviness of legs, very difficult walking (especially going up or down stairs), legs are so heavy, feel like lead.

Trembling of limbs, legs give way.

Lower limbs ache all night, preventing sleep.

Legs do not go right in walking.

Little dropping of right leg.

Very restless with the legs.

Numbness in left leg from knee to hip, feeling as if paralyzed.

Longing to stretch legs.

The pain seems to tighten the whole body, especially the feet and thighs.

|| Rheumatic pains in muscles of legs.

Many years since had a leg amputated just above ankle; after healing it began to swell, end of stump turned black, severe pains in muscles and bones, and ultimately a pimple appeared on stump, which broke and discharged for some time; all this has been reproduced.

During a terrific thunderstorm, very sharp pains in knees shot upwards; pains < by stretching.

Aching pain in legs, with inability to keep them still in bed, < when giving up control of himself, as when trying to sleep (> after Lil. tigr.).

Weak kneed when getting up from a chair.

When walking, pain in left knee, that caused it to give way, letting her down.

Trembling in legs from knees down, left leg trembles most, burning in feet.

Legs dead and heavy, throbbing from knees down.

Coldness of legs up to knees, also of hands and forearms.

Short pulling pains in knees, toes, ankle joints and hands.

Drawing sensation under knees and in ankles.

Contraction of muscles under left knee and in left calf.

Cramps in soles and calves at night.

Cramp in left calf, afterwards in right leg between knee and thigh.

Kind of cramp in left calf at night, muscles knotted, > stretching; not cramp, but knotting.

Ankles turn easily when walking.

|| Sudden intense pain in left ankle, back or joint, on

going to bed, could not move limb or body without screaming; could find no position of comfort.

| Burning of feet, wants them uncovered and fanned.

Both feet somewhat swollen; dropsy of feet.

Sore feeling under left foot.

Edema of feet followed and > by diarrhea.

Cold feet with chills all over body.

Small sharp pain in soles when first stepping on them in morning, not felt any other time.

|| Swelling and itching in soles, itching between toes, and pulling pains extending up to knees; itching, painful, papulous eruption around waist, and hivelike eruption wherever flesh is pressed on.

|| Tenderness of soles so that he could not stand on them at all and had to walk on his knees.

| Soreness in ball of foot under toes.

Great toe sore, right one worst; pains shooting through toes when sitting still.

Pain, swelling and inflammation of right great toe.

|| Cold and sweaty feet.

Great toe covered with scales like tetters.

|| Old foot sweats, < during winter, for seven years.

Corns very tender:

| Almost entire loss of nervous force in legs and arms; exhausted by slightest effort.

|| Pain like rheumatism along right side, right hip, left leg (upper, lower left); pains drawing, < in dampness; left leg swollen near knee.

|| Stiffness throughout body and joints.

||Deformity of finger joints, large, puffy knuckles, swelling, stiffness and pain of both ankles; great tenderness of heels and balls of feet; the swellings of all affected joints were puffy like wind galls; general condition < inland, > near shore.

Numb sensation in left arm, hand and leg; left leg. goes to sleep.

Eruption under and on toes and on hands and feet.

Right knee painful, red and swollen.

Synovitis of left wrist, dorsal aspect, tendons attacked being the extensor proprius policis and indicis.

Acute pain in the tendo Achillis, left foot and along the inner border of the right tibia. The part is edematous and very sensitive.

The rheumatic symptoms in the extremities are of extreme intensity.

A man with clonic spasms, the legs suddenly shot up from the bed.

Feet always wet with perspiration.

Rest, Position, Motion—

Rest: little darting pains in left shoulder.

Lying down: vertigo slightly >; on ear, aching in cartilage; cough <.

Lying on back or either side when coughing: rattling, wheezing or whistling.

Lying on stomach: cough >.

Lying on either side: contents of lower part of chest and abdomen seem to press upon each other.

Cannot lie on left side for any considerable length of time.

Can only sleep on back, with hands over head.

Sleeps on her knees, with face forced in pillow.

Must lie on face and protrude tongue; larynx stopped so that no air could enter.

Could find no position of comfort; intense pain in left ankle, back of joint.

Sitting still: pains shooting through toes.

Sitting up in bed: faint suffocative sensation.

Stooping: vertigo; cannot rise again without violent pain in region of kidneys; impossible, pain in hip.

Leaning head forward: tight band across forehead <.

Desire to throw head back; drawing in cords of neck.

Head drawn backwards.

Leaning body very far back: can only pass stool.

Drawing up knees: clawing in stomach <; menstrual colic.

Must rise and double up: pain in pit of stomach.

Thrusting tongue in cheek brought on coughing.

Applied right hand to pit of stomach and left to lumbar region: intense agonizing pain in solar plexus.

Cannot hold paper long: numb pain in left arm.

When closing hands: pain in them.

Slight exertion: palpitation; heat; tendency to perspire.

Motion: vertigo <; of left leg, pain in uterus <; of arm causes pain in upper right lung; sharp pain at apex of heart <; least, pain in chest <; of arms, pains in chest <; soreness of left shoulder-blade; of head causes pain in neck; of shoulders, neck or arms, pain in shoulders; < of elbow, sharp pain.

Getting up from a chair: weak kneed.

Getting up: as if bones were out of joint; shakes herself to get them into place.

Cannot keep still: restlessness, > by clutching hands.

Inability to keep legs still in bed: aching pain.

Continual rubbing of head in pillow, and rolling from side to side: cerebral suffering.

Attempt to raise arm: discomfort and irritability.

When rolling eyes: neuralgic pains <.

Could not move limb or body without screaming: intense pain in left ankle, back of joint.

Stretching: tenderness of spinal column; pains in knees <; cramp in calf <.

When first stepping on soles: small sharp pains.

Had to walk on his knees: tenderness of soles.

Walking: pain passed from left ovary to groins; pain in uterus <; aching in left lung; difficult, pain in hip; pains from hips down to knees; heaviness in limbs; legs do not go right; pain in left knee; ankles turn.

Going up and down stairs: difficult from heaviness of legs.

Extremely sensitive, swollen bunions, worse on left foot, puffed, very red, feet hot; in the centre there is a spot as if blood had collected, which is very sore; itching very annoying, must remove shoes to rub them, which relieves for the time; very sensitive to pressure; flesh feels as if cracked open; in the evening, after being on the feet all day, almost unendurable; worse on warm days; feet swollen and tender.

Nerves—

Intense nervous sensibility, respecting touch of garment or a lock of hair by any one not en rapport.

Starts at slightest sound.

Unusually active, going as if on wings.

Restlessness, cannot keep still, but feels greatly relieved by clutching hands very tight.

|| Consumptive languor; great general depression of vitality.

| Very tired.

Faintness early in morning with no appetite.

Sensation as if she would faint, followed by a great heat down spine and between shoulders.

Trembling all over, great nervousness and profound exhaustion.

Great general subjective trembling, even tongue felt trembling.

Sensation of creeping things throughout body continually.

Quivering sensation, with tingling and numbness.

Tonic spasm, rigid extension of arms and legs, the hands everted, palms outward, thumbs down, fingers clawlike.

Epileptiform spasms with foaming at mouth, rigidity of body and limbs; violent regurgitation at heart with absence of mitral cluck.

Opisthotonos.

State of collapse, nearly gone; wants to be fanned all the time, wants more air; cold and pulseless, with cold perspiration; throws off all covers.

Risus sardonicus.

Medorrhinum, in the same sphere, is characterized by great disturbance and irritability of the nervous system from center to periphery. Its pains are intolerable, tensive, shooting, neuralgic. It produces tension, involuntary tension, which cannot be relaxed except by voluntary effort of the will. Its nerves are easily shocked, it is easily startled at the slightest sound. Its restlessness is > by clutching the hands very tight. Its nerves quiver, tingle, tremble and produce spasms. It is also cold, yet throws the cover off and wants to be fanned. It is < by warmth, even when too cold to be fanned. It is < by warmth, even when too cold to touch, as in collapse. It is also < by wet, damp, drafts and thunder storms. As to time, it is worse from daylight to sunset; worse mornings and bright evenings. Its functional disturbance covers a long period before organic destruction begins. Its general condition is > near the seashore and < inland.

Sleep—

Sleepy, yawning, chilly; sleepy but cannot sleep.

Spasmodic yawning, cannot suppress it; followed by spasm of glottis.

Asleep, but hears everything, answers questions as if she was awake. Nightmare.

Bites tip of tongue in sleep.

Feels as if she would have nightmare.

Sleeps at night on her knees, with face forced in pillow; kneeling position.

Can only sleep on back with hands over head; if she lies on either side, the contents of lower part of chest and abdomen seem to press upon each other and cause discomfort.

When asleep day or night, no matter how short a time, profuse perspiration on face and neck.

Sleep with wearing dreams of walking; waking with impression that she had slept for hours, although it was only thirty minutes.

Such restless nights and terrible dreams of ghosts and dead people, she dreads night to come.

Dreams: horrid; painful; exhausting; that she is drinking.

Woke at night and saw a woman of pleasant face, dressed in grey, standing by bedside, wiping a tumbler; she backed from me miles away, becoming very small.

Wakeful; slept towards morning.

Great restlessness at night, sleepy but could not sleep,

|| Becomes wide awake at 6 P.M. and continues so till 12, with entire passivity of brain and cessation of thought; slight restlessness.

Restless sleep, talking and tossing all night, with copious sweat of head, neck and chest, had to dry her hair several times in the night.

Slept well but woke at an early hour with a frightened sensation as if something dreadful had happened; the weight on the head was heavy, and great heat in it; could not rest in bed; felt as if she must do something to rid her mind of this fearful torture; for two hours was in this state of mind; she struggled against it; fought with what seemed to be the adversary; scolded herself for her weakness; all to no purpose, and grew weak with the effort; she cannot describe the mental agony she endured.

Time—

Aggravation from daylight to sunset; always brighter in evening.

Morning: soreness and crawling in left nostril; bad taste; tongue thickly coated; foul breath; gleety discharge; soreness of heart; small sharp pains in soles when first attempting to step on them; early faintness.

10 A.M.: chill, chattering, shivering.

10:30 A.M.: headache <; fever with thirst.

11 A.M.: pain in region of suprarenal capsules.

From 10 to 11 A.M.: cold feet and legs.

From 10 A.M. to 12: nervous during fever, moving fingers.

From 10 A.M. to 1P.M.: fever and malaise <.

From 10:30 A.M. to 12:30 P.M.: thirst during chill.

At 11 A.M.: chill, beginning with great coldness of fingers and toes; fever, preceded by cold feet.

At 2 P.M.: feet cold first, after chill excessive languor.

At 5 P.M.: chill, followed by fever and slight sweat; next day same, but slighter.

From midnight to 3 A.M.: fever, with nervous restlessness.

Day: frequent and intense erections.

Afternoon: fever.

After 5 or 6 P.M.: cannot retain urine more than an hour.

6 P.M.: became wide awake until 12 P.M.

Evening: sharp pain through temples; itching <.

Night: headache; aching in cartilage of ear; intense and frequent erections; cannot retain urine; dryness, soreness and choking very severe; incessant dry cough; cough <, causing retching; sensation of a boil coming on back of hand; aching in legs; cramp in soles and calves; restless sleep; rapid pulse; sweats.

Temperature and Weather—

In sun, walking: left lung becomes very hot.

Too much heat: < urination in bed at night.

After getting warm in bed: when urinating, must do so every hour rest of night.

Entering warm room: cough.

Wants hands fanned and uncovered.

Wants to be fanned all the time, wants more air, state of collapse; hands and feet must be fanned.

Sensitive to drafts of air, takes cold easily.

When wind blows on parietal bone: pain.

Salt water bathing: sore throat and cold in head <.

After getting wet: chill, followed by fever and slight sweat.

Damp weather: pains in limbs >.

Getting cold: incontinence of urine.

Craving for ice: during kidney attack.

Piece of ice cools chest for an instant, then it is hotter.

Inland: chronic rheumatism in joints <, > near shore.

Fever—Creeping chills running down back and all over body in a zigzag course.

Chills: up and down back; several times a day; 10 A.M., some chattering and shivering; at 10:30 A.M., fever with thirst, began in fingers and toes; from 10:30 to 12:30, thirst during chill, none during fever; from 10 to 11 A.M., cold feet and legs, from 10 to 12, nervous during fever, moving fingers; at 11 A.M., beginning with great coldness of fingers and toes; at 2 P.M., feet cold first, after chill excessive languor; at 5 P.M., followed by fever and slight sweat (after getting wet); repeated next day, but slighter.

Shivering chills, with boring pains in chest.

Cold hands, with coldness extending all over body.

Coldness of legs up to knee, also of hands and forearms.

Flashes of heat alternating with chills.

Coldness: right hand, then left; a slight flush of heat succeeded, then sensation of a foreign substance in right eye, then in left.

Must be fanned all the time, throws clothes off, yet surface is cold; burning, mostly subjective, of hands and feet, wants them uncovered and fanned.

Great general internal heat after dinner, as if blood was boiling hot in veins, same after slight exertion.

Great burning heat all over body, with flashes of heat in face and neck.

Fever: with or without thirst; with gushes of perspiration on face, followed by languor; with nervous restlessness from midnight to 3 A.M.; at 11 A.M. preceded by cold feet; fell asleep during fever; after fever, sweat on palms, feet and legs; with rapid pulse at night; in afternoon; and malaise < from 10 to 1

Hectic fever; every afternoon.

Great tendency to perspire on exertion; sensitive to cold.

|| Profuse sweat about neck.

Night sweats.

|| Chills for four months every day, commencing from 3 to 4 P.M.; chill with headache, thirst, nausea, sometimes vomiting; fever with headache, thirst, nausea, principally on head and neck; pains from waist downwards; frequent urination, dark colour; frequent, tasteless eructations; constipation; bad taste in mouth in morning.

|| Chill came first at night, afterwards at various hours; for instance, on two consecutive days at 2 P.M., then two days at 3, 4, 5 and 6 each, then at 7 P.M., where it remained for two weeks; chill commenced in small of back, running up and down, lasted about an hour, and as it ceased, profuse and frequent urination appeared and continued during fever; congestion of chest simulating pneumonia during fever, causing great alarm; great renal distress during paroxysm; thirst during fever for hot drinks; fever continued for six or eight hours; profuse sweat after fever; great nervousness during paroxysm, was sure he would die; intolerance of noise; irritable.

Attacks,, Periodicity—

In close succession: pains in ear.

Alternately: flashes of heat and chills.

Several times during day: sudden attacks of vertigo; chill up and down back.

Takes half hour to empty bladder.

Every day for four months: chills commencing from 3 to 4 P.M.

Every afternoon: hectic fever; about 5 P.M., oppression of breathing.

Nightly: passes enormous quantity of urine in bed.

Chill came first at night, afterwards at various hours; on two consecutive days at 2 P.M., then two days at 3, 4, 5, 6 each, then 7 P.M., where it remained for two weeks.

For six or eight hours: fever.

For forty-eight hours: violent retching and vomiting.

For three nights: cannot sleep, pain in carbuncular boils.

For several days: entire loss of smell.

For three days: intense headache, inflammation of eyes.

For six days: child hard of hearing.

For a whole week: heat in medulla and spine.

Six months after chancrelike ulcer on prepuce there came for several months successive crops of vesicles on prepuce.

For ten months: gonorrhea.

For seven years: < during winter, old standing foot sweats.

For twenty years: gleety gonorrheal discharge.

Locality and Direction—

Right: neuralgia in temple; in eye; headache in temple; as of a worm crawling in ear; soreness of concha; quick, darting pains in ear; fever-blisters near corner of upper lip; neuralgia of upper and lower jaw; hard swelling in upper jaw; as of a tumor in side of abdomen; tensive pain in side of abdomen; darting pain from centre of ovarian region to lower edge of liver; cutting in lower abdomen, running into spermatic cord; testes very tender, distinct bubbling sensation in kidney; sensation of three bubbles in renal region; heavy, drawing, wandering pains in arm and hip; tense pain passing diagonally in ovary; small chancres on edges of labia; pain in upper part of lung; pain in right shoulder as though it came from left darting pain from centre of lung to lower edge of liver; cold pain in lung; sharp stitching pain in bottom of lung; lung cold; sharp pain along edge of sternum; mild heat spreading over right side; pain in bottom of lung; sensation of enlarged gland in side of neck; pain under scapula; throbbing and thumping in region of suprarenal capsule, seeming to come from just below fifth rib; creeping chills in region of kidney; rheumatic pain in shoulder and arm; severe pain from abscess of liver, extending to shoulder and down elbow; crampy pain in first and second fingers of hand; dropping of leg; cramp in leg; between knee and thigh; soreness of great toe; pain, swelling and inflammation of great toe; pain like rheumatism along nape, whole side, hip, upper leg. Left: neuralgia in temple and eye; aching over eye; pain in parietal bone; tensive pains in side of head; ptosis of outer end of upper lid; pulling pain in lower lid; itching, aching or boring pain in ear; ringhole in ear sore; soreness of outer wing of nostril; crawling in nostril; fever sore on lower lip near commissure; swelling in region of submaxillary gland; mild cramp in calf; hot swelling on side of anus; heavy, drawing, wandering pains in calf; great deal of pain in ovary; ovary seemed enlarged; soreness and nervous pain in a spot on side of uterus; swelling of breast; oppression < on side; sharp pain in bottom of lung; aching in back of lung; an old sore spot in top of lung aroused; fatigue of lung; walking in sun, lung becomes excessively hot; pain in upper chest; aching in lung under scapula; sharp pain in edge of sternum and lung; lung very painful, feels drawn towards right side; side of chest from top of lung to waist hot as fire; bottom of lung sore to pressure; dull, heavy pain at top of lung; intense boring below scapula; sore spot size of silver dollar begins at top of lung, extends through to lower part of back; after having slept on side, soreness of heart; great pain in cardiac plexus, extending to arm; intense pain in side of chest; pain from sore spot below scapula to heart; dull pain in heart, with pain in arm; burning in arm; sensation of an abscess in chest; great soreness of muscles of lower chest; ribs sore to touch; occasional creeping sensation in region of kidney; pain in region of kidney darting over hip; rheumatic pain in top of shoulder; itching eruption on shoulder; pain commencing under scapula, running down arm to little finger; forearm and hand numb; pain in arm and sensation in hand as if swollen; numbness down arm; numb pain in arm; sensation of a boil coming on back of hand; pains across middle knuckles of hand; middle finger swollen; sharp pain over hip; numbness of leg, pain in knee when walking; trembling in leg; contraction of muscle under knee and in calf; knotting of muscle in calf; sudden intense pain in ankle, back of joint; sore swelling under foot; pains like rheumatism in lower leg; leg swollen near knee; numb sensation in arm, hand and leg; leg goes to sleep; itching sometimes confined to side.

From without inward: pain in right ear.

First right hand cold, then left.

From left to right: pain in shoulders; burning and itching of hands.

Sensations—

Of falling; as if intoxicated; as if occiput was enlarged; head as if tightening; as of a tight band across forehead; as if front half of brain would come through forehead; as if skin was drawn tight; as if she would go crazy; as of three points of tension in head, as if large cords were drawn to each; as if tensive pains would break; as if head had been struck; as if occipital protuberances were enlarged; as if eyes were pulling out of head; as if she stared at everything; as if eyes protruded; as of sand under lids; as of sticks in eyes, lids and inner canthi; as of a cool wind blowing in eyes; as if upper lid had a cartilage in it; as if a tube went through head; as if parchment was drawn over ear; as of a worm crawling in right ear, as if it commenced boring in anterior wall of auditory canal; as if mucous membrane of nose was hypertrophied; as of a centipede crawling in left nostril; mouth as if burnt; throat as if scraped; as of a paper of pins in pit of stomach that seemed to force themselves through flesh; as if heart palpitated in pit of stomach; as if a lump in stomach; cramps in stomach as from wind; sensation in liver as if caused by icy cold insects with claws; as of a heavy weight in lower abdomen; as of a tumor in right side of abdomen; pressure as of a hard, biconvex body in abdomen; beating as of a pulse in abdomen; as if there was a large lump on posterior surface of sphincter ani; as of passage of calculus in ureter; after urinating, a feeling as if something more remained in urethra; as if a sac was distended in left ovary and if pressed would burst; pain in left groin as if leg pushed something; left ovary as if enlarged; as if she must press ovary; cutting as if with knives in pelvic region; pain as if menses were coming on; choking as if epiglottis was closed; as if lining of larynx and pharynx was torn off; larynx as if ulcerated; as of a lump in larynx; as if thorax was too full; as if larynx would be torn to pieces; as if bronchial tubes were enlarged; as if lining membrane was a loose fold of tissue; chest as if painfully contracted; lung as if beaten or bruised; as if her breath was fanning a blistered sore in lung; as if there was a cavity extending from side to side in chest, filled with burning air, which dilated in puffs in all directions; pain in right shoulder as though it came from left straight through; left lung as if collapsed or paralyzed; as if lung was drawn up in hand and let loose; left lung as if drawn toward right side as if something had grown to sore spot in front of chest and was drawing back; heart as if large; as of a cavity where heart ought to be; pain as if radiating in different parts of left side of chest; as if heart was swollen; as of an abscess on left chest; between pectoralis major and minor; as of an enlarged gland in right side of neck, under upper part of sterno-cleido-mastoid; pains in shoulders as if bones would be crushed; as of water dropping out of a bottle in lumbar region; pricking in left little finger as if asleep; left hand as if swollen; as if a boil was coming on back of hand; left leg as if paralyzed; creeping chills in region of right kidney, as if caused by icy cold insects with claws; as if she would faint; as of creeping things throughout body; as if she would have nightmare; as if contents of lower part of chest and abdomen seemed to press upon each other; as of a foreign substance in right eye, then in left; as if blood was boiling hot in veins; as if she had taken a severe cold; sore all over as if bruised; as if all bones were out of joint.

Pain: in forehead; in temples; over eyes; in centre of brain; in left parietal bone; circling through head and around crown; in back of head; in right eye; in eyes; up Eustachian tube and out of both ears; in renal region; at end of penis; in left ovary; in lower abdomen; in upper part of right lung; in right shoulder; in left upper chest through to shoulders; from upper lung to sore spot below left scapula; in heart and lungs; in heart from sore spot below left scapula to heart; in left arm; through chest and mammæ; in nape and between scapulas, running on to either side, shoulder and down to lumbar region; in back between scapula?; under right scapula; straight through from left to right shoulder; in region of left kidney; in lumbar portion of spine; in back of hips, running around abdomen and down limbs; in sacrum and coccyx; commencing under left scapula, running down arm to little finger; in left arm; when bending middle finger of left hand; in both legs, from hips down to knees; in left knee; of right great toe; from waist downwards.

Intolerable pains: in carbuncular boils.

Intense, agonizing pain: in solar plexus.

Terrible pains: all through head; in liver.

Intense pain: in head, in cerebral region; in stomach and upper abdomen; in abdomen; in heart; in left ankle, back of joint.

Awful pain: in middle lobes.

Violent pain: in region of kidneys.

Extreme pain: in urethra.

Intense, excruciating neuralgic pains: in pelvic region.

Intense neuralgic pains: from teeth to head.

Severe pain: in back of head; all over head; from abscess of liver to right shoulder and elbow; in ureters; on deglutition; from abscess extending to right shoulder and down to elbow; in muscles and bones of stump of amputated leg.

Sharp pain: through temples; in occiput; in bottom of left lung; along right edge of sternum, changing to left edge and then into lung; around heart, thence to head; at apex of heart; in elbow; over left hip; in knees.

Great pain: in chest; in cardiac plexus, extending to left arm and throat.

Hard pain: in frontal region.

Tearing pains: in abdomen.

Sharp, cutting pain: across root of penis.

Sharp, shooting pains: in swelling in region of submaxillary glands.

Short, shooting pains: in breasts.

Acute, sharp, quick, or dull quick pain in heart.

Quick, darting pain: in right ear.

Darting pain: from centre of right ovarian region to lower edge of liver; in abdomen; through scapulae; through lung, which makes her start; from centre of right lung to lower edge of liver; over left hip.

Boring pain: in left ear; intense, in chest and below left scapula.

Shooting pains: through toes; about three inches long in various directions and all over body.

Cutting: in right lower abdomen, running into spermatic cord; in pelvic region.

Neuralgia: in temples and parietal bone; in left eye; around middle part of cranium; in eyeballs; of right upper and lower jaws to temple; in head.

Sharp, stitching pain: in bottom of right lung; over surface of both lungs.

Sharp, needlelike pains in rectum.

Terrible, bearing down, laborlike pains: during menses.

Intense menstrual and renal colic.

Intense burning pain: in head.

Grasping pains: in liver and spleen.

Contracting pain: from superior angles of scapulae, passing to seventh dorsal vertebra and down same to ninth.

Dull, pinching pain: in region of suprarenal capsules.

Cramping pain: in first and second fingers of right hand.

Gnawing, aching pain: in abdomen.

Short, pulling pains: in knees, toes, ankle joints and hands.

Pulling pain: in left lower lid from outer canthus; in sacrum and pubic region; extending up to knees.

Heavy, drawing, wandering pains: in right arm, right hip and left calf.

Drawing pains: in every direction of chest; on back of hand, from every direction; in limbs.

Rheumatic pains: in top of left shoulder; in right shoulder and arm; in hands; across middle knuckles of left hand; of legs; in muscles of legs; along right nape, whole right side, right hip, left leg.

Most distressing aching: in bones.

Severe aching pain: in left ovary.

Dull, heavy pain: at top of left lung.

Dull pain: in broad ring around head; in cerrebellum; in epigastric region; in left heart.

Small, sharp pain: in soles.

Little darts of pain: in left shoulder.

Cramps: in stomach; in soles and calves; in right leg between knee and thigh.

Mild cramp: in left calf.

Clawing: in stomach; like cold insects in right kidney.

Gnawing feeling: in stomach.

Painful shock: at base of each lung.

Tensive pain: in left side of head as far back as parietal eminence and to middle of crown; in right side of abdomen; all over body from head to foot.

Tense pains: diagonally in right ovary.

Numb pain: in left arm.

Cold pain: in right lung and liver.

Weak, stiff aching: in back.

Heavy throbbings: in heart; all over body.

Painful tenesmus: of bladder and bowels.

Painful eruption: around waist.

Burning pain: in lower part of back; in hips.

Smarting: of eyelids.

Burning heat: from liver round to back; in left ovary; in back of neck and down spine.

Burning glow: in cerebellum and down spine.

Burning: in both nostrils; in pit of stomach; on urination; in meatus; over chest; in heart, through to back and down into left arm; of hands, in palms; soles of feet; in chest.

Heat: in temporal region; under lids; in abdomen; in left ovary; in chest; in left side of chest from top of lung to waist; of heart; from chest through to back of shoulder; in medulla and spine; down spine and between shoulders.

Flushes of heat: in face and neck.

Soreness: of edges of eyelids; of outer wing of left nostril; in left nostril; of teeth; of mouth; of pharynx; of throat; through urethra; of testes; in one spot in lower part of uterus; of nipples; of breasts; of larynx; in heart, chest and mammae; in ball of foot under toes; of great toe; all over body.

Excoriated sensation: in glottis.

Sore feeling: throughout chest; under left foot.

Sore spot: on top of left lung, size of silver dollar, begins at top of left lung and like a red hot bolt extends through to lowerpart of back.

Slight pain: in bottom of right lung.

Pricking sensation: all over body.

Tingling: through body.

Tenderness: of brain; of spine, from cerebellum to kidneys; of testes; of breasts; of spinal column; of soles; of heels and balls of feet.

Hot numbness: of backs of hands.

Simmering: in head.

Dragging: of testes.

Constricted sensation: at bottom of both lungs.

Contracting, drawing and relaxing: in region of kidneys.

Contraction: extending from eyes and meeting in brain; down whole length of spine; of muscles under left knee and in left calf.

Contractive stiffness: extending from spine to head and seeming to thicken scalp.

Drawing: in cords of neck; under knees and in ankles.

Discomfort: in left forearm and hand; in chest and abdomen from lying on side.

Distress: in renal region.

Bursting sensation: in heart.

Stiffness: in jaws and tongue; of pharynx; throughout body and joints of both ankles.

Stuffed feeling: in chest.

Suffocative sensation: in thorax.

Pressure: back of eyes; in vertex; in lower abdomen; in bladder.

Oppression: of chest; of heart.

Weight: in vertex.

Heavy feeling: in head; in limbs.

Tightness: extending from eyes and meeting in brain, extends down whole length of spine; in stomach.

Twitching and drawing in: of limbs and cords of neck. Throbbing and thumping: in region of right suprarenal capsule.

Throbbing: in temporal region; in sides of stomach; in region of liver; from knees down.

Pulsation: in ears.

Bubbling sensation: in right kidney.

Fluttering: about heart.

Quivering: in body.

Trembling: at pit of stomach; of limbs; in legs from knees down; all over; of tongue.

Tickling: in ears; under upper part of sternum.

Singular sensation: through chest.

Sensation of action: in bones of nose.

Restlessness: at night.

Numbness: down left arm; of left middle finger; in left leg from knees to hip; in left arm, hand and leg; through body.

Lightness: of head.

Sinking and agonizing sickness: at stomach.

Deathly feeling: in kidneys.

Sinking sensation: under sternum.

Faintness: early in morning.

Weakness: after nocturnal emission.

Fatigue: of left lung.

Dryness: of eyelids; of mouth; of throat; of larynx; of glottis.

Creeping sensation: in region of left kidney.

Itching: of scalp; in nose; of eyebrows; over left eye; of ears; in occiput; in cerebellum and medulla; in base of brain; in eyeballs; in left ear; in cartilage of ear; across kidneys; in sacrum and down back of legs to feet; in back part of left lung; in left lung under scapula; in bones of arm; in hip joints and knees; in lower limbs; of vagina and labia; of eruption on left shoulder; in side of elbow joints; of hands; at roots of and between fingers; in soles; between toes; of eruption around waist; all over body; of eruption on limbs; from knees up, on forearms and around waist.

Chilliness: when bladder is too full.

Cold numbness: on outer side of arms, just below elbow.

Coldness: of end of nose; of right arm; extending all over body; of legs up to knees; of hands and forearms; of fingers and toes.

Tissues—

Great heat and soreness, with enlargement of lymphatic glands all over body.

Sensation as if she had taken a severe cold, with most distressing aching in bones; throat very sore and swollen, deglutition of either liquids or solids impossible.

There is scarcely a spot on body from head to foot but what is full of pain, of tensive and letting go character, accompanied by heat; this heat is a sensation, burning hot, but not perceived on surface by touch.

Sore all over as if bruised.

The pains seem to tighten the whole body, especially feet and thighs.

Feeling as if all the bones were out of joint in getting up; shakes herself to get them into place.

Obstinate rheumatism.

| Sequelae of acute articular rheumatism; walks leaning on a cane, bent over; muffled in wraps to ears, looking like a broken down man apparently soon to fall into his grave.

Carbuncular boils that seem small, discharge slowly and show dark red streaks; pains are intolerable, could not sleep for three nights.

Leukemia, of Grauvogl and Virchow, occurring in children of sycotic parents.

A girl of 17, of tubercular history, with the same rheumatic order of symptoms, with epistaxis, hemoptysis, albuminuria, endocarditis, with suffocative attacks and violent palpitations ended in permanent disablement.

Glandular enlargement in various parts of the body, with rachitis, is traced to hereditary gonorrhea; patients are better at the seaside.—*Gilbert.*

Wildes thinks that the suppression of favus when derived from gonorrhea in the father leads to hydrocephalus, capillary bronchitis, obstinate teething diarrheas and cholera infantum; if derived from the grandfather, suppression leads to consumption and lingering diseases.

Fiery red rash developing about the anus in babies a few days old; constipation with hard dry stools; when the nurses say "Baby's water scalds it terribly," the indications for Medorrhinum are clearight He regards the latent and gonorrheal taint as the true explanation of many of the disease manifestations included by Hahnemann under psora. Among other diseases he traces vascular meningitis and cerebro-spinal meningitis in infants to the same source.

Burnett appears to confirm this as he traces gout and some forms of rheumatism to a sycotic origin.

Sycotic children (born so), when one or both parents have gonorrhea, have cholera infantum, marasmus, are pining children.

Noeggerath says latent gonorrhea in husband may cause in wife acute and chronic perimetritis, oöphoritis; if impregnation results, abortion follows, or only one child is born; exceptionally two or three.

I have traced epithelioma, phthisis, cauliflower excrescences, sterility, and erosions to a sycotic origin; pernicious anemia often has gonorrhea as its base; suppressed gonorrhea may produce iritis, syphilis produces it without suppression.

The suppression of the external manifestations of gonorrhea seems first to involve the central nervous system functionally, and is much later in attacking the organism destructively.

Touch. Passive Motion. Injuries—

Touch: soreness of right concha; soreness of vesicles on prepuce; nipples and breasts very tender; chest sore; small spot below left scapula very sensitive; chest sensitive; whole length of backbone, also ribs of left side and lumbar vertebrae sensitive; of garment, or lock of hair, nervous sensibility.

Pressure: of eyelids together causes neuralgic pains in eyeballs; on left ovary; could not bear; bottom of left lung sore; on spine, pain in kidneys and hips <; on flesh causes hivelike eruptions.

Rubbing: intense itching in nose.

Scratching: red spots on limbs itch.

Motion of cars: headache and diarrhea.

Straining when lifting causes lumbago.

Skin—

Great yellowness of skin.

Intense and incessant itching, fugitive, < towards night, sometimes confined to left side.

Itching all over body, most on back, vagina and labia, and < thinking of it.

Intense itching all over body, would scratch till it bled, but no relief; no visible eruption.

Pricking sensation all over body.

Red spots itching when scratched and on undressing at night, on limbs, particularly from knees up, on forearms and around waist.

|| Copper coloured spots (syphilitic) remaining after eruptions, turn yellow brown and detach in scales, leaving skin clear and free.

Small, pedunculated warts, with pin heads like small button mushrooms on various parts of body and thighs.

Itching: intense, incessant, fugitive; of vulva, vagina; frequently erratic, changes place, but not > by scratching; < towards night; < when thinking of it.

An eruption of roseolous patches appeared on the body, abdomen and chest, so exactly like those of typhoid that the possibility of this was discussed.

Girl of eleven had been treated by many physicians with salves and ointments to the general impairment of her health. Face mottled with a profusion of red scurfy sores; eyelids involved and nearly denuded of lashes; hairy scalp one diffuse mass of thick yellow scabs, from beneath which oozed a highly offensive mixture of ichor and sebum. Passing down neck, back, perineum and involving genitals and pubes was a fiery red band as broad as a child's hand, oozing a pale yellow serum, which caused the clothing to stick to the body. Told the mother he could cure the case but it would certainly get worse the first three months. Medorrhinum cm. was given, one dose dry on the tongue. The external appearance grew rapidly worse, but appetite, sleep and general health steadily improved, and in nine months she was completely cured.— *Wildes.*

Child of six since infancy horribly disfigured with tinea capitis. Scalp a mass of dense crusts exuding a fetid ichoright The only semblance of hair being a few distorted stumps ending in withered roots. One dose cured in a few months, and at the time of writing patient was a healthy and extremely talented young lady, and the possessor of a luxurient head of chestnut hairight— *Wildes.*

Characteristics—

For the constitutional effects of maltreated and suppressed gonorrhea, when the best selected remedy fails to relieve or permanently improve.

For persons suffering from gout, rheumatism, neuralgia and diseases of the spinal cord and its membranes—even organic lesions ending in paralysis—which can be traced to a sycotic origin.

For women, with chronic ovaritis, salpingitis, pelvic cellulitis, fibroids, cysts, and other morbid growths of the uterus and ovaries, especially if symptoms point to malignancy, with or without sycotic origin.

For scirrhus, carcinoma or cancer, either acute or chronic in development, when the symptoms correspond and a history of sycosis can be traced.

Bears the same relation in deep-seated sycotic chronic affections of spinal and sympathetic nervous system that Psorinum does to deep-seated affections of skin and mucous membranes.

Children, pale, rachitic; dwarfed and stunted in growth (Baright c.); mentally, dull and weak.

Great heat and soreness, with enlargement of lymphatic glands all over body. Spinal curvatures or more or less pronounced traces of rachitis.

Consumptive languor; fatigue; great general depression of vitality.

Pains: arthritic, rheumatic, a sequel of suppressed gonorrhea (Daph. od., Clem.); constricting, seem to tighten the whole body (Cac.); sore all over, as if bruised (Arn., Eup.).

Trembling all over (subjective), intense nervousness and profound exhaustion.

State of collapse, wants to be fanned all the time (Carbo v.); craves fresh air; skin cold, yet throws off the covers (Camph., Sec.); cold, and bathed with cold perspiration (Ver.).

Insatiate craving: for liquor, which before she hated (A. S. A. R.); for salt (Cal., Nat.); for sweets (Sulph., Tub.); for beer, ice, acids, oranges, green fruits, coffee grounds.

Nocturnal enuresis: passes enormous quantity of ammoniacal, high-coloured urine in bed every night; < by overwork or overplay, extremes of heat or cold; when with a history of sycosis the best selected remedy has failed to cure.

Intensely restless and fidgety legs and feet.

Burning of hands and feet, wants them not only uncovered, but fanned (Lach., Sulph.).

Relations–

Antidoted by: Nux vom., nervous and general symptoms and the aggravations from an overdose or too frequent, repetition; Ipecac (dry cough).

Compatible: Aloe, Sulph., Tuber, (especially early morning diarrhea, stool driving out of bed).

Compare: Pic. ac., Gels., inability to walk, legs tire and give out; priapism; Camph., Secale, Tab., Veright (in collapse, skin cold, covered with cold sweat, throws off all covering); Amb., Anac., Cal., Can. I., Con., Cup., Stram., Val., Ziz. (as if in a dream).

Aggravation: when thinking of it (Helon., Ox. ac.); heat, covering; stretching out; leaning head forward; thunderstorm; least movement; sweets; salt bathing; early morning (three to four A.M.); common to this remedy and all sycotics; in the mountains; in the sun; warmth of bed; entering a warm room; from warmth, even when cold to the touch; from daylight to sunset (rev. of syph., which is worse from sunset to sunrise).

Amelioration: at the seashore; lying on the face or stomach; damp weather (Caust., Nux); by leaning far back (constipation, can only pass stool in this position).

In summer, 1875, I had an obstinate case of acute articular rheumatism in a man aet. 60, from June llth to September 5th; he suffered excruciating agony from neuralgia. After a desperate battle for life the first week of September, he was relieved, and arose from his bed a wreck. It was expected that time and out-door life and the best hygienic measures would restore him. But weeks and months passed without change; he walked the streets leaning on a cane, bent over, muffled in wraps to his ears, and looking like an old man about to fall into the grave. Three months after my attendance I saw him pass my office, and considering his previous good health and robust frame the question arose: Why does he remain in this condition? Is there any miasm hereditary or acquired uncured to explain the obstinacy of the case? Could it be a gonorrheal taint ? For reasons unnecessary to mention I could not ask him.

Dr. Swan's suggestion now occurred to me:

An obstinate case of rheumatism might be due to latent gonorrhea, and Medorrhinum high will cure it; in many cases where improvement reaches a certain stage, and then stops, Medorrhinum has removed the obstruction and the case progressed to a cure; and this too in cases where gonorrhea appeared to be a most unlikely cause, teaching us, if anything, the universality of latent gonorrhea and the curative power of the dynamic virus.

His wife consulted me on other matters, and said "her husband was as well as could be expected considering his age; she believed he would not do anything more, as he regarded his feeble state due to his age." However, he came next day, and I gave him three doses of Medorrhinum, to be taken every morning; within ten days he returned feeling Well and looking well. I then gave him one dose to be taken after some time; this was the last prescription he has required. Within the month, after the Medorrhinum, he dropped his cane and muffler, walked the street erect with a firm step a perfectly well man, having increased in weight from 140 to 212 pounds.

PSORINUM

In the subsequent list of antipsoric remedies no isopathic remedies are mentioned, for the reason that their effects upon the healthy organism have not been sufficiently ascertained. Even the itch miasm (psorinum), in its various degrees of potency, comes under this objection. I call psorin a homeopathic anti-psoric, because if the preparations of psorin did not alter its nature to that of a homeopathic remedy it never could have any effect upon an organism tainted with that same identical virus. The psoric virus, by undergoing the processes of trituration and shaking, becomes just as much altered in its nature as gold does, the homeopathic preparations of which are not inert substances in the animal economy, but powerfully acting agents.

Psorinum is a similimum of the itch virus. There is no intermediate degree between idem and similimum; in other words, the thinking man sees that similimum is the medium between simile and idem. The only definite meaning which the terms 'isopathic and aequale' can convey is that of similimum; they are not idem.

Hitherto syphilis alone has been to some extent known as such a chronic miasmatic disease, which when uncured ceases only with the termination of life. Sycosis (the condylomatatous disease), equally ineradicable by the vital force without proper medicinal treatment, was not recognized as a chronic miasmatic disease of a peculiar character, which it nevertheless undoubtedly is, and physicians imagined they had cured it when they had destroyed the growth upon the skin, but the persisting dyscrasia occasioned by it escaped their observation.

Incalculably greater and more important than the two chronic miasms just named, however, is the chronic miasm of psora, which, whilst those two reveal their specific internal dyscrasia, the one by the venereal chancre, the other by the cauliflower-growths, does also, after the completion of the internal infection of the whole organism, announce by a peculiar cutaneous eruption, sometimes consisting of only a few vesicles accompanied by intolerable voluptuous tickling itching (and a peculiar odor), the monstrous internal chronic miasm—the psora, the only real fundamental cause and producer of all the other numerous, I may say innumerable, forms of disease, which under the names of nervous debility, hysteria, hypochondriasis, mania, melancholia, imbecility, madness, epilepsy and convulsions of all sorts, softening of the bones (rachitis), scoliosis and cyphosis, caries, cancer, fungus hematodes, neoplasms, gout, hemorrhoids, jaundice, cyanosis, dropsy, amenorrhea, hemorrhage from the stomach, nose, lungs, bladder and womb, of asthma and ulceration of the lungs, of impotence and barrenness, of megrim, deafness, cataract, amaurosis, urinary calculus, paralysis, defects of the senses and pains of thousands of kinds, etc., figure in systematic works on pathology as peculiar, independent diseases.

Characteristics—

Especially adapted to the psoric constitution.

In chronic cases *when well selected remedies fail to relieve or permanently improve* (in acute diseases, Sulph.); when Sulphur seems indicated but fails to act.

Lack of reaction after severe acute diseases. Appetite will not return.

Children are pale, delicate, sickly. Sick babies will not sleep day or night but worry, fret, cry (Jalap.); child is good, plays all day; restless, troublesome, screaming all night (rev. of, Lye.).

Great weakness and debility; from'loss of animal fluids; *remaining after acute diseases;* independent of or without any organic lesion, or apparent cause.

Body has a filthy smell, even after bathing.

The whole body painful, *easily sprained and injured.*

Great sensitiveness to cold air *or change of weather.*

Stormy weather he feels acutely; feels restless for days before or during a thunderstorm (Phos.); dry, scaly eruptions *disappear in summer, return in winter.*

Ailments: from suppressed itch or other skin diseases when Sulphur fails to relieve; severe, from even slight emotions; never recovered from typhoid.

Feels unusually well day before attack.

Extremely psoric patients; nervous, restless, easily startled.

All excretions—diarrhea, leucorrhea, menses, perspiration— have a carrion-like odor.

Anxious, full of fear; evil forebodings.

Religious melancholy; very depressed, sad suicidal thoughts; despairs of salvation (Mel.), of recovery.

Despondent: fears he will die; that he will fail in business; during climaxis; making his own life and that of those about him intolerable.

Driven to despair with excessive itching.

Headache: preceded, by flickering before eyes; by dimness of vision or blindness (Lac d., Kali bi.); by black spots or rings.

Headache: *always hungry during; > while eating* (Anac., Kali p.); from suppressed eruptions, or suppressed menses; > by nosebleed (Mel.).

Hair, dry, lustreless, tangles easily, glues together (Lye.). Plica polonica (Baright, Sars., Tub.).

Scalp: dry, scaly or moist, fetid, suppurating eruptions; oozing a sticky, offensive fluid (Graph., Mez.).

Intense photophobia, with inflamed lids; cannot open the eyes; lies with face buried in pillow.

Ears: humid scurfs and soreness on and behind eirs; oozing and offensive viscid fluid (Graph.).

Otorrhea: thin, ichorous, horribly fetid discharge, like decayed meat; chronic, after measles or scarlatina.

Acne: all forms, simplex, rosacea; < during menses, from coffee, fats, sugar, meat; when the best selected remedy fails or only palliates.

Hungry in the middle of the night; must have something to eat (Cina, Sulph.).

Eructations tasting of rotten eggs (Arn., Ant. t., Graph.).

Quinsy: tonsils greatly swollen; difficult, painful swallowing; burns, feels scalded; cutting, tearing, intense pain to ears on swallowing (painless, Baright c.); profuse, offensive saliva; tough mucus in throat, must hawk continually. To not only > acute attack but *eradicate the tendency.*

Hawks up cheesy balls, size of a pea, of disgusting taste and carrion-like odor (Kali m.).

Diarrhea: sudden, imperative (Aloe, Sulph.); stool watery, dark brown, *fetid; smells like carrion;* involuntary, < at night from 1 to 4 A.M.; after severe acute diseases; teething; in children; when weather changes.

Constipation: obstinate, with backache; from inactivity of rectum; when Sulphur fails to relieve.

Enuresis: from vesical paresis; during full moon obstinate cases, with a family history of eczema.

Chronic gonorrhea of year's duration that can neither be suppressed nor cured; the best selected remedy fails.

Leucorrhea: large, clotted lumps of an intolerable odor; violent pains in sacrum; debility; during climaxis.

During pregnancy: most obstinate vomiting, fetus moves too violently; when the best selected remedy fails to relieve; to correct the psoric diathesis of the unborn.

Profuse perspiration after acute diseases, *with relief of all suffering* (Calad., Nat. m.).

Asthma, dyspnea: < in open air, sitting up (Lauright); > *lying down* and keeping arms stretched far apart (rev. of Ars.); despondent, thinks he will die.

Cough returns every winter.

Hay fever: appearing regularly every year the same day of the month; with an asthmatic, psoric or eczematous history. Patient should be treated the previous winter to eradicate the diathesis and prevent summer attack.

Cough: after suppressed itch, or eczema; chronic of years' duration; < mornings on waking and evenings on lying down (Phos., Tub.); sputa green, yellow or salty mucus; pus-like; coughs a long time before expectorating.

Skin: abnormal tendency to receive skin diseases (Sulph); eruptions easily suppurate (Hep.); *dry, inactive, rarely sweats;* dirty look, as if never washed; coarse, greasy, as if bathed in oil; bad effects from suppression by Sulphur and Zinc ointments.

Sleepless from intolerable itching, or frightful dreams of robbers, danger, etc. (Nat. m.).

Psorinum should not be given for psora or the psoric diathesis, but like every other remedy, upon a strict individualization—the, totality of the symptoms—and then we realize its wonderful work.

Relations—

Antidoted by Coffea, Nux v. (if < when too frequently repeated or over-dose).

Compatible: Carb. v., Cinchona, Opium, Sul., Tub. (if want of susceptibility to medicinal action).

Followed well by Alum., Boright, Hep., Lye., Sul., Tub.

Complementary: Sul., Tub.; after Lact. ac. and Nux v. (vomiting of pregnancy); after Arn., Bellis, Ham. (in traumatic affections of the ovaries); Sulph. follows Psor. in mammary cancer.

Inimical: Apis, Crot., Lach. and the serpent poisons.

Compare: Cham., Jalap (sick babies, fret day and night); (happy all day, scream at night) (Lye.) cry all day, sleeps at night; nervous effects of electric storms (Phos., X-ray); Gels., Lac d., Kali bi. (headache preceded by dim vision and dark spots); Anac., Kali phos. (headache with hunger > while eating); Mel. (headache relieved by nose-bleed); Baryt. c., Lyc.,Sars., Tub. (plica polonica); Kali mur. (offensive cheesy balls from the throat); Cal., Nat. muright (all symptoms > by lying down and keeping arms stretched far apart; (Ars., must sit up and lean forward); Phos., Tub. (cough and affections of the respiratory tract < mornings on waking, and evenings lying down); Graph., Hep., Sil. (eruptions and slight injuries of the skin easily suppurating); Dig. (drinking < cough); Bry., Nat., Mal. (earthy, sallow, greasy face); Puls., Tub. (erratic shifting pains < from fats and pastry < evenings); Sang., Tub. (sensation as if tongue were burned); Ars., Bap., Pyr. (sensation as if parts were separated, Ars. body at waist, Bap. the brain and limbs); Kali c., Pyr. Tub. (profuse sweat during convalescence); Amb., Caps., Cin., Laur., Op., Val. (lack of susceptibility to best selected remedy); Gels., Kali iod., Sab., Cin. n. (hay-fever); Cina, Chin, s., Ign., Lye., Sul., Tub. (hungry at night, can't sleep until they eat).

Ars., Rhus, X-ray, Tub. causes: mental emotions, or mental labor; overlifting; suppressed eruptions; weather changes; electric storms; traumatism; sprains and dislocations.

Mind—

Thoughts vanish after overlifting.

Memory weak, cannot remember; does not even know his room.

Thoughts which he cannot get rid of constantly reappear in his dreams

Dull all forenoon, disinclined to work.

Dull, stupid, foggy, as after a debauch, on awaking in night; dizziness, he falls down.

As if stupid in left half of head, morning.

Mental labor causes: fulness in head; intense headache; throbbing in brain; pain in left temple.

| Very disagreeable mood; impatient; extremely ill-humored.

| Irritable, peevish, passionate, noisy; nervous, easily startled; restless, hands tremble.

| | Intolerably self-willed, annoys those about him; a boy, suffering from an eruption.

| She is very irritable, easily angered; always thinks of dying.

Vacillating, fearful; mania.

| Anxiety, with oppression of chest.

| | Anxious, full of fear, melancholic; evil forebodings. Great fear of death; anxiety about heart and dyspnea, with attacks of pain in chest.

| | Believe the stitches in heart will kill him if they do not cease.

| Restlessness: with eruption, in a child; with oppression of chest.

| Sentimental: full of spleen, very low-spirited.

| Discouragement.

| His ideas are sad and joyless.

| | Very depressed, sad, suicidal thoughts.

| | Depressed in spirits and hopeless.

Melancholy, sorrowful, despairing.

| Desparing mood; fears he will fail in business.

| | Much depression on account of an eruption on dorsum of hand which appears over night.

| Greatest despondency, making his own life and that of those about him intolerable; dry cough; evening fever.

| Is so downhearted she could commit suicide, then is so full of phantasms.

Great depression of mind during climaxis, with chronic abdominal disorders.

Hypochondriasis, with hemorrhage from rectum.

| Religious melancholy. (Melilotus.)

| Despairs of recovery; thinks he will die; hopeless; especially after typhus, > from nosebleed.

| | Melancholy after suppressed itch; emaciated, pale, earthy complexion, weakness of limbs; flushes of heat and pal-

pitation prevent sleep; sleep comes toward morning; would like to stay in bed until midday; aversion to work, indifference, weeping; seeks solitude, despairs of recovery; she is irritable and forgetful.

|| Feels the greatest anguish in head, with a whirling before eyes every day, from 5 A.M. until 5 P.M., since two years; walks up and down his room wringing his hands and moaning continually, "Oh, such anguish! Oh, such anguish!" only when he takes his meals he ceases moaning; appetite is good.

|| Has been nervous about nine months; was obliged to abandon all business; has taken much quinine and other drugs; a very disagreeable feeling about head; mental depression; thinks he will not recover; has lost all hope; cannot apply his mind to business; confusion of senses, he cannot reckon; attacks of numbness of legs and arms, left side<; < on going to bed; formication and crawling, with pricking and smarting on scalp, and some on extremities; tongue white.

|| Driven to despair with excessive itching.

Every moral emotion causes trembling.

Severe ailments from even slight emotions.

Disturbances of the mind and spirit of all kinds.

Melancholy by itself, or with insanity, also at times alternating with frenzy and hours of rationality.

Anxious oppression, early on awaking.

Anxious oppression in the evening after going to bed.

Anxiety, several times a day (with and without pains), or at certain hours of the day or of the night; usually the patient then finds no rest, but has to Şun hither and thither, and often falls into perspiration.

Melancholy, palpitation and anxiousness cause her at night to wake up from sleep (mostiy just before the beginning of the menses).

Mania of self-destruction (spleen).

A weeping mood; they often weep for hours without knowing a cause for it.

Attacks of fear; *e. g.*, fear of fire, of being alone, of apoplexy, of becoming insane, etc.

Attacks of passion, resembling frenzy.

Fright caused by the merest trifles; this often causes perspiration and trembling.

Disinclination to work, in persons who else are most industrious; no impulse to occupy himself, but rather the most decided repugnance thereto.

Excessive sensitiveness.

Irritability from weakness.

Quick change of moods; often very merry and exuberantly so, often again and, indeed, very suddenly, dejection; *e. g.*, on account of his disease, or from other trifling causes. Sudden transition from cheerfulness to sadness, or vexation without a cause.

Numbness and giddiness of the head; the patient can neither think, nor accomplish any mental labor.

She cannot control her thoughts.

At times she seems to be deprived of thought; she sits there as if she were absent.

The head feels benumbed and drowsy in the open air.

Sensorium—

Vertigo; mornings, objects seem to go around with him; with headache; eyes feel pressed outward; with confusion and drawing in forehead, with roaring in ears.

Great dulness of head; he fears inflammation of brain; nosebleed relieves.

Fulness and heaviness in head.

Vertigo; the patient reels in walking.

Vertigo, on closing the eyes, everything around him seems to turn; he is then attacked with nausea.

Vertigo; on turning briskly he almost falls over.

Vertigo attacking him with a jerk in the head; he loses his senses for a moment.

Vertigo, accompanied with frequent eructations.

Vertigo, on looking down upon the floor, or on looking up.

Vertigo, in walking along a road in a plain, which is not enclosed on either side.

Vertigo; she appears to herself either too large or too small; other objects, likewise, appear either too large or too small.

Vertigo Resembling a swoon.

Vertigo, causing a loss of consciousness.

Inner Head—

Frontal headache, with sensation of weakness in forehead.

Headache by sweat at night.

Pain as if brain had not room enough in forehead, when rising in morning, a forcing outward; < after washing and eating.

Pressing headache in small spots in forehead and temples, < left side; feels intoxicated, stupid.

Morning headache, with pressing in forehead; stupefaction, staggering; eyes feel sore.

Sensation as from a heavy blow received on forehead awakens him; 1 A.M.

|| Surging, drawing and digging in forehead with vertigo.

|| Pain beginning over left eye and goes to right; < from hour to hour, then diarrhea and nausea, finally bloody vomiting; dizziness, obliges her to lie down; blur, and blue stars before eyes: veins of temples much distended; day before headache inordinate appetite; also during first hours of pain; < and brought on by change of weather, so that even in middle of night she is awakened by pain and always knows there has been a change; soreness of stomach, sensitive to touch and pressure of clothes; catamenia regular.

| Headache preceded by: flickering before eyes; dimness of sight or spots; spectres; objects dancing before eyes, black spots or rings.

|Headache from repelled eruption.

Pressing headache, especially unilateral.

Cramplike contractive headache.

Like hammers striking head from within outward; all through head as from a hammer.

Fulness of head during mental labor.

Fulness in vertex as if brain would burst, with formication in head, followed by heavy sleep.

Pain in back of head as if sprained; pressure in right side of occiput as if luxated.

Pain from right to left as if a piece of wood was laid on back of head.

|| Is always very hungry during headaches.

|| Congestion of blood to head immediately after dinner.

| Great congestion of brain, relieved nosebleed.

Congestion to head, heat; awakened at night stupefied; could not recollect; after sitting still awhile had to rise to collect his senses.

|| Congestion to head, cheeks and nose red and hot; eruption on face reddens; great anxiety every afternoon after dinneright Fifth month of pregnancy.

Vertigo: reeling while walking.

Vertigo: when closing the eyes, everything seems to turn around with him; he is at the same time seized with nausea.

Vertigo: on turning around briskly, he almost falls over.

Vertigo, as if there was a jerk in the head, which causes a momentary loss of consciousness.

Vertigo with frequent eructations.

Vertigo even when only looking down on the level ground, or when looking upward.

Vertigo while walking on a road not enclosed on either side; in an open plain.

Vertigo: she seems to herself now too large, now too small, or other objects have this appearance to her.

Vertigo: resembling a swoon.

Vertigo, passing over into unconsciousness.

Dizziness; inability to think or to perform mental labor.

Her thoughts are not under her control.

She is at times quite without thought (sits lost in thought).

The open air causes dizziness and drowsiness in the head.

Everything at times seems dark and black before his eyes, while walking or stooping, or when raising himself from a stooping posture.

Rush of blood to the head.

Heat in the head (and in the face).

A cold pressure on the top of the head.

Headache, a dull pain in the morning immediately on waking up, or in the afternoon when walking rapidly or speaking loudly.

Headache on one side, with a certain periodicity (after 28, 14 or a less number of days), more frequently during full moon, or during the new moon, or after mental excitement, after a cold, etc.; a pressure or other pain on top of the head or inside of it, or a boring pain over one of the eyes.

Headache daily at certain hours; *e. g.*, a stitching in the temples.

Attacks of throbbing headache (*e. g.*, in the forehead) with violent nausea as if about to sink down, or, also, vomiting; starting early in the evenings repeated every fortnight, or sooner or later.

Headache as if the skull were about to burst open.

Headache, drawing pains.

Headache, stitches in the head (passing out at the ears).

Roaring noise in the brain, singing, buzzing, humming, thundering, etc.

Rush of blood to the head.

Sometimes he sees everything dim or black on walking or stooping, or raising the head from stooping.

Rush of blood to the head.

Heat in the head and in the face.

Feeling of cold pressure on the head.

Dull headache in the morning, on waking up, or in the afternoon, either on walking fast or speaking loud.

Headache, twinges in the head (coming out by the ears); usually in walking, especially in walking and taking exercise after eating.

Headache, shooting pains in the head coming out by the ears; they often see everything black. Din in the brain, singing, humming, noise, thunder, etc.

Stupefying, pressing, morning headache; > relieved by sweat at night.

Pain from right to left, as if piece of wood were laid on back of head.

Headache preceded by dim vision or dark spots before eyes; extreme dullness, fears inflammation of brain; > by nosebleed followed by darkness before eyes. Cured.—Haynel.

Outer Head—

| Hair: dry, lustreless; tangles easily; glues together; must comb it continually.

|| A man, aet. 28, dark complexion, dark brown hair, had a spot on left frontal region, commencing at edge of hair and extending upward three-fourths of an inch; the skin covering spot was many shades whiter than the surrounding skin, and the lock of hair growing on it had turned perfectly white; after Psoright hair and spot became natural colour.

|| Sensation as if head was separated from body.

Averse to having head uncovered; wears a fur cap in hot weather.

Viscid sweat about head.

Whole head burns.

Pustules, boils on head, mostly scalp, which looks dirty and emits an offensive odor.

| | Moist, suppurating, fetid, also dry eruptions on scalp.

| Scurfy eruption of children; large yellow vesicles around and between scabs.

| Profusely suppurating fetid eruption on head; rawness and soreness behind ears.

Large humid blotches on head, with scabby eruptions on face.

Pustules and boils on head, containing large quantities of pus; severe itching, causing child to scratch so violently that blood flows; formation of thick, dirty, yellow scabs, which when removed show a raw surface from which a yellow lymph exudes, which makes the linen stiff; after removal new scabs form; eruption spreads on nape of neck, scalp and most of forehead; the eruption is of very offensive odor; such large quantity of lymph is exuded that head seems to stick to pillow; child very restless, scratches head violently, and if prevented becomes irritable and screams; large pustules on arms and body, which show no tendency to heal.

| Eruption on head, particularly on occiput, completely hiding scalp from view; profuse exudation, soiling pillow at night and causing excoriation of skin of nape of neck; offensive smelling; innumerable lice.

| Humid, scabby itching; offensive smelling eruption on head, full of lice; glandular swellings.

| Head so covered with eruptions that no part of scalp was visible.

| Eruption on head: with swelling of glands; with urticaria.

| | Tinea capitis et faciei.

| Crusta serpiginosa.

The scalp full of dandruff, with or without itching.

Eruption on the head, tinea capitis, malignant tinea with crusts of greater or less thickness, with sensitive stitches when one of the places becomes moist; when it becomes moist a violent itching; the whole crown of the head painfully sensitive to the open air; with it hard swellings of the glands in the neck.

The hair of the head as if parched.

The hair of the head frequently falls out, most in front, on the crown and top of the head; bald spots or beginning baldness of certain spots.

Under the skin are formed painful lumps, which come and pass away, like bumps and round tumors.

Feeling of contraction in the skin of the scalp and the face.

The hairy scalp is covered with scales, with or without itching.

Eruptions on the head, scald, malignant scabs (the crust being more or less thick), with shooting pains when a liquid is oozing out; intolerable itching during the wet stage; the whole top of the head painfully affected by the open air; at the same time hard glandular swellings on the back part of the neck.

Hair feels as if it were dried; hair falling out abundantly, especially on the forepart and on the top of the head, or in the centre of the crown, or baldness of some places.

Painful tubercles on the skin of the head, coming and going, like boils; round tumors; in rare cases they terminate in suppuration.

Sensation of constriction in the skin of the head and face.

Eyes and Sight—

Aversion to light.

|| Great photophobia, walks with eyes bent upon ground; scurfy eruption on face.

| Photophobia: when walking in open air; with inflammation of lids.

| Fiery sparks before eyes.

| Objects seem to tremble for a few moments and get dark.

| Confusedness before eyes after anxiety.

Vision blurred; black spots before eyes; flickering; dancing about of objects.

| Darkness before eyes and ringing in ears.

Amnaurosis, with scabby eruption on occiput and ears.

| Serous choroiditis; some ciliary congestion and great haziness of vitreous, so that optic nerve was only discerned with great difficulty and then was found decidedly hyperemic, as was the whole fundus; headache, especially in morning; constant profuse sweating of palms of hands.

|| Lids spasmodically closed; intense photophobia and profuse flow of hot tears; much pustular eruption on face; large brown scab on right eye, from beneath which pus pours forth abundantly when touched; bowels costive; appetite poor and only for dainties. Pustular keratitis.

| Recurrent pustular inflammation of cornea and conjunctiva; chronic form; scrofulous basis.

Pterygium.

Eyes feel tired in evening.

| Lachrymation.

Stitches in eyes.

Soreness of eyes and burning, must close them frequently.

Heat and redness of eyes with pressing pains.

Burning, pressing pains in eyes.

| Heat, redness and pressure in eyes; tendency to catarrhal inflammation; lids slightly agglutinated during morning.

| Inflammation of eyes with burning.

Eyes water, inflamed; hurt so she can scarcely open them; pains over eyebrows, down nose, also back of head; complained mostly of head.

Right eye inflamed, pressure as from foreign body when lids are closed.

| Ophthalmia, with pressing pains, as if sand were in eyes.

|| Right eye red, internally and externally; vesicles on cornea; eruption on head.

| Acute ciliary blepharitis; internal surface of lid chiefly affected; photophobia; strumous diathesis, with unhealthy, offensive discharges.

Ciliary blepharitis right to left, < morning and during day; chronic cases; subject to exacerbations.

| Scrofulous inflammation of eyes; ulceration of cornea.

| Rheumatic, chronic and blepharophthalmia. Eyes become gummy.

| Inflammation of lids, internal surface much congested; great photophobia, cannot open eyes, lies on face.

Eyelids: swollen; inflamed; bloated; child rubs eyes; puffy; greatly swollen, closely pressed together; thickened; tendency to styes; itching, especially in canthi; herpetic eruption; scrofulous inflammation, covered with thick crusts, whole body covered with branlike tetter.

Eyes much inflamed, left more than right; supra-orbital pain; profuse lachrymation; intolerance of light, must bury face in pillow; tear-sac very sensitive.

The right eye feels as if moulding away.

Pressive pain on the eyes, especially late in the evening; he must shut them.

He cannot look long at anything, else everything flickers before him; objects seem to move.

The eyelids, especially in the morning, are as if closed; he cannot open them (for minutes, sometimes even for hours); the eyelids are heavy as if paralyzed or convulsively closed.

The eyes are most sensitive to daylight; they are pained by it, it makes them smart, and they close involuntarily.

Sensation of cold in the eyes.

The canthi are full of pus-like mucus (eye-gum).

The edges of the eyelids full of dry mucus.

The meibomian glands round the edges of one of the eyelids are inflamed, either one or more (stye).

On the edges of the eyelids, inflammation of single meibomian glands or of several of them.

Inflammation of the eyes, of various kinds.

Yellowness around the eyes.

Yellowness of the white of the eye.

Dim, opaque spots on the cornea.

Dropsy of the eye.

Obscuration of the crystalline lens, cataract; squinting.

Far-sightedness; he sees far in the distance, but cannot clearly distinguish small objects held close.

Short-sightedness; he can see even small objects by holding them close to the eye, but the more distant the object is, the more indistinct it appears, and at a great distance he does not see it.

False vision; he sees objects double, or manifold, or only the one-half of them.

Before his eyes there are floating as it were flies, or black points, or dark streaks, or networks, especially when looking into bright daylight.

The eyes seem to look through a veil or a mist; the sight becomes dim at certain times.

Night-blindness; he sees well in daytime, but, in the twilight, he cannot see at all.

Blindness by day; he can only see well during the twilight.

Amaurosis; uninterrupted dimness of vision increased finally even to blindness.

Hearing and Ears—

Singing, cracking, humming, buzzing and ringing in ears with hardness of hearing.

Sensation as if he heard with ears not his own.

Severe pain in ear, confined him to bed for four days; ear swollen; thought pain would drive him crazy.

| Discharge of reddish earwax or fetid pus.

|| Otorrhea: with headache; thin, ichorous and horribly offensive, like rotten meat; very offensive, purulent (watery, stinking diarrhea); brown, offensive, from left ear, for almost four years; chronic cases following scarlet fever.

| Ulceration of membrana tympani.

| Itching in ears; child can hardly be kept from picking or boring in meatus.

| Meatus externus scabby.

| External ears raw, red, oozing, scabby; sore pain behind ears.

Soreness of whole external ear, with abundant yellow, offensive smelling discharge; severe itching < in evening and lasting till midnight, preventing sleep and nearly driving him crazy; loss of appetite; great despondency.

Herpes from temples over ears to cheeks; at times throws off innumerable scales; at others shows painful rhagades with yellow discharge, forming scurfs; fetid humor; itching intolerable.

|| Right ear a mass of crusts and pus, the crusts extended behind auricle to occiput upward upon parietal bone nearly to vertex, forward to right ear and over cheek; upon edge of region involved small vesicles filled with clear fluid, which became yellow, then crusted, and pus flowed from beneath crusts.

Humid soreness behind ear.

|| Scurfs on ears, and humid scurfs behind ear.

Scabby eczema behind right ear came out, curing child's old dry deafness.

| Pustules: on and behind concha; behind left ear.

The hearing is excessively irritated and sensitive; she cannot bear to hear a bell ring without trembling; he is thrown into convulsions by the beating of the drum, etc.; many sounds cause pains in the ear.

There are stitches in the ear, outwardly.

Crawling sensation and itching in the ear.

Dryness in the ear; dry scabs within, without any earwax.

Running from ear of thin, usually ill-smelling pus.

Pulsation in the ear.

Various sounds and noises in the ear.

Deafness of various degrees even up to total deafness, with or without noise in the ear; occasionally worse, according to the weather.

Swelling of the parotid glands.

A brown-coloured offensive discharge from the left ear for four years.

Ears: pain in ear so severe as to confine him to bed for five days. External ear much swollen. Thought the pain in his ear would make him insane. Soreness in jaw, right side, around the ear; could not use his mouth, because of the contraction and pain; could scarcely crowd his fingers between his teeth.

Ears: man, aged 40, discharge of reddish cerumen from left ear < at night; had troubled him for many years. Sensation of valve opening and shutting in left ear < in afternoon. Buzzing in ear which stopped suddenly and was followed by violent itching. Dull, heavy pain in base of brain in afternoon, with sensation as though skin of abdomen was greatly relaxed and drawn down. Face sallow and greasy. Many pustules on skin and neck, which itch intensely and bleed easily when scratched.—*G. A. Whippy.*

Nose and Smell—

Loss of smell; with coryza.

Smell of blood.

Soreness of nose; nose sensitive when inhaling air.

Boring, stinging in right nostril, followed by excessive sneezing.

Burning followed by thin nasal discharge, which relieves.

|| Dry coryza with stoppage of nose.

|| Septum narium inflamed, with white, suppurating pustules.

Tough mucus in nose; feels like a plug there; it nauseates him; > when stooping.

Catarrh, with cough and expectoration of yellow-green mucus.

|| Bloody, purulent discharge from nose.

|| Chronic catarrh; dropping from posterior nares, so as to awaken him at night; hawking quantities of lumpy mucus gave temporary relief from feeling of fullness; mucus in nose would dry like white of egg, needed to be forcibly removed.

|| Pain in liver, < from sneezing.

| Acne rosacea.

Epistaxis, more or less profusely, more or less frequently.

The nostrils as it were stopped up.

Sensation of dryness in the nose, troublesome even when the air passes freely.

Polypi of the nose (usually with the loss of the power of smelling); these may extend also through the nasal passages into the fauces.

Sense of smell, weak, lost.

Sense of smell perverted.

Too violent sensation of smell, higher and highest sensitiveness for even imperceptible odors.

Scabs in the nose; discharge of pus or hardened clots of mucus.

Fetid smell in the nose.

Nostrils frequently ulcerated, surrounded with pimples and scabs.

Swelling and redness of the nose or the tip of the nose, frequent or continual.

Coryza at once, whenever she comes into the open air; then usually a stuffed coryza while in her room.

Dry coryza and a stuffed nose often, or almost constantly, also sometimes with intermissions.

Fluent coryza at the least taking of cold, therefore mostly in the inclement season and when it is wet.

Fluent coryza, very often, or almost constantly, also in some cases uninterruptedly.

He cannot take cold, even though there have been strong

premonitory symptoms of it, simultaneously with other great ailments from the itch malady.

Chronic catarrh: constant dropping from posterior nares awakens patient at night; hawking quantities of lumpy mucus with temporary > from sensation of fulness; mucus in nose would dry like white of an egg, needing to be forcibly removed. Psorinum 200th cured.

Face—

Face: pale, yellow, sickly; broad blue rings around eyes; bluish appearance; burning heat and redness; swollen, with eruption.

|| Painful tension and pressure in right zygoma, towards ear.

Cheek bones pain as if ulcerated.

|| Pain as if lame in condyle of jaw.

|| Sweat of face with general heat.

| Much roughness of skin of face; eruption on forehead between eyes; stools very offensive. Eczema. Scrofulous ophthalmia.

| Scabby face; especially cheeks from ears; lips and eyelids swollen, sore about eyes.

| Crusta lactea on face and scalp, especially over either ear and cheek, exfoliating numerous scabs, or it cracks and discharges a yellow, fetid humor.

|| Moist scab behind ears with dry tetter on back of head, on both cheeks extending upward to eyes and downward to corners of mouth, reddish, very closely packed, millet-seed-like, itching, dry pimples, with frequent loose stools; a child one and a half years old.

|| An offensive-smelling, crusty eruption extending over whole face for three months, had completely closed eyes.

|| Eruption on face of a child; whole face covered with a crust, lips and eyelids swollen, aversion to light, large moistening spots on head and behind ears.

| Humid eruptions on face; whole face covered with hu-

mid scurfs or crusts, with swelling of lips and eyelids and humid soreness behind ears.

Pimples on forehead.

Red, small pimples on face, especially on nose, chin and middle of cheeks.

| Closely packed, itching pimples on both cheeks from eyes to corners of mouth.

| Ulcers in face.

| Coppery eruption on face.

| Tinea faciei.

| Lips: painful; swollen, particularly upper; dry; burning; brown and black, dry; ulcerated; swollen and covered with scurfs.

| Corners of mouth sore, often ulcerated; sycotic condylomata.

Soreness of jaw, right side, around ear; could not open wide enough to admit fingers.

Submaxillary and lingual glands swollen, sore to touch; at same time suppurating pustules on same place.

Paleness of the face during the first sleep, with blue rings around the eyes.

Erysipelas on the face.

Frequent redness of the face, and heat.

Yellowish, yellow colour of the face.

Sallow yellowish complexion.

Gray, yellow colour of the face.

Painfulness of various spots on the face, the cheeks, the cheek-bones, the lower jaw, etc., when touched; while chewing, as if festering inwardly; also like stitches and jerks; especially in chewing there are jerks, stitches and a tension so that he cannot eat.

Under the nose or on the upper lip, long-lasting scales or itching pimples.

The red of the lips is quite pale.

The red of the lips is dry, scabby, peeling off; it chaps.

Swelling of the lips, especially of the upper lip.

The inside of the lips is lined with little sores or blisters.

Cutaneous eruptions of the beard and of the roots of the hairs of the beard, with itching.

Eruptions of the face of innumerable kinds.

Glands of the lower jaw swollen, sometimes passing over into chronic suppuration.

Glandular swellings down the sides of the neck.

TEETH AND GUMS.—Stitching in teeth from one side to other, radiating to head, with burning in right cheek, which is swollen.

Sensation of soreness of teeth.

Stinging in teeth (while eating).

|| Looseness of teeth; they feel so loose, fears they may fall out, < from touch, especially from teeth.

| Toothache: < at night and from cold; > from warmth.

| Gums: ulcerated, bleeding.

Gums bleeding at a slight touch.

Gums, the external or the internal, painful, as if from wounds.

Gums, with erosive itching.

Gums, whitish, swollen, painful on touching.

Gums, recession, leaving the front teeth and their roots bare.

Gnashing of the teeth during sleep.

Looseness of the teeth, and many kinds of deterioration of the teeth, even without toothache.

Toothache of innumerable varieties, with varying causes of excitation.

She cannot remain in bed at night, owing to toothache.

Taste and Tongue—

| Loss of taste with coryza.

Taste: bitter, goes off when eating or drinking; foul, much

mucus in mouth; > in fresh air; bitter with yellow-coated tongue; flat, sticky, dinner tastes oily.

Tongue: dry, tip feels burnt as far as middle, he has hardly any taste; tip very dry, as if burnt, painful; white, yellow; thickly coated with whitish-yellow slime; ulcerated.

On the tongue, painful blisters and sore places.

Tongue white, coated white or furred white.

Tongue pale, bluish white.

Tongue full of deep furrows; here and there, as if torn above.

Tongue dry.

Sensation of dryness on tongue, even while it is properly moist.

Stuttering, stammering; also at times sudden attacks of inability to speak.

Mouth—

Adhesion of tough mucus to posterior surface of soft palate, necessitating hawking.

Tough mucus in mouth of a foul, nauseous taste, teeth stick together as if glued.

Dryness of mouth; burning.

Tickling, burning; mouth inflamed, sore, < from warm food; not annoyed by cold food.

Blisters inside lower lips; burning, painful.

| Ulcers in mouth.

On the inside of the cheeks painful blisters or sores.

Flow of blood from the mouth; often severe.

Sensation of dryness of the whole internal mouth, or merely in spots, or deep down in the throat.

Fetid smell from the mouth.

Burning in the throat.

Mouth inflamed and sore; < from warm food, but not annoyed by cold.

Constant flow of saliva, especially while speaking, particularly in the morning.

Continual spitting of saliva.

Insipid, slimy taste in mouth.

Intolerably sweet taste in the mouth, almost constantly.

Bitter taste in the mouth, mostly in the morning.

Sourish and sour taste in the mouth, especially after eating, though the food tasted all right.

Putrid and fetid taste in the mouth.

Bad smell in the mouth, sometimes mouldy, sometimes putrid like old cheese, or like fetid foot-sweat, or like rotten sour-krout.

Throat—

| Accumulation of mucus in throat and mouth.

Tough mucus in throat, hawking. Typhoid.

|| Sensation of a plug or lump in throat impeding hawking.

| Dryness in throat with thirstlessness.

|Dryness; scraping sensation in throat.

|| Throat burns, feels scalded.

|| Tension and swollen feeling in throat.

Difficult swallowing, throat feels swollen.

Pain when swallowing saliva.

|| Cutting tearing pain in throat on swallowing.

11 Steam arising from fat causes immediate constriction of throat and chest.

Severe angina; on right side an ulcer, with a sore pain deep inside and burning in fauces.

Tonsilitis; submaxillary glands swollen; fetid otorrhea.

Ulcerated sore throat.

Ulcers on right side, with deep-seated pain and burning in fauces.

Frequently mucus deep down in the throat (the fauces), which he has to hawk up with great exertion and expectorate frequently during the day, especially in the morning.

Frequently inflammation of the throat, and swelling of the parts used in swallowing.

Appeite, Thirst, Desires, Aversions—

Good appetite, with daily attacks of anxiety, easily satisfied; great hunger, even after a hearty meal; canine hunger preceding attacks (diarrhea).

| Diminished appetite: after typhus; but great thirst; during convalescence.

|| Thirst: during dinner; with dryness of throat; especially for beer, mouth feels so dry.

Desire for acids.

Loathing of pork.

Ravenous hunger at midnight, waking from sleep.

Eating and Drinking—

While eating ceases complaining.

|| Immediately after dinner, congestion of blood to head.

|| Pain in chest extending to shoulder, < after cold drinks.

| Drinking causes cough.

Hiccough, Belching, Nausea and Vomiting—

Eructations: sour, rancid; tasting and smelling like rotten eggs; room is filled with an offensive odor. Arn., Graph., Ant. t. Arn.— especially in A.M.; Ant. t.—at night; Graph, in A.M. only, after rising, disappearing on rinsing the mouth.

|| Waterbrash when lying down, > on getting up.

| Nausea: with poor appetite; in morning; with backache, after suppressed itch; morning with pain in small of back; all day, with vomiting.

Vomiturition, followed by vomiting, first of blood, then of sour, slimy fluid.

Constant nausea during the day, with inclination to vomit; a kind of vomiting of sweet mucus every morning at ten and in evening.

Vomiting of sour mucus in morning before eating.

Eructations, with the taste of the food, several hours after eating.

Eructations, empty, loud, of mere air, uncontrollable, often for hours, not infrequently at night.

Incomplete eructation, which causes merely convulsive shocks in the fauces, without coming out of the mouth; spasmodic straining in the esophagus.

Eructation, sour, either fasting or after food, especially after milk.

Eructation, which excites to vomiting.

Eructation, rancid (especially after eating fat things).

Eructation, putrid or mouldy, early in the morning.

Frequent eructations before meals, with a sort of rabid hunger.

Heart-burn, more or less frequent; there is a burning along the chest, especially after breakfast, or while moving the body.

Water-brash, a gushing discharge of a sort of salivary fluid from the stomach, preceded by writhing pains in the stomach (the pancreas), with a sensation of weakness (shakiness), nausea causing as it were a swoon, and gathering of the saliva in the mouth, even at night.

The ruling complaints in any part of the body are excited after eating fresh fruit, especially if this is acidulous, also after acetic acid (in salads, etc.).

Nausea early in the morning.

Nausea even to vomiting, in the morning immediately after rising from bed, decreasing from motion.

Nausea always after eating fatty things or milk.

Vomiting of blood.

Hiccough after eating or drinking.

Swallowing impeded by spasms, even causing a man to die of hunger.

Spasmodic, involuntary swallowing.

Scrobiculum and Stomach—

Stitching pain in pit of stomach.

|| Weakness of stomach.

|| Frequent oppression of stomach, especially after eating.

Cramps in stomach.

| Dyspepsia; eructations, flatus and stools like spoiled eggs.

|| Gastric bilious affections.

Frequent sensation of fasting and of emptiness in the stomach (or abdomen), not unfrequently with much saliva in the mouth.

Ravenous hunger (canine hunger), especially early in the morning; he has to eat at once else he grows faint, exhausted and shaky (or if he is in the open air he has to lie straight down).

Ravenous hunger with rumbling and grumbling in the abdomen.

Appetite without hunger; he has a desire to swallow down in haste various things without there being any craving therefor in the stomach.

A sort of hunger; but when she then eats ever so little, she feels at once satiated and full.

When she wants to eat, she feels full in the chest and her throat feels as if full of mucus.

Want of appetite; only a sort of gnawing, turning and writhing in the stomach urges her to eat.

Repugnance to cooked, warm food, especially to boiled meat, and hardly any longing for anything but rye-bread (with butter), or for potatoes.

In the morning, at once, thirst; constant thirst.

In the pit of the stomach there is a sensation of swelling, painful to the touch.

Sensation of coldness in the pit of the stomach.

Pressure in the stomach or in the pit of the stomach, as from a stone, or a constricting pain (cramp).

In the stomach beating and pulsation, even when fasting.

Spasm in the stomach; pain in the pit of the stomach as if drawn together.

Griping in the stomach; a painful griping in the stomach; it suddenly constricts the stomach, especially after cold drinking.

Pain in the stomach, as if sore, when eating the most harmless kinds of foods.

Pressure in the stomach, even when fasting, but more from every kind of food, or from particular dishes, fruit, green vegetables, rye-bread, food containing vinegar, etc.

During eating, feels dizzy and giddy, threatening to fall to one side.

After the slightest supper, nocturnal heat in bed; in the morning, constipation and exceeding lassitude.

After meals, anxiety and cold perspiration with anxiety.

During eating, perspiration.

Immediately after eating, vomiting.

After meals, pressure and burning in stomach, or in the epigastrium, almost like heartburn.

After eating, burning in the esophagus from below upward.

Feels shaky and exhausted; wants food continually, or else gets cold and wet all over.

Hypochondria—

|| Deep-seated stitching, pressing pain in region of liver, < from external pressure and lying on right side; pain hinders sneezing, laughing, yawning, coughing, deep inspiration and walking.

Stinging, sharp pain in region of liver and spleen.

| Chronic hepatitis.

Stitches in spleen, > when standing; < when moving, and continuing when again at rest.

| Chronic induration of spleen.

Abdomen–

| Bloated abdomen.

|| Flatulency with disorders of liver.

Constant feeling of emptiness and looseness in abdomen; sensation as if intestines were hanging down.

| Pains in abdomen after eating; flatulency and tendency to diarrhea; > when flatus passes.

Pain in abdomen while riding.

Cutting pain in intestines.

| Colic: removed by eating; > passing fetid flatus.

Painful bearing down, with painful burning micturition.

Stinging, sharp pains in inguinal glands.

Pain through right groin when walking.

Lumps in right groin, preventing stooping.

| Inguinal hernia; hernial sac infiltrated.

| Chronic abdominal affections.

Abdominal affections during climaxis, with a high degree of ill-humor.

After meals, distension of the abdomen.

After meals, very tired and sleepy.

After meals, as if intoxicated.

After meals, headache.

After meals, palpitation of the heart.

Alleviation of several, even remote, complaints from eating.

The flatus does not pass off but moves about, causing many ailments of body and spirit.

The abdomen is distended by flatus, the abdomen feels full, especially after a meal.

Sensation as if the flatus ascended; followed by eructations—then often a sensation of burning in the throat, or vomiting by day or by night.

Pain in the hypochondria when touched, and in motion, or also during rest.

Constricting pain in the epigastrium, immediately under the ribs.

Cutting pains in the abdomen, as if from obstructed flatus; there is a constant sensation of fulness in the abdomen—the flatus rises upwards.

Cutting pains in the abdomen almost daily, especially with children, oftener in the morning than in other parts of the day, sometimes day and night without diarrhea.

Cutting pains in the abdomen, especially on the one side of the abdomen, or the groin.

In the abdomen qualmishness, a sensation of voidness, disagreeable emptiness, even immediately after eating, he felt as if he had not eaten anything.

From the small of the back, around the abdomen, especially below the stomach, a sensation of constriction as from a bandage, after she had had no stool for several days.

Pain in the liver, when touching the right side of the abdomen.

Pain in the liver, a pressure and tension—a tension below the ribs on the right side.

Below the last ribs (in the hypochondria), a tension and pressure all over, which checks the breathing and makes the mind anxious and sad.

Pain in the liver, stitches; mostly when stooping quickly.

Inflammation of the liver.

Pressure in the abdomen as from a stone.

Hardness of the abdomen.

Crampy colic, a grasping pain in the bowels.

In colic, coldness on one side of the abdomen.

A clucking, croaking and audible rumbling and grumbling in the abdomen.

So-called uterine spasms, like labor pains, grasping pains often compelling the patient to lie down, frequently quickly distending the abdomen without flatulence.

In the lower abdomen, pains pressing down towards the genitals.

Inguinal hernias, often painful while speaking and singing.

Swellings of the inguinal glands, which sometimes turn into suppuration.

Stool and Rectum—

Emission of hot, fetid, sulphurous flatus; smelling like rotten eggs.

Stool: normal, but passed in a great hurry, with quantities of flatus; can hardly reach the water-closet. (Aloe.)

Griping and desire for stool while riding.

| Diarrhea, preceded by colic.

| Frequent thin stool, with eruption on head.

Green bilious diarrhea, mixed with mucus; soft, voided with difficulty from weakness.

Stool: dark brown, very fluid and foul-smelling; having the smell of rotten eggs; mostly in children in their first or second summer; green mucus, or bloody mucus; smells like carrion, < at night; frequent, liquid; involuntary; nearly painless.

|| Semiliquid, brownish, indelible, insufferably nasty; passed during sleep, at 1 and 4 A.M., with undigested food. Infantile diarrhea.

|| *Horribly offensive,* nearly painless, almost involuntary, dark and watery stool; only at night and most towards morning.

| | *Involuntary stool* during sleep.

|| Boy, act. four months, whitish bad-smelling diarrhea; constantly crying, with drawing up of knees as if in pain; rattling cough, cries all night; acts as if he had earache in left ear, from which there was a slight discharge; seldom urinates; after second dose, sixteen hours after first, broke out all over his head and face, with a small pimply eruption, a vesicle at the apex of each pimple, which exuded lymph which dried in a

thick brown scab, which gradually fell off in a day or two, and in two weeks left the skin perfectly clean.

| Diarrhea: after severe acute disease; at night; early in morning; when rising in morning; in childbed; when weather changes (general condition).

Before stool: griping pains about navel.

| Cases which do not respond promptly to the indicated remedy, the children having dirty, yellow, greasy skin, with a partially developed eruption on forehead and chest, with constant fretting and worrying.

| Lienteria.

| Chronic diarrhea; offensive stools.

| Cholera infantum; stools dark brown, watery, of an intolerably offensive odor; liquid, mucous or bloody and excessively fetid.

Cholera infantum in summer; nervous and restless at night, awake at night as if frightened, or cry out during sleep; then two or three nights afterwards, they begin with diarrhea; stools are profuse and watery, dark brown or even black in colour, very offensive, almost putrid in odor, < at night.

Cholera.

| Soft stool: passed with difficulty; from weakness.

| Obstinate constipation: with coryza and obstruction of nose; pain in small of back; blood from rectum; due to torpor of rectum; lasting three or four days, due to inactivity of rectum; stool on third or fourth day was accompanied by severe pains which induced patient to withhold effort as much as possible.

|| Sensitive hemorrhoidal pain in rectum.

| Unpleasant burning in rectum.

Soreness in rectum and anus while riding.

|| Hemorrhage from rectum; in old women large quantities of blood discharged at once, with constipation and hypochondriasis.

Burning hemorrhoidal tumors.

Prolapsus recti, with burning.

Stool: normal, but imperative; passed in a great hurry, with large quantities of flatus; can scarcely reach the toilet.

Prolapsus recti, with intense burning of parts.

Constipation: delayed stools sometimes for several days, not infrequently with repeated ineffectual urging to stool.

Stools hard, as if burnt, in small knots, like sheep-dung, often covered with mucus, sometimes also enveloped by veinlets of blood.

Stools of mere mucus (mucous piles).

Passage of round worms from the anus.

Discharge of pieces of tape-worm.

Stools, in the beginning very hard and troublesome, followed by diarrhea.

Very pale, whitish stool.

Gray stools.

Green stools.

Clay-coloured stools.

Stools with putrid, sour smell.

At the stools, cutting pains in the rectum.

Stools show diarrhea for several weeks, months, years.

Frequently repeated diarrhea, with cutting pains in the abdomen, lasting several days.

After stool, especially after a softer, more copious evacuation, great and sudden prostration.

Diarrhea soon weakening, that she cannot walk alone.

Painless and painful hemorrhoidal varices on the anus, in the rectum (blind piles).

Bleeding hemorrhoidal varices on the anus or in the rectum (running piles), especially during stools, after which the hemorrhoids often pain violently for a long time.

With bloody discharges in the anus or in the rectum, ebullition of blood through the body and short breathing.

Formication and itching formication in the rectum, with or without the discharge of ascarides.

Itching and erosion in the anus and the perineum.

Polypi in the rectum.

Cholera infantum: obstinate, which seemed to defy the best selected remedy. Stool very thin and watery; dirty, greenish, smelled like carrion. Child very fretful, had no sleep for two days and nights. Psorinum 4 cm., one dose. In two hours child went to sleep, and in four hours was well, without a repetition.— *W. A. Hawley.*

Urinary Organs—

|| Involuntary urine, cannot hold it; vesical paresis. Typhus.

|Enuresis: wets bed at night; again during full moon; obstinate cases.

|| Scanty urination nearly every half hour, with burning in urethra and in condylomata.

Urine: dark brown, with reddish sediment; loaded with pus; frequent, scanty; burning and cutting in urethra; thick whitish; turbid; red deposit; cuticle forms on surface; profuse.

During micturition, anxiety, also at times prostration.

At times too much urine is discharged, succeeded by great weariness.

Painful retention of urine (with children and old people).

When he is chilled (feels cold through and through), he cannot urinate.

At times, owing to flatulence, she cannot urinate.

The urethra is constricted in parts, especially in the morning.

Pressure on the bladder, as if from an urging to urinate, immediately after drinking.

He cannot hold the urine for any length of time, it presses on the bladder, and passes off while he walks, sneezes, coughs or laughs.

Frequent micturition at night; he has to get up frequently at night for that purpose.

Urine passes off in sleep involuntarily.

After urinating, the urine continues to drip out for a long time.

Whitish urine, with a sweetish smell and taste, passes off in excessive abundance, with prostration, emaciation and inextinguishable thirst (diabetes).

During urination, burning, also lancinating pains in the urethra and the neck of the bladder.

Urine of penetrating, sharp odor.

The urine quickly deposits a sediment.

The urine discharged is at once turbid like whey.

With the urine there is discharged from time to time a red sand (kidney grits).

Dark-yellow urine.

Brown urine.

Blackish urine.

Urine with blood particles, also at times complete hematuria.

Male Sexual Organs—

Excessive, uncontrollable sexual instinct.

| Aversion to coition; impotence; want of emission during coitus.

| Absence of erections; parts flabby, torpid.

Prostatic fluid discharged before urinating.

Drawing pains in testicles and spermatic cords.

Inflamed ulcer on glans, with swelling arid heaviness of testicles.

|| After suppressed gonorrhea; rheumatism, lameness; conjunctivitis, with granulations; intense photophobia; pain darting around, through head; other eye sensitive to light.

| Chronic painless discharge from urethra, leaving yellow stain upon linen.

|| Gleet of twelve years' duration.

|| Seven large, moist, itching, occasionally burning

condylomata on prepuce; every night nocturnal enuresis; during day must urinate nearly every half hour; urination scanty and accompanied by burning in urethra and condylomata; lips ulcerated, particularly at corners of mouth; in several localities, but particularly in popliteal spaces, dry, herpetic eruption, not itching.

| | Sycotic excrescence on edges of prepuce, with itching and burning.

| | Boy, aet. 7, suffering since birth; r-sided inguinal hernia, about three inches of intestine descending to testicle through widely opened inguinal canal; upon applying a bandage severe inflammation of tunica vaginalis occurred, which yielded to Pulsat., bat returned every time bandage was applied; child gradually grew miserable and thin and lost all appetite; fever set in, and a large amount of water collected in tunica vaginalis; as the case improved a painful, burning, itching excoriation with acrid discharge appeared upon inner surface of prepuce and upon corona glandis.

Hydrocele.

| |Hydrocele, caused by repeated inflammation, in consequence of pressure from a truss.

Discharge of prostatic fluid after urination, but especially after a difficult stool (also almost constant dripping of the same).

Nocturnal passage of semen, too frequent, one, two or three times a week, or even every night.

Nightly discharge of the genital fluid in women, with voluptuous dreams.

Nocturnal pollutions, even if not frequent, yet immediately attended with evil consequences.

Semen passes off. almost involuntarily in daytime, with little excitation, often even without erection.

Erections very frequent, long continuing, very painful, without pollutions.

The semen is not discharged, even during a long continued coition and with a proper erection, but it passes off afterwards in nocturnal pollutions or with the urine.

Accumulation of water in the tunica vaginalis of the testicle (hydrocele).

There is never a complete erection, even with the most voluptuous excitement.

Painful twitches in muscles of the penis.

Itching of the scrotum, which is sometimes beset with pimples and scabs.

One or both of the testicles chronically swollen, or showing a knotty induration *(Sarcocele).*

Dwindling, diminution, disappearance of one or both testicles.

Induration and enlargement of the prostatic gland.

Drawing pain in the testicle and the spermatic chord.

Pain as from contusion in the testicle.

Lack of the sexual desire in both sexes, either frequent or constant.

Uncontrollable, insatiable lasciviousness, with a cachectic complexion and sickly body.

Sterility, impotence, without any original organic defect in the sexual parts.

Female Sexual Organs—

|| Left ovary indurated after a violent knock; followed by itching eruption on body and face.

|| Knotty lump above right groin; even a bandage hurts.

Pinching in pubic region in women.

Cutting in left loin; cannot walk without assistance.

|| Metrorrhagia.

Menses delayed and scanty.

Amenorrhea: in psoric subjects when tetter is covered by thick scurfs; with phthisis.

|| Dysmenorrhea near climaxis.

|| Menstrual disorders during climaxis.

|| Leucorrhea, large lumps, unbearable in odor; violent pains in sacrum and right loin; great debility.

| Ulcers of the labia.

Disorders of the menstrual function; the menses do not appear regularly on the twenty-eighth day after their last appearance, they do not come on without other ailments and not at once, and do not continue steadily for three or four days with a moderate quantity of healthy coloured, mild blood, until on the fourth day it imperceptibly comes to an end without any disturbance of the general health of body and spirit; nor are the menses continued to the forty-eighth or fiftieth year, nor do they cease gradually and without any troubles.

The menses are slow in setting in after the fifteenth year and later, or after appearing one or more times, they cease for several months and for years.

The menses do not keep their regular periods, they either come several days too early, sometimes every three weeks, or even every fortnight.

The menses flow only one day, only a few hours, or in imperceptibly small quantities.

The menses flow for five, six, eight and more days, but only intermittently, a little flow every six, twelve, twenty-four hours, and then they cease for half or whole days, before more is discharged.

The menses flow too strongly for weeks, or return almost daily (bloody flux).

Menses of watery blood or of brown clots of blood.

Menses of very fetid blood.

Menses accompanied with many ailments, swoons or (mostly stitching) headaches, or contractive, spasmodic, cutting pains in the abdomen and in the small of the back; she is obliged to lie down, vomit, etc.

Polypi in the vagina.

Leucorrhea from the vagina, one or several days before, or soon after, the monthly flow of blood, or during the whole time from the one menstrual discharge to the other, with a diminution of the menses, or continuing solely instead of the menses; the flow is like milk, or like white, or yellow mucus, or like acrid, or sometimes like fetid, water.

Pelvic tumor, pronounced malignant by Dright Macdonald; after opening abdomen refused to remove it on account of adhesions; urine loaded with pus; stool involuntary and horribly offensive, nurses could not endure it. Psor. 30 cured.—S. -S. *Mofatt*.

A lady, 32, had severe fever, temperature from 103 to 105, attended with headache, backache and cramps in muscles of limbs, with severe abdominal and pelvic pains, the result of instrumental abortion. As the acute symptoms passed off, there was a great fear and mental restlessness, which Aconite failed to relieve.

Each evening at 6, would become restless and break out in profuse icy cold sweat, continued all night, very exhausting, not > by external heat. As evening approached, great fear of the on-coming cold sweat and icy chilliness. With the cold copious sweat was a foul taste and very offensive odoright Psorinum dmm., one dose dry on tongue >.

Parturition. Pregnancy. Lactation—

| During pregnancy: fetus moves too violently; abdomen tympanitic; nausea; vomiting; obstinate cases.

|| Mammae swollen, painful; redness of nipples, burning around them.

|| Pimples itching violently, about nipples; oozing a fluid. Second month of pregnancy.

|| Mammary cancer.

Dwindling of the breasts, or excessive enlargement of the same, with retroceding nipples.

Erysipelas on one of the breasts (especially while nursing).

A hard, enlarging and indurating gland with lancinating pains in one of the mammae.

Itching, also moist and scaly eruptions around the nipples.

Premature births.

During pregnancies great weariness, nausea, frequent vomiting, swoons, painful varicose veins on the thighs and the legs, and also at times on the labia, hysteric ailments of various kinds, etc.

Mrs. H. E. L., aged 56, had an attack of acute peritonitis two years ago, involving especially the right lower abdomen; has never been well since, having persistent attacks of pain in right inguinal region, so severe that her attending physician always resorted to Morphine.

The concomitant symptoms were easily controlled, but on their disappearance the attacks of pain increased in frequency and violence. Physical examination revealed adhesive bands, which contracted the vagina, and involved the right broad ligament and right ovary, which was apparently firmly bound down to the side of the pelvis. The pain was aggravated by moving the limb; walking; standing erect; lying on the painful side. After attempting in vain for months to relieve the localized pain by the careful selection of a remedy, with only temporary relief, certain to be followed by a more severe relapse, in desperation Psorinum was given; the pains disappeared and have never returned, notwithstanding the pathological diagnosis.

A lady, 32, had severe fever, temperature from 103 to 105, attended with headache, backache and cramps in muscles of limbs, with severe abdominal and pelvic pains, the result of instrumental abortion. As the acute symptoms passed off, there was great fear and mental restlessness, which Aconite failed to relieve.

Each evening at 6, would become restless and break out in profuse icy-cold sweat, continued all night, very exhausting, not > by external heat. As evening approached, great fear of the on-coming cold sweat and icy chilliness. With the cold, copious sweat, was a foul taste and very offensive odor. Psorinum dmm., one dose dry on tongue >

Voice and Larynx. Trachea and Bronichia—

| Hoarseness; when talking, phlegm sticks in larynx.

| Talking is very fatiguing.

|| Voice weak, trembling.

| Suffocative and crawling sensation in larynx, producing a paroxysmal, dry, hacking cough.

Tickling, throat as if narrowing, must cough to relieve it.

|| For eleven years hay fever, coming on about 20th of August.

Hoarseness, after the least amount of speaking; she must vomit in order to clear her voice.

Hoarseness, also sometimes aphony (she cannot speak loud but must whisper), after a slight cold.

Constant hoarseness and aphony for years; he cannot speak a loud word.

uppuration of the larynx and the bronchia (laryngo-bronchial phthisis).

Hoarseness and catarrh very often, or almost constantly; his chest is continually affected.

Cough; there is frequently an irritation and a crawling in the throat; the cough torments him, until sweat breaks out upon the face (and upon the hands).

Respiration—

| Short breath or want of breath.

|| Convalescents go out for a walk, instead of being invigorated return home in order to get breath or to lie down so they can breathe more easily, feel < instead of > from being in open air.

Chest expands with great difficulty; cannot get breath.

Anxious dyspnea, with palpitation and pain in cardiac region.

| *Dyspnea: < when sitting up to write, > when lying down,* congestion to head after dinner, great despondency; < *the nearer arms are brought to body.*

Must keep arms spread wide apart.

| Asthma, as if he would die; precursor of hydrothorax.

Stitches from behind forward, in chest and back, when breathing.

Want of breath in open air, must hurry.

Obstruction of the breath, with stitching pains in the chest at the slightest amount of walking, he cannot go a step farther (angina pectoris).

Asthma, merely when moving the arms, not while walking.

Attacks of suffocation especially after midnight; the patient has to sit up, sometimes he has to leave his bed, stand stooping forward, leaning on his hands; he has to open the windows, or get out into the open air, etc.; he has palpitations; these are followed by eructations or yawning, and the spasm terminates with or without coughing and expectoration.

Palpitation with anxiety, especially at night.

Asthma, loud, difficult, at times also sibilant respiration.

Shortness of breath.

Asthma, on moving, with or without cough.

Asthma, mostly while sitting down.

Asthma, spasmodic; when she comes into the open air it takes her breath.

Asthma, in attacks, lasting several weeks.

Cough—

Cough: from tickling in larynx; dry, hard, caused by tickling in trachea; in evening with pains in chest and throat, passing off when she is quiet; produced by talking; with sensation of weakness in chest; dry, with sensation of heaviness in chest; dry, with soreness under sternum, with stitches in chest; dry, with constricting pain in chest; < mornings when awaking and evenings on lying down; coughs a long time before expectorating; periodic attacks; chronic, spasmodic; of twenty-five years duration.

|| Severe, dry cough with oppression of chest and pain

as if everything in chest were raw and scratched; fever in evening; great depression of spirits, making life burdensome to him.

|| Cough, causing tearing from centre of chest to throat, all on right side; cough < at night; urine escapes when coughing.

An old, dull cough, palpitation and a fixed pain in chest disappear, the entire feeling is better, only the lower white of eye turns red and ulcers form on it, eye waters, without pain, with photophobia, > in fresh air.

|| Dry cough, pain in the chest for last three months, a constricting pressure at fourth and fifth ribs near sternum, excessive irritability and ill-humor.

|| Cough with expectoration; asthma, thinks he will die.

Cough with expectoration of green mucus, nearly like matter; especially in morning when waking and in evening when lying down, with nausea; it sticks firmly and he can only expectorate with difficulty.

|| Cough with salty-tasting, green and yellow expectoration; oppression of chest; gradual loss of strength; after suppressed itch.

| Expectoration: of blood with hot sensation in chest; yellowish-green.

| Chronic blennorrhea of lungs, threatening phthisis. Drinking causes cough.

|| Cough aggravates pain in liver and pain in chest extending to shoulder.

Cough; frequent irritation and crawling in the throat; the cough torments him, until perspiration breaks out on his face (and on his hands).

Cough, which does not abate until there is retching and vomiting, mostly in the morning or in the evening.

Cough, which terminates every time with sneezing.

Cough mostly in the evening after lying down and whenever the head lies low.

Cough, waking the patient up after the first brief sleep.

Cough, especially in the night.

Cough, worst after awaking in the morning.

Cough, worst after eating.

Cough, at once with every deep breath.

Cough, causing a sensation of soreness in the chest, or at times stitches in the side of the chest or the abdomen.

Dry cough.

Cough, with yellow expectoration resembling pus, with or without spitting of blood.

Cough, with excessive expectoration of mucus and sinking of the strength (mucous phthisis) .

Attacks of spasmodic cough (whooping cough).

Inner Chest and Lungs—

Oppression: in chest; anxious, every morning; with cough.

Pressure on chest.

Burning pressing pain in chest.

Pain in chest, great anxiety by spells.

|| Constriction of chest when inhaling steam from fat.

Excruciating pains in chest.

Cutting as of knives in chest.

Feels as if everything were torn in chest.

Whole chest feels sore.

At times bruised, suppurative pain through whole chest, extending towards right shoulder and becoming fixed there; < after frequent coughing; after cold drinks.

|| Pain in chest, as if raw, as from subcutaneous ulceration.

Ulcerative pain in chest under sternum.

|| Stitches: in sternum, with backache; from behind forward in chest and back when breathing; in right side of chest when breathing; in chest (left side).

Sharp pain, right side, opposite tenth rib.

|| Fixed pain in right side of chest.

Pains in right side of chest < from motion, laughing, coughing, with sweat.

|| Chest pains from coughing.

|| Pains in chest grow more severe two or three times a day, begin with chilliness and trembling, followed by heat one hour in duration; great anxiety of heart and mind with fear of death, dyspnea and restlessness; attacks pass off with sour, clammy sweat and chilliness; sweat however occurs every night independent of attack.

|| Hot sensation in chest.

|| Tedious recovery in pneumonia.

|| Dull pressure in right side of chest, extending thence over whole chest, < bending forward in writing, not by motion or deep inspiration; dry cough with expectoration of small lumps of mucus; speaking affects him very much; great prostration after preaching, so that he must rest a long time to recuperate; voice is not husky, but it requires all his strength to get through with his work; chest narrow, shoulders projecting. Phthisis.

|| Pain in chest comes by fits; great anxiety; a feeling of ulceration under sternum; chest inflates only with much exertion; coughs a long time before beginning to expectorate. Phthisis pulmonalis.

Suppuration of lungs. Phthisis pulmonalis.

| Chronic blenorrhea of lungs.

| Hydrothorax.

Chest symptoms > when lying down.

Violent, at times unbearable, stitches in the chest at every breath; cough impossible for pain; without inflammatory fever (spurious pleurisy).

Pain in the chest on walking, as if the chest was about to burst.

Pressive pain in the chest, at deep breathing or at sneezing.

Often a slightly constrictive pain in the chest, which, when it does not quickly pass, causes the deepest dejection.

Burning pain in the chest.

Frequent stitches in the chest, with or without cough.

Violent stitches in the side; with great heat of the body, it is almost impossible to breathe, on account of stitches in the chest with hemoptysis and headache; he is confined to his bed.

Rush of blood to the chest.

Heart, Pulse and Circulation—

| | Stitches in cardiac region, low gurgling extending towards heart, for a moment breathing is impossible.

| Pain in heart > when lying down, thinks the stitches will kill him if they continue.

| | Gurgling (gluckern) in region of heart, particularly noticeable when lying.

Palpitation: with anxiety; mental disquietude, dislike for work; from coughing; in those suffering from hepatic disorders.

| Dyspnea: with palpitation; with pain in cardiac region.

Sounds of heart indistinct; bellows' murmur with first sound.

| | Stenosis of left osteum venosum; purring in region of apexr; cyanotic lips; dyspnea and shortness of breath when walking in open air; > lying down.

| | Rheumatic pericarditis; pulse 144; skin dry; pain in head and limbs, but more particularly in shoulder; dyspnea, with pain in region of heart; effusion, indistinct heart sounds; bellows' murmur with first sound; inability to lie down.

| Pericarditis of psoric origin; > lying quietly.

Pulse: weak, feeble; irritable, indicating return of abscesses on neck.

Neck and Back—

Painful stiffness of neck, soreness and tearing on bending backward.

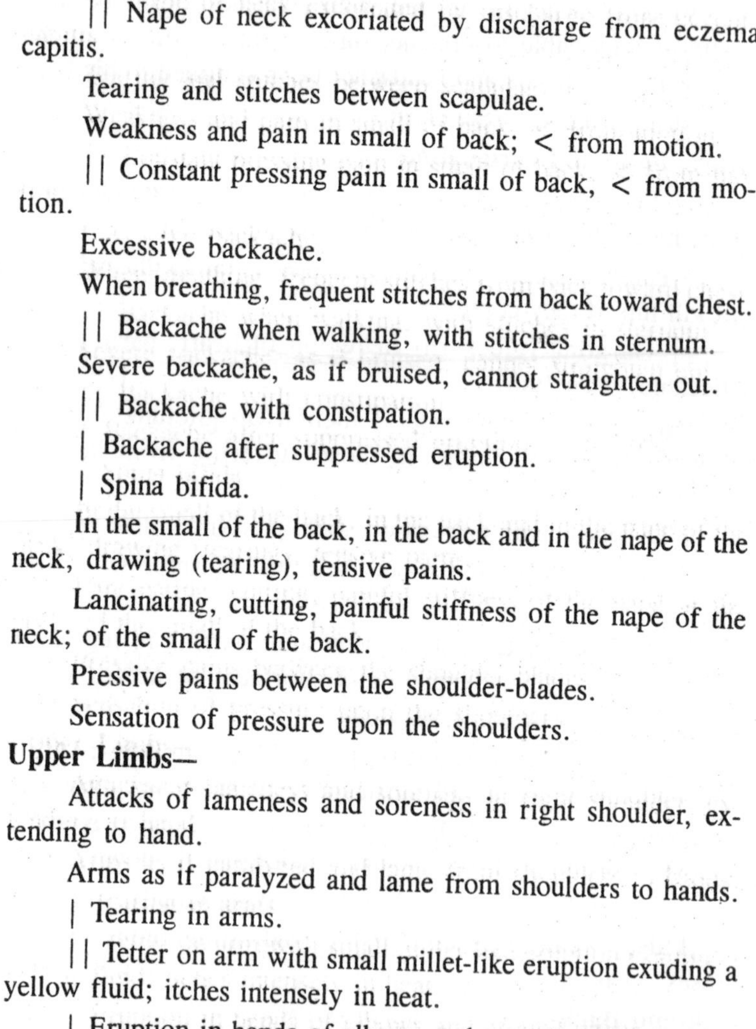

Glands of neck swollen on both sides, painful to touch, as if bruised; pain extends to head.

|| Herpetic eruption on side of neck extending from cheek.

|| Nape of neck excoriated by discharge from eczema capitis.

Tearing and stitches between scapulae.

Weakness and pain in small of back; < from motion.

|| Constant pressing pain in small of back, < from motion.

Excessive backache.

When breathing, frequent stitches from back toward chest.

|| Backache when walking, with stitches in sternum.

Severe backache, as if bruised, cannot straighten out.

|| Backache with constipation.

| Backache after suppressed eruption.

| Spina bifida.

In the small of the back, in the back and in the nape of the neck, drawing (tearing), tensive pains.

Lancinating, cutting, painful stiffness of the nape of the neck; of the small of the back.

Pressive pains between the shoulder-blades.

Sensation of pressure upon the shoulders.

Upper Limbs—

Attacks of lameness and soreness in right shoulder, extending to hand.

Arms as if paralyzed and lame from shoulders to hands.

| Tearing in arms.

|| Tetter on arm with small millet-like eruption exuding a yellow fluid; itches intensely in heat.

| Eruption in bends of elbows and around wrists.

|| Itchlike eruption on wrists with tearing in limbs.

|| Dry tetter on wrists with rheumatism in limbs.

| Trembling of hands.

| | Swelling and tension of backs of hands and of fingers.

| Malignant boil; on hand a cone-shaped scab the size of a quarter of a dollar on a base as large again, bluish-red and strongly demarcated, where scab extends over ring there is another moist, white ring which forms a new scab; much tension and burning.

| Pustules on hands, near finger-ends suppurating.

| | Copper-coloured eruption or red blisters on backs of hands.

| Itching between fingers; vesicles.

| | Herpes in palms of hands; itching tetter.

| Sweaty palms, especially at night.

Small warts size of pin's head on left hand.

Nails brittle.

Itch: in axillal; bends of elbows; arm; forearm; elbow and wrist; hands; finger joints.

Arthur D., aged 21, has had for two months a papular eruption on his hands, forearms, between his fingers, in the popliteal and elbow flexures, with intolerable itching; bleeding and burning after scratching. Great thirst for cold water in large quantities. Itching < at night, when warm in bed; sweats easily and profusely; very weak and emaciated; is anxious regarding his condition. Psorinum cm., one dose, cured.

E. M., aged 8, a papular vesicular eruption over entire body, but < in the flexures of joints, on hands and wrists, and between fingers; in palms, which resembled eczema; the itching was intolerable; scratched until it bled, which > itching, and he would sleep; < at night on undressing and in bed; night sweats without relief; face sallow, pale; tongue coated dirty white; great thirst for cold water; offensive odor from body. Was attended with periostitis on right tibia, resulting in abscess. After removal of sequestrum, under Psorinum, completely recovered.

M. V. had chronic eczema on legs, of twenty years' standing. Had been treated by specialists, and spent months in various hospitals, with all kinds of external applications, without relief. The front of left leg, from knee to ankle, covered with thick whitish crusts, and the skin drawn and wrinkled. At the edges of the crusts the skin was red and irritable. White bran-like scales shed in large quantities, during sleep, by scratching or rubbing the leg; underlying surface red, angry looking, bleeding; with intolerable itching. Psorinum 200, one dose dry on tongue, effected a permanent cure.

Child, aged 3, had milk crusts since three months old; was emaciated, with enlarged cervical glands, and a sickly, puny appearance; the whole scalp was involved, and emitted an offensive odoright The hair was matted, impossible to keep it clean; bowels constipated, never moving without artificial aid. Psorinum 200, one dose, produced severe <, then a permanent cure.

Lower Limbs—

Pain in hip-joints as if dislocated, < when walking, with weak arms.

Sciatic pains; tension down to knee while walking.

|| Ischias: sciatica.

Paralysis of legs from suppression of eruption on arms.

|| Purpura on inner side of thigh.

|| Old itch eruption on inner side of thigh and in popliteal space.

|| Knees give way under him.

|| Dry herpes, especially in bend of knees.

|| Eruption about joints makes walking difficult, as if encased in armor.

| Pain in knee caused by a fall a year ago.

| Chronic gonitis.

Pains in legs, especially in tibiæ and soles after too much exercise in walking, with a peculiar restlessness in legs, so that he frequently changes position, passing off after rising.

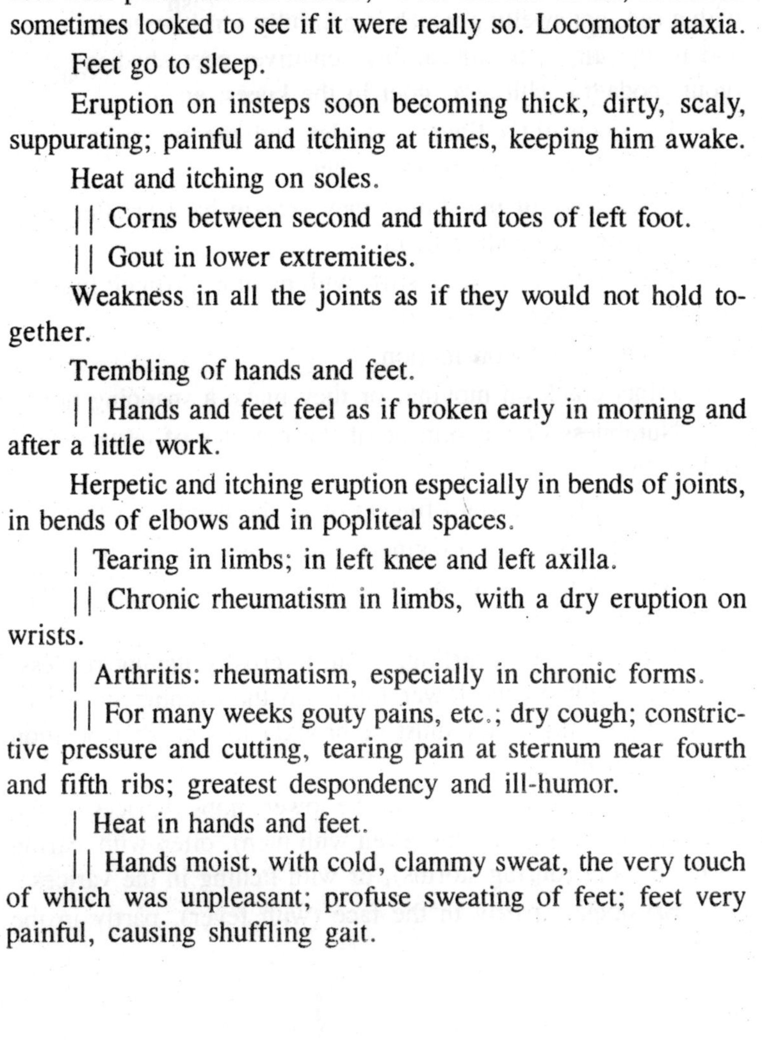

| Oozing blisters on legs, from small pustules, increasing in size, with tearing pains.

|| Vesicles becoming ulcers, on feet,

| Ulcers: on legs usually about tibiae and ankles or other joints; ulcers are indolent, slow to heal; on lower legs with intolerable itching over whole body; on feet.

|| Large swelling about ankle.

|| For four or five weeks, feeling when walking as if left foot were pulled around inward; < for last two weeks, so that he sometimes looked to see if it were really so. Locomotor ataxia.

Feet go to sleep.

Eruption on insteps soon becoming thick, dirty, scaly, suppurating; painful and itching at times, keeping him awake.

Heat and itching on soles.

|| Corns between second and third toes of left foot.

|| Gout in lower extremities.

Weakness in all the joints as if they would not hold together.

Trembling of hands and feet.

|| Hands and feet feel as if broken early in morning and after a little work.

Herpetic and itching eruption especially in bends of joints, in bends of elbows and in popliteal spaces.

| Tearing in limbs; in left knee and left axilla.

|| Chronic rheumatism in limbs, with a dry eruption on wrists.

| Arthritis: rheumatism, especially in chronic forms.

|| For many weeks gouty pains, etc.; dry cough; constrictive pressure and cutting, tearing pain at sternum near fourth and fifth ribs; greatest despondency and ill-humor.

| Heat in hands and feet.

|| Hands moist, with cold, clammy sweat, the very touch of which was unpleasant; profuse sweating of feet; feet very painful, causing shuffling gait.

| | Carries; rachitis.

In the limbs, drawing (tearing), tensive pains, partly in the muscles and partly in the joints (rheumatism).

In the periosteum, here and there, especially in the periosteum of the long bones, pressive-drawing pains.

Stitching pains in the fingers or toes.

Stitches in the heels and soles of the feet while standing.

Burning in the soles of the feet.

In the joints a sort of tearing, like scraping on the bone, with a red, hot swelling which is painfully sensitive to the touch and to the air, with unbearably sensitive, peevish disposition (gout, podagra, chiragra, gout in the knees, etc.).

The joints of the fingers, swollen with pressive pains, painful when touching and bending them.

Thickening of the joints; they remain hard swollen, and there is pain on bending them.

The joints, as it were, stiff, with painful, difficult motion, the ligaments seem too short.

Joints, painful on motion.

Joints crack on moving, or they make a snapping noise.

Numbness of the skin or of the muscles of certain parts and limbs.

Dying off of certain fingers or of the hands and feet.

Crawling or also pricking formication (as from the limbs going to sleep) in the arms, in the legs and in other parts (even in the finger-tips).

A crawling or whirling, or an internally itching restlessness, especially in the lower limbs (in the evening in bed or early on awaking); they must be brought into another position every moment.

Varices, varicose veins in the lower limbs (varices on the pudenda), also on the arms (even with men), often with tearing pains in them (during storms), or with itching in the varices.

Erysipelas, partly in the face (with fever), partly in the

limbs, on the breast while nursing, especially in a sore place (with a pricking and burning pain).

Whitlow, paronychia (sore finger with festering skin).

Chilblains (even when it is not winter) on the toes and fingers, itching, burning and lancinating pains.

Corns, which even without external pressure cause burning, lancinating pains.

Boils (furuncles), returning from time to time, especially on the nates, the thighs, the upper arms and the body. Touching them causes fine stitches in them.

Ulcers on the thighs, especially, also upon the ankles and above them and on the lower part of the calves, with itching, gnawing, tickling around the borders, and a gnawing pain as from salt on the base of the ulcer itself; the parts surrounding are of brown and bluish colour, with varices near the ulcers, which, during storms and rains, often cause tearing pains, especially at night, often accompanied with erysipelas after vexation or fright, or attended with cramps in the calves.

Tumefaction and suppuration of the humerus, the femur, the patella, also of the bones of the fingers and toes (spina ventosa).

Thickening and stiffening of the joints.

Eruptions, either arising from time to time and passing away again; some voluptuously itching pustules, especially on the fingers or other parts, which, after scratching, burn and have the greatest similarity to the original itch-eruption; or nettle-rash, like stings and water-blisters, mostly with burning pain; or pimples without pain in the face, the chest, the back, the arms and the thighs; or herpes in fine miliary grains, closely pressed together into round, larger or smaller spots of mostly reddish colour, sometimes dry, sometimes moist, with itching, similar to the eruption of itch and with burning after rubbing them. They continually extend further to the circumference with redness, while the middle seems to become free from the eruption and covered with smooth, shining skin (herpes circinatus). The moist herpes on the legs are called salt rheum; or crusts raised above the surrounding skin, round in form, with deep-red, painless borders, with frequent violent stitches on the parts of the skin not yet affected; or small, round spots on the skin, covered with bran-like, dry scales, which often peel off and are again renewed without sensation; or red spots on the skin, which feel dry, with burning pain; somewhat raised above the rest of the skin.

Freckles, small and round, brown or brownish spots in the face, on the hands and on the chest, without sensation.

Liver spots, large brownish spots which often cover whole limbs, the arms, the neck, the chest, etc., without sensation or with itching.

Yellowness of the skin, yellow spots of a like nature around the eyes, the mouth, on the neck, etc., without sensibility.

Warts on the face, the lower arm, the hands, etc.

Encysted tumors (wens) in the skin, the cellular tissue beneath it, or in the bursæ mucosæ of the tendons (exostosis), of various forms and sizes, cold without sensibility.

Glandular swellings around the neck, in the groin, in the bend of the joints, the bend of the elbow, of the knee, in the axillæ, also in the breasts.

Watery swelling, either of the feet alone, or in one foot, or in the hands, or the face, or the abdomen, or the scrotum, etc., alone, or again cutaneous swelling over the whole body (dropsies).

Attacks of sudden heaviness of the arms and legs.

Attacks of paralytic weakness and paralytic lassitude of the one arm, the one hand, the one leg, without pain, either arising suddenly and passing quickly, or commencing gradually and constantly increasing.

Sudden bending of the knees.

Children fall easily, without any visible cause. Also similar attacks of weakness with adults, in the legs, so that in walking one foot glides this way and the other that way, etc.

While walking in the open air sudden attacks of faintness, especially in the legs.

While sitting the patient feels intolerably weary, but stronger while walking.

The predisposition to spraining and straining the joints at a misstep, or a wrong grasp, increases at times even to dislocation; *e. g.*, in the tarsus, the shoulder-joint, etc.

The snapping and crackling of the joints at any motion of the limb increases with a disagreeable sensation.

The going to sleep of the limbs increases and follows on slight causes; *e. g.*, in supporting the head with the arm, crossing the legs while sitting, etc.

The painful cramps in some of the muscles increase and come on without appreciable cause.

Slow, spasmodic straining of the flexor muscles of the limbs.

Sudden jerks of some muscles and limbs even while walking; *e. g.*, of the tongue, the lips, the muscles of the face, of the pharynx, of the eyes, of the jaws, of the hands and of the feet.

Tonic shortening of the flexor muscles (tetanus).

Involuntary turning and twisting of the head, or the limbs, with full consciousness (St. Vitus' Dance).

Sudden fainting spells and sinking of the strength, with loss of consciousness.

Attacks of tremor in the limbs, without anxiety. Continuous, constant trembling, also in some cases beating with the hands, the arms, the legs.

Attacks of loss of consciousness, lasting a moment or a minute, with an inclination of the head to the one shoulder, with or without jerks of one part or the other of the body.

Almost constant yawning, stretching and straining of the limbs.

Increasing susceptibility of straining a joint, even by a very slight muscular effort, by light mechanical labor, on stretching the arms above the head for the purpose of reaching something elevated, on lifting light things, on turning the body quickly, on rolling something, etc. This, often slight, straining or extending the muscles sometimes induces the most violent diseases, swoons, hysterics, complaints of all degrees, fevers, hemoptysis, etc., whereas a person that is not affected with psora is able to lift any burdens he pleases, without any inconvenience.

Rest, Position, Motion—

Sitting aggravates dyspnea (asthma) and pain in heart; these and other ailments are > while lying down.

Many ailments are < or come on when riding in a carriage, and when exercising in open air, and > by rest and in room.

Rest: stitches in spleen.

Lying down: waterbrash; cough <; chest symptoms >; pain in heart >; gurgling in region of heart; pericarditis better.

Lies in same position in morning as when he fell asleep.

Lies on face: inflammation of eyes.

Lying on right side: pain in region of liver <.

Must lie down: dizziness; to breathe more easily.

Cannot lie down: rheumatic pericarditis.

Cannot straighten out: backache.

Changes position: restlessness in legs.

Sitting up to write: dyspnea <.

The nearer arms are brought to body, dyspnea <.

Bending forward: pressure in chest <.

Bending backward: painful stiffness of neck.

Stooping: tough mucus in nose; lumps in groin prevent.

Had to rise at night to collect his senses.

Getting up: waterbrash >.

Standing: stitches in spleen >.

Morning: stitches in spleen <; pain in chest <; does not < pressure in chest; pains in small of back <.

Exertion: causes perspiration; eczematous eruption; urticaria.

Slightest exercise: profuse perspiration.

Walking: pain in region of liver hinders; pain through groin; cannot walk without assistance; cutting in left loin; shortness of breath in open air; backache; pain in hip joints <: tension to knees; difficult, eruptions above joints, as if left foot were pulled around inward; profuse sweat with debility.

Nerves—

| Nervous, restless, easily startled.

|| Subsultus tendinum.

| Malaise: feels tired out.

| Constantly tired and sleepy; very little labor exhausts him; exhausted after riding in a wagon.

Looks pale, exhausted and thinner than usual.

|| Very weak and miserable after suppressed itch.

Weakness; of all the joints of the body as if they would not hold together.

| Loss of strength, with cough, with oppression of chest.

|| Trembling and chilliness, with attacks of pain in chest.

Stormy weather affects him.

|| Debility: independent of any organic disease; loss of appetite; tendency to perspiration on exertion and at night; after acute diseases; after protracted diseases or loss of fluids; after typhus, with despair of recovery; thinks he is very ill when he is not; appetite will not return; in the evil consequence of suppressed itch, especially after large doses of sulphur.

After typhoid, diphtheria, pneumonia.

(Kali c. after parturition or abortion.)

| Constantly increasing debility, with abdominal affections.

|| A man, aet. 21, was obliged to run until nearly exhausted; although strong and well before, he now became weak, perspiring easily and had severe pain in right side, < by coughing, laughing, motion.

Frequent attacks of epilepsy; religious melancholy (improved).

Epilepsies of various kinds.

Burning pains on the whole right side of body; felt as if the right side of the head and right eye would burst, was so painful and swollen.

Mright C., 43, spare, dark. Hypochondriacal. Nervous for nine months. Had to give up business. Took much quinine and many other drugs, without >. Complains of very disagreeable feeling about the head, great mental depression; thinks he will never recover; hopeless and despondent. Cannot apply his mind to business. Seems confused; cannot reckon. Numbness of legs and arms < on left side; < going to bed, formication and crawling, with pricking and smarting on scalp and on extremities. Tongue coated white. After three months' treatment remained stationary. It was then ascertained that he sweated very easily on least exertion, and somewhat at night, with great loss of memory. Psorinum 400 soon caused marked improvement and enabled him to return to business.—*J. B. Bell.*

Sleep—

| Sleepy by day; sleepless at night, from intolerable itching; dyspnea; congestion to head.

| Sleepless after 12 P.M., from congestion to head.

|| Child apparently well, but at night would twist and turn and fret from bedtime till morning and next day be as lively as ever.

| Sick babies will not sleep at night, but worry and fret and cry. (See Jalapa.)

Dreams: anxious; vivid, continue after waking; of robbers, danger, traveling, etc.

On waking: cannot get rid of the one persistent idea.

|| In morning lies in same position as when he fell asleep.

Night-mare; he usually suddenly awakes at night from a frightful dream, but cannot move, nor call, nor speak, and when he endeavors to move, he suffers intolerable pain, as if he were being torn to pieces.

Sleepiness during the day, often immediately after sitting down, especially after meals.

Difficulty in falling asleep, when abed in the evening; he often lies awake for hours.

He passes the nights in a mere slumber.

Sleeplessness, from anxious heat, every night, an anxiety which sometimes rises so high that he must get up from his bed and walk about.

After three o'clock in the morning, no sleep, or at least no sound sleep.

As soon as he closes his eyes, all manner of fantastic appearances and distorted faces appear.

In going to sleep, she is disquieted by strange, anxious fancies; she has to get up and walk about.

Very vivid dreams, as if awake; or sad, frightful, anxious, vexing, lascivious dreams.

Loud talking, screaming, during sleep.

Somnambulism; he rises up at night, while sleeping with closed eyes, and attends to various duties; he performs even dangerous feats with ease, without knowing anything about them when awake.

Attacks of suffocation while sleeping (nightmare).

Early on awaking, dizzy, indolent, unrefreshed, as if he had not done sleeping and more tired than in the evening, when he lay down; it takes him several hours (and only after rising) before he can recover from his weariness.

After a very restless night he often has more strength in the morning, than after a quiet sound sleep.

Various sorts of severe pains at night, or nocturnal thirst, dryness of the throat, of the mouth, or frequent urinating at night.

Time—

Aggravations in the evening and before midnight.

Morning: left half of head stupid; vertigo; when rising, forcing outward in head; headache <; eyes slightly agglutinated; ciliary blepharitis <; nausea towards stools; early, diarrhea; when rising, diarrhea; cough < when awaking; hands and feet, as if broken.

Forenoon: dull.

Day: ciliary blepharitis worse; nausea and vomiting; sleepy.

Evening: fever; eyes feel tired; itching in ear <; vomiting; cough; chilliness in upper arm and thighs, as if he should lose his senses; heat, with delirium, itching and heat in eyes.

Night: feels dull, stupid; dropping from posterior nares awakens him; toothache <; stools <; stools only; diarrhea; nervous, restless; awakens as if frightened; wets bed; cough <; sweaty palms; perspiration; sleepless; child twists, turns and frets; heat; terrible itching of whole body; screaming.

Temperature and Weather—

Great sensitiveness to cold air or change of weather; wears a fur cap, overcoat or shawl, even in hottest summer weather.

Aggravation from sudden changes of weather.

Feels a restlessness in his blood days before and during a thunderstorm.

Cough: returns every winteright.

Air: nose sensitive when inhaling.

Open air: when walking, photophobia; taste >; feels <; cough >; shortness of breath; itching >.

Averse to having head uncovered.

While in bed: itching of body.

Warmth: toothache >; of body causes itching; intolerable itching.

Warm food: inflamed mouth <.

Summer: cholera infantum; dry scaly eruption disappeared.

Cold: toothache <; drinks, < pain in chest; weather, dry scaly eruption returned.

Change of weather: headache caused and made <; diarrhea.

Washing: > pressure in head.

Increasing susceptibility to colds, either of the whole body (often even from repeatedly wetting the hands, now with warm water, then with cold, as in washing clothes), or only susceptibility of certain parts of the body, of the head, the neck, the chest, the abdomen, the feet, etc., often in a moderate or slight draft, or after slightly moistening these parts; even from being in a cooler room, in a rainy atmosphere, or with a low barometer.

So-called weather prophets; *i. e.,* renewed severe pain in parts of the body which were formerly injured, wounded, or broken, though they have since been healed and cicatrized; this renewed pain sets in, when great changes of the weather, great cold, or a storm are imminent, or when a thunderstorm is in the air.

Fever—

| Chilliness in evening on upper arms and thighs, with thirst; drinking causes cough, then heat and cough, with oppression of chest; and trembling, with attack of pain in chest.

The more intense the pain the more he sweats. Tibia.

| Internal shivering, creeping chills and icy-cold feet. Heat: at night and dryness in mouth; in afternoon or evening, feels as if he would lose his senses, with thirst; in evening, with delirium, great thirst, followed by profuse sweat; when riding in a carriage; sudden over whole body, with trickling perspiration all over face.

| Sweats easily, weak.

Sweat: profuse; cold, clammy from least exertion; profuse when-taking slightest exercise; when walking; at night; on face, palms of hands and perineum when moving about; profuse sour, clammy, with faint oppression of chest after chill and heat; after typhus; colliquative.

Sweat: profuse at 3 A.M.

|| When taking a walk profuse sweat with consequent debility, taking cold easily.

Sweat at night > headache.

|| Profuse sweating relieves all the complaints; chronic diseases. (Calad.)

Profuse night sweats of phthisis.

| Want of perspiration; dry skin.

Typhus: picks bedclothes, reaches for objects in air; profound debility.

|| After ague colour of face worse.

Painful sensation of cold in various parts.

Burning pains in various parts (frequently without any change in the usual external bodily temperature).

Coldness, repeated or constant of the whole body, or of the one side of the body; so also of single parts, cold hands, cold feet which frequently will not get warm in bed.

Chilliness, constant, even without any change in the external bodily temperature.

Frequent flushes of heat, especially in the face, more frequently with redness than without; sudden, violent sensation of heat during rest, or in slight motion, sometimes even from speaking, with or without perspiration breaking out.

Warm air in the room or at church is exceedingly repugnant to her, makes her restless, causes her to move about (at times with a pressure in the head, over the eyes, not infrequently alleviated by epistaxis).

Rushes of blood, also at times a sensation of throbbing in all the arteries (while he often looks quite pale, with a feeling of prostration throughout the body).

Perspiration comes too easily from slight motion; even while sitting, he is attacked with perspiration all over, or merely on some parts; *e. g.*, almost constant perspiration of the hands and feet, so also strong perspiration in the axilla? and around the pudenda.

Daily morning sweats, often causing the patient to drip, this for many years, often with sour or pungent-sour smell.

One-sided perspiration, only on one side of the body, or only on the upper part of the body, or only on the lower part.

Intermittent fever, even when there are no cases about, either sporadic or epidemic, or endemic; the form, duration and type of the fever are very various; quotidian, tertian, quartan, quintan or every seven days.

Every evening, chills with blue nails.

Every evening, single chills.

Every evening, heat, with rush of blood to the head, with red cheeks, also at times an intervening chill.

Intermittent fever of several weeks' duration, followed by a moist itching eruption lasting several weeks, but which is healed again during a like period of intermittent fever, and alternating thus for years.

The more intense the pain, the more profuse he sweats (Tilia).

Perspiration, cold and hot alternately, appeared about 3 A.M.

Attacks, Periodicity—

Every other day: headache, thirst, cold.

Nearly every half hour: urination.

Two or three times a day: pains in chest grow severe.

1 A.M.: sensation as of a heavy blow on forehead, diarrhea.

Immediately after dinner: congestion of blood to head.

Every morning at ten: oppression.

Every afternoon: great anxiety.

Every day, from 5 A.M. until 5 P.M.; anguish in head.

Every night: nocturnal enuresis; sweat.

Day before headache: inordinate appetite.

For three or four days: constipation.

During full moon: wets bed.

For four or five weeks: feeling when walking as if left foot were pulled around inward.

Nine months: has been nervous.

For four years: discharge from ear.

For eleven years on 20th of August: hay fever.

Twelve years' duration: gleet.

For twenty-five years: cough.

Locality and Direction—

Right: pressure in side of occiput; large brown scab on eye; eye inflamed; ear a mass of crusts; eczema behind ear cured deafness; stinging in nostril; soreness of jaw; burning in cheek; ulcer on side of throat; pain through groin; lumps in groin; inguinal hernia; knotty lump over groin; violent pain in loin; tearing in side from cough; pain extending to shoulder; stitches in side of chest; sharp pain opposite tenth rib; fixed pain in side of chest; dull pressure in chest; lameness and soreness in shoulder; small vesicles behind ear.

Left: half of head stupid; pains in temple; numbness of arm and leg; pressing headache <; pain over eye; spots on frontal region much whiter than surrounding skin; discharge from ear; pustules behind ear; ovary indurated after violent knock; cutting in loin; stitches in chest; stenosis of osteum venosum; small warts on hand; as if foot was pulled inward; corns between toes; tearing in knee; in axillae.

From right to left: pain in occiput; ciliary blepharitis.

From left to right: pain in eyes.

From within outward: as of hammers striking head.

From behind forward: stitches in chest.

Sensations—

As if stupid in left half of head; eyes as if pressed outward; as if brain had not room enough in forehead; as if brain would protrude; back of head as if sprained; right side of occiput as if luxated; as if piece of wood were lying across back of head; as if head were separated from body; as of a foreign body under eyelid; as if sand were in eyes; as if he heard with ears not his own; cheek bones as if ulcerated; condyle of jaw as if lame; tongue as if burnt; teeth as if glued together; as if a plug in throat; as if intestines were hanging down; as if frightened; throat as if narrowing; asthma as if he would die; as if everything in chest were raw and scratched; as if everything were torn in chest; glands of neck as if bruised; back as if bruised; arms as if paralyzed; hip joint as if ulcerated; joints as if encased in armor; as if left foot were pulled around inward; as if joints would not hold together; hands and feet as if broken; as if he would lose his senses.

Pain: in left temple; in chest; over left eye to right; in back of head; over eyebrows; down nose; in liver; in cheek bones; in condyle of jaw; in throat; in chest extending to shoulder;, in small of back; in abdomen; through right groin; in rectum; in cardiac region; in chest and throat; in heart; in head and limbs; in hip joint; in knee; in legs.

Excruciating pains: in chest.

Intense pain: in head.

Violent pains: in sacrum and right loin.

Severe pain: in left ear; in limbs.

Sharp pain: right side opposite tenth rib.

Anguish: in head.

Cutting, tearing pain: in throat.

Cutting pains: in intestines; in urethra; in loin.

Tearing: from centre of chest to throat; in neck; between scapulae; in arms; in limbs; in legs; in left knee and left axilla.

Cutting: in chest.

Stitches: in heart; in eyes; in teeth; in spleen; in chest and back; in sternum; in right side of chest; in cardiac region; between scapulas; from back towards chest.

Stitching pain: in pit of stomach; in region of liver.

Throbbing: in brain.

Fixed pain: right side of chest.

Griping pains: about navel.

Cramps: in stomach.

Cramplike contractive pain: in head.

Ulcerative pain: in chest under sternum.

Suppurative pain: through whole chest.

Pinching pain: in pubic region.

Constricting pain: in chest.

Boring: in right nostril.

Digging: in forehead.

Drawing: in forehead; in testicles and spermatic cords.

Pressing pain: in small spots in forehead and temples; in eyes; in region of liver; in small of back.

Sore pain: behind ears.

Burning pressing pain: in chest.

Stinging: in right nostril; in teeth; in region of liver and spleen; in inguinal glands; in many parts of skin.

Burning of eyes; in nose; of face; in right cheek; of blisters on inside of lower lip; of throat; in fauces; in rectum; in urethra; in condylomata; of excrescences on prepuce; around nipples.

Smarting: on scalp.

Soreness: of eyes: of stomach; behind ears; of external ear; of nose; of jaw; of teeth; of mouth; in rectum and anus; under sternum; of whole chest; in neck; in right shoulder.

Rawness: behind ears.

Hot sensation: in chest.

Pricking: on scalp.

Heat: of eyes; of hands and feet.

Rheumatism: in limbs.

Constricting pressure: at fourth and fifth ribs near sternum; at sternum.

Constriction: of throat and chest.

Pressure: in right side of occiput; in right zygoma; on chest; in right side of chest.

Heaviness: of head; of testicles; in chest.

Tension: in right zygoma; in throat; of hands and of fingers; of boil on hand; down to knees.

Fulness: in head; in vertex.

Oppression: of chest; of stomach.

Singing: in forehead.

Tired feeling: in eyes.

Dullness: of head.

Painful stiffness: of neck.

Lameness: of shoulders and arms.

Numbness: of legs and arms.

Weakness: in forehead; of stomach; in chest; in small of back; in joints.

Trembling: of hands; of feet.

Restlessness: in legs.

Dryness: of tongue; of mouth; of throat.

Tickling: in throat; in larynx; in trachea.

Crawling: on scalp; in larynx.

Formication: on scalp; in head.

Itching: eruption on head; in canthi; in ears; of external ear; of pimples of cheeks; of excrescence on prepuce; of pimples around nipples; of tetter on arm; of body in bed; between fingers; tetter on palms; intolerable over whole body; of eruption on instep; on soles; inner angles of eyes; condylomata; of herpes.

Disagreeable sensation of dryness over the whole body (also in the face, around and in the mouth, in the throat or in the nose, although the breath passes freely through it).

Tissues—

Thinner than usual, pale, exhausted.

Great emaciation, in children; they are pale, delicate, sickly, will not sleep day or night, but worry, fret and cry, or child is good, plays all day, is restless, troublesome, screaming all night.

Glandular swellings with eruption on head.

All excretions, diarrhea, leucorrhea, menstrual flow and perspiration, have a carrion-like odor

Body has a filthy smell even after a bath.

Whole body painful, easily sprains and hurts himself.

Rheumatism and arthritis.

Deeply penetrating ichorous ulcers.

Caries; rachitis; dropsy.

The joints are easily sprained or strained.

Increasing disposition to *strains* and to *overlift* oneself even at a very slight exertion of the muscles, even in slight mechanical work, in reaching out or stretching for something high up, in lifting things that are not heavy, in quick turns of the body, pushing, etc. Such a tension or stretching of the muscles often then occasions long confinement to the bed, swoons, all grades of hysterical troubles, fever, hemoptysis, etc., while persons who are not psoric lift such burdens as their muscles are able to, without the slightest after effects.

The joints are easily sprained at any false movement.

In the joint of the foot there is pain on treading, as if it would break.

Softening of the bones, curvature of the spine (deformity, hunchback), curvature of the long bones of the thighs and legs *(morbus anglicus,* rickets).

Fragility of the bones.

Touch. Passive Motion. Injuries—

Touch: stomach sensitive; lingual glands sore; teeth <; vesicles sore.

Pressure: stomach sensitive; pain in region of liver <; from a truss; inflammation.

Bandage: caused inflammation of tunica vaginalia.

Rubbing: causes small vesicles to arise.

Riding: pain in abdomen; griping and desire for stool; soreness in rectum and anus; in a wagon, exhausted; sweat.

Violent knock: left ovary indurated.

Fall: caused pain in knee.

Painful sensitiveness of the skin, the muscles and of the periosteum on a moderate pressure.

Intolerable pain in the skin (or in the muscles, or in the periosteum) of some part of the body from a slight movement of the same or of a more distant part; *e, g.*, from writing there arises a pain in the shoulder or in the side of the neck, etc., while sawing or performing other hard labor with the same hand causes no pain; a similar pain in the adjacent parts, from speaking and moving the mouth; pain in the lips and in the back at a slight touch.

Skin—

| Abnormal tendency to receive skin diseases.

|| Large suppurating pustules on hands, particularly near ends of fingers; had eight or ten within a few weeks, itching of body particularly while in bed.

| Skin inactive; want of perspiration.

| Itching: when body becomes warm; and stinging in many parts at same time; intolerable, < in bed and from warmth; scratches until it bleeds; over whole body, when rubbed, small papules and vesicles arise; between fingers; in knee joints; in bends of knees; terrible, of whole body at night, preventing sleep.

|| A girl, aet. 18, sallow complexion but cleanly appearance; constant irritation of the different parts of body, day and night, compelling her to scratch; numerous pediculi corporis cling to neck, back and shoulders; menstruation had never occurred; anxious, depressed and tearful; inner angles of eyes filled with gummy mucus, heat and itching in them, in evening; corners of mouth sore.

|| Skin has a dirty, dingy look, as if patient never washed; in some places looks coarse as if bathed in oil; sebaceous glands secrete in excess; body always smells dirty.

| Skin dirty, greasy looking, with yellow blotches here and there.

|| Severe pains in limbs and dark, burning spots, so that skin of whole body except face resembled that of a mulatto; itch had been suppressed five times.

|| Scaly condition of skin of whole body; skin has a dirty, tawny colour, although carefully kept; much itching causing desire to scratch, which gave but temporary relief; some months back instep showed signs of eruption, which soon became a thick, dirty-looking mass of scales and pus, painful and violently itching; at times pain kept her awake at night; disease of at least a-dozen years' standing.

Rash on back and neck.

Urticaria with eruptions on head.

Fine, red eruption, forming small white scales.

Dry and scaly eruption, with little pointed vesicles around reddened edges, disappearing during summer, but reappearing when cold weather comes on.

Eczematous eruption after any severe exertion, accompanied by sensation of tension and swelling on fingers, dorsum of hands, nape of neck and towards ears; slightly elevated blotches upon an erysipelatous, swollen, hard base; eruption of numberless small vesicles; face in several places affected; eyelids swollen; intolerable itching, disturbing sleep; fingers so swollen that they cannot be flexed; after several days desquamation in very fine scales occurred.

|| Eczema behind ears, on scalp and in bends of elbows and armpits, accompanied by abscesses affecting bones; nothing relieved, but the eruption disappeared, to reappear again, years after, on wrists; there was then a patch on each wrist as large as a half dollar, with intense itching, preventing sleep, with constant desire to scratch.

Eruption of small vesicles, quickly filling with a yellow lymph, painful, like sores, to touch, drying up after a few days, on forehead and several places on face, also behind right ear.

| Moist herpes after suppressed scabies; intolerable itching when getting warm; < before midnight and in open air.

| Herpes: with itching and burning; with biting-itching, with meal-dust, humid.

| Herpetic eruptions.

On face, hand and back, also on legs, an itchlike eruption appears and the eyes agglutinate so that they cannot be opened.

|| Itch: dry on arms and chest, most severe on finger joints; followed by boils; inveterate cases with symptoms of tuberculosis; in recent cases, with eruptions in bends of elbows and around wrists; repeated outbreak of single pustules after main eruption seems all gone.

After suppressed itch: urticaria in attacks, after every ex ertion; tuberculosis; single pustules often appear.

| Consequences of itch suppressed by sulphur ointment.

|| Psoriasis; psoriasis syphilitica.

Copper-coloured pustules, no itching.

Pustules on forehead, chin and chest.

|| Pustules or boils on head, particularly on scalp; scalp had a dirty look and emitted an offensive odor; fine, red eruption, forming small white scales; pustules on hands.

|| Burning itching pustule after vaccination.

| Eruptions bleed easily and constantly tend to suppurate.

| Crusty eruptions all over body.

| Crusta serpiginosa.

| Pemphigus.

|| Retrocession of eruption.   Measles.

| Ulcers: deep, penetrating, ichorous; on face and legs; old, with fetid pus; violently itching; scrofulous, with swelling of bones.

|| Moist, itching condylomata.

|| Suppressed eruptions.

Dryness of the (scarf) skin either on the whole body with inability to perspire through motion and heat, or only in some parts.

Sensation of dryness over the whole body, also in the face, at the mouth and in the mouth, in the throat or in the nose, although the air passes freely (especially upon the hands, the external side of the arms and legs, and even in the face; the skin is dry, rough, parching, feels chapped, often scaly like bran).

Eczema: something more than a year since a young lady came under my observation who had one of the worst cases I ever saw. At 15 years I remember her as attractive and brilliant, with a fine head of hair and one of the most perfect complexions, or skins, I ever saw. Upon questioning her I learned: Family history negative. Had been in every way in perfect health. At 14 years was vaccinated, 'worked' well, six months later attended a school exhibition one very cold night in winter and face was considerably exposed. Next morning awakened, face greatly swollen, intensely red, almost unbearable itching. Eyes suffused and injected, ears double their normal size. Very little constitutional disturbance. Called an allopathic physician who employed local and internal measures with little immediate result. Soon papules were formed, many of which became vesicular and not a few pustular; discharge of a thick, dirty fluid which stained and stiffened linen. Hair was cut close and 'locals' applied here also. Week after week she had slight improvements and aggravations. She was of strong allopathic faith, yet after three years of arsenic, potash, cathartics, zinc and a dozen other local applications she sought homeopathic treatment. Appeared to improve for a time, then as bad as ever, and finally returned to allopathy; finding no relief, employed some patent, remedies with apparent transitory improvement. She was now, at the time I saw her, taking nothing at all, had suffered for six years, and was still as bad as ever, or even slightly worse. I found her in mind, though naturally bright and cheerful, very despondent, with even suicidal thoughts, complete despair of recovery. Hair dry and without lustre, eyes somewhat suffused and injected, which condition attends a sort of incipient asthmatic affection, making its appearance each fall;

some hoarseness. Face, neck and much of body was coarse, rough and of a dirty brown colouright Does not perspire at all. Eruption behaves much the same as at first and above described, itching intolerably, better by gentle scratching which is continued until it bleeds. Between points of eruption skin is much indurated. Eruption surrounded by bluish circle; pruritus worse at night, when undressing, and by warmth of bed. Desquamation is so great that the sheet was each morning shaken and scales swept away. I went to work with a faint heart, feeling that I was somewhat lacking in uncommon and peculiar symptoms. I prescribed Psorinum 200 (B. & T.), a powder each night dry on tongue, for a week.

Eruption in bends of elbows and knees; dry, scaly and small pointed vesicles around the reddened joints; disappeared entirely in summer and reappeared when cold weather set in; violent itching < by warmth of bed or by scratching. Psorinum 42 m., two doses, at six weeks intervals, cured. No return the following winter.

A teething baby, nine months old, had eczema, beginning at outer angle of right eye and spreading over entire face. First a raised inflamed base of a tawny red, then scattered pustules which coalesced to form large crusts, from which oozed an zoily, yellow, viscid discharge, cracks upon ears with a similar discharge. Graphites cm. was given without result; then Sulphur, but the eruption spread until the cheeks were a mass of crusts. It then appeared on back and arm and one leg, and here gave off fine bran-like scales. The scalp soon became involved and covered with crusts a quarter of an inch thick, Psorinum cm., one dose, which < for a week, then improvement began and went on to a perfect cure; notwithstanding the eruption of three teeth.

A man, aged 80, suffered with eczema since 18 years old, which appeared soon after vaccination. A very troublesome cough had annoyed him for months, for which I was called to attend him.

Cough < at night, on lying down and on rising in the

morning. Coughs long before expectorating. Sputa yellowish, salty, puriform. Sensation of pressure on chest; requires great effort to expand lungs. Chest painful, < after coughing; mucous rales over both lungs. Loss of appetite. Eczema always < in winter; intense itching < nights. The eczema had been suppressed by local treatment, and cough developed. Psorinum crn. Within 48 hours cough and chest symptoms improved, but the eczema reappeared over the body, with intense itching. Improving in health, but still has some eczema which gives him little trouble.—*Chapman.*

Mrs. M., aged 72, tissues enormously distended with dropsy, unable to lie down for nine weeks from dyspnea. Legs from ankles to crest of ilium and arms from wrist to elbows covered with a dirty, scaly eruption, itching violently < at night, could not avoid scratching, which gave no relief until it caused bleeding. All forms of external applications had been used in a vain effort to suppress the eruption. Psorinum 52m. one powder in four teaspoonfuls of water, given in four doses, half hour intervals, and six powders of placebo, one each night, gave prompt relief, and the patient was able to walk in two weeks. One week later another dose was required, as there was a slight return of the eruption on the ankles; this completed the cure.—*Hawley.*

Eczema Rubrum: Mrs. G., aged 71, face red and swollen, almost erysipelatous. in appearance. Heat of fire caused torture when it touched her face; always sits with her back to the fire. Cold air > bathing <, must dry face with great care. Burning and itching intolerable; cannot sleep; sits all night by an open window gently rubbing face with a handkerchief. Scratching increases burning and itching; mental excitement, of which she has much, greatly < Psorinum 500 cured in one month.

A woman had attacks of terrible itching of skin without eruption through three periods of gestation. In the last she complained of the same itching, when Dr. Lippe advised Psorinum. In two days erysipelas appeared. Her face was very much swollen.

PYROGEN (A Product of Sepsis)

For sapremia or septicemia: puerperal or surgical; from ptomaine or sewer gas infection; during course of diphtheria, typhoid or typhus; *when the best selected remedy fails to > or permanently improve.*

The bed feels hard (Arn.); *parts lain on feel sore and bruised* (Bapt.); rapid decubitus (Carb. ac.).

Great restlessness; must move constantly to > the soreness of parts (Arn., Bellis, Eup.).

Tongue: *large, flabby;* clean, smooth as if varnished; fiery red; dry, cracked, articulation difficult (Crot., Ter.).

Taste: *sweetish; terribly fetid;* pus-like; as from an abscess.

Vomiting: persistent; brownish; coffee-ground; offensive, stercoraceous; with impacted or obstructed bowels (Op., Plb.).

Diarrhea: horribly offensive (Psoright); brown or black (Lep.); painless, involuntary; uncertain, when passing flatus (Aloe, Olean.).

Constipation: with complete inertia (Op., Sanic.); *obstinate from impaction, in fevers;* stool, large, black, carrion-like; *small, black balls,* like olives (Op., Plb.).

Fetus: or secundines retained, decomposed; dead for day, black; horribly offensive discharge; 'never well since' septic fever, following abortion or confinement. To arouse vital activity of uterus.

Lochia; thin, acrid, brown, very fetid (Nit. ac.); suppressed, followed by chills, fever and profuse fetid perspiration.

Distinct consciousness of a heart; it feels tired; as if enlarged; purring, throbbing, pulsating, constant in ears, preventing sleep; cardiac asthenia from septic conditions.

Pulse abnormally rapid, out of all proportion to temperature (Lil.)

Skin: pale, cold of an ashy hue (Sec.); obstinate, varicose, offensive ulcers of old persons (Psor.).

Chill: *begins on the back,* between scapulae; severe, *general, of bones and extremities;* marking onset of septic fever; temperature 103 to 106; heat sudden, skin dry and burning; pulse rapid, small, wiry, 140 to 170; cold clammy sweat follows.

In septic fevers, especially puerperal, Pyrogen has demonstrated its great value as a homeopathic dynamic antiseptic.

Relations—

Antidote: Nux vomica for the agg. from over-action of a single dose or for bad effects of repeated doses; Rhus, Eup. peright for the aching, restlessness and bone pains.

Compatible: Arn., Bap., Rhus, Eup. peright in typhoid and other fevers with muscle soreness, bed feels hard. Ars., Ech.. Lach., Malar, (the vegetable Pyrogen), Ant. t., Bapt., Brom., Lye., Phos., fan-like motion of Alse nasi. Bry., cough < by motion and in warm room. Ipec., uterine hemorrhage (if Ipec. fails when apparently well selected). Bap., Psor, offensive diarrhea. Lept., Psor., black stools. Opium, Plumb., Sanic., constipation, hard black balls. Nit. ac., Sec., thin, offensive lochia. Phos., water is vomited as soon as warm in stomach. Bell., Melil., throbbing, bursting headache. Carbo v., Ech., Psoright, offensive varicose ulcers of old people. Hep., Sil., Calc. sulph., tendency to profuse suppuration. Sulph., Psor., patient continually relapsing after the apparent simillimum.

Aggravation: motion, moving the eye; in a warm room; rising from lying or sitting up (cough relieved by sitting up; < by lying down, Clarke).

Amelioration: heat, hot bathing or drinking hot water; binding affected part tightly; stretching out limbs; walking, changing position.

Mind—

Loquacious; can think and talk faster than ever before (S).

Irritable (S).

Delirious on closing eyes; sees a man at foot of bed. Whispers; in sleep.

Sensation as if she covered the whole bed; knew her head was on pillow, but did not know where the rest of her body was.

Feels when lying on one side that she is one person, and another person when turning on the other side.

Sensation as though crowded with arms and legs.

Hallucination that he is very wealthy; remaining after fever.

Increased buoyancy of spirits, although he felt ill.

Great depression.

Muttering delirium.

Anxiety, restlessness.

The muttering delirium sets in early, leading to unconsciousness and death.

The signs of infection are horror, delirium, stupefaction.

Brain active during the night, could not sleep, was making speeches and writing articles.

Head—

Staggers as if drunk on rising in morning (S).

Dizziness on rising up in bed.

Pains in both mastoids, < right; dull throbbing in mastoid region (S).

Great throbbing of arteries of temples and head; every pulsation felt in brain and in ears, the throbbings meet on top of brain (S).

Painless throbbing all through front of head; sounds like escaping steam (S).

Frightful throbbing headache > from tight band.

Excruciating, bursting, throbbing headache with intense restlessness (often accompanied with profuse nose-bleed, nausea, and vomiting).

Sensation as if a cap were on.

Rolling of head from side to side.

Forehead bathed in cold sweat.

Throbbing of carotids and vessels of the neck; a distinct, wave-like throb from the clavicles upwards.

Child with cerebro-spinal meningitis was so sick that at one time it seemed as though she could not recover; there was automatic motion of the right arm and right leg; rolling the head from side to side; this kept up until it would turn her around from left to right till her feet would get on the pillow or touch the head-board; she was brought out of this condition with Pyrogenium.

Dull headache.

Cerebral symptoms are not usually severe, but there is often a low form of delirium.

Dizziness, headache.

Heavy headache, uncomfortable.

Morning headache.

Pulsation felt in head, painless throbbing.

Eyes—

Left eyeball sore, < looking up and turning eye outward (S).

Projecting eyes.

Lids seem dry and roughened as if filled with sand; mucus collecting in inner canthi; agglutinated and crusty borders on waking in the morning.

Sticky and inflamed eyes.

Intense photophobia, lies with fists pressed tight in eyes.

Phlyctenular keratitis, both eyes < by light.

Ears—

Loud ringing, like a bell, in left ear; ringing and roaring in right ear < at night.

Ears cold.

Ears red, as if blood would burst out of them.

Sound as of escaping steam, a puffing, purring sound.

Loud ringing in right ear lasting but a few minutes.

Nose—

Nose-bleed; awakened by dreaming of it and found it was so.

Sneezing: every time he puts hands from under covers; at night.

Nostrils closing alternately (S).

Cold nose.

Fan-like motion of alae nasi.

Sneezing at night, nostrils closing and alternating from side to side.

Thick, gluey discharge from nose < right.

Face—

Face: burning; yellow; very red; pale, sunken, and bathed in cold sweat; pale, greenish, or chlorotic.

Circumscribed redness of cheeks.

Hectic flush in afternoon and evening, coming on regularly at 3 or 4 P.M. and lasting till midnight; then face covered with large drops of cold perspiration.

Face assumes a pinched and anxious expression.

Mouth—

Tongue: coated white in front, brown at back; yellowish brown, bad taste in morning (S).

Tongue: coated yellowish grey, edges and tip very red; large, flabby; yellow brown streak down centre.

Tongue clean, smooth, and dry; first fiery red, then dark red and intensely dry; smooth and dry; glossy, shiny as if varnished; dry, cracked, articulation difficult.

Tongue dry and not a particle of moisture on it. Has had no thirst since she has been sick. Bitter taste in the mouth; tongue dry down the center.

Taste: took one dose of Pyrogen cm. (Swan) in the afternoon. During the evening a terribly fetid taste, as if mouth and throat were full of pus, which lasted 24 hours; sensation as of a broken abscess in the mouth. A nauseating, offensive taste in morning, for many days during proving.

Tongue dry and brown.

Bad taste in the mouth.

Sticky saliva.

Pasty, furred tongue.

Throat—

Diphtheria with extreme fetor.

Relaxed throat.

Elongated uvula.

Ulcerated tonsils.

Larynx—

Usually cough.

Coughing when expiring. .

Cough attended with rusty expectoration.

Laryngitis.

Cough every time I move or turn over in bed.

Coughed up yellow sputa through the night.

Cough severe after rising.

Coughing, spitting up large masses of phlegm from larynx.

Cough < by motion.

Cough more in a warm room.

Coughing causes pain in back of head.

Burning in larynx and bronchi on coughing.

Cough up yellow sputa through the night.

Appetite—

No appetite or thirst (19th day). Complete loss of appetite.

Great thirst for small quantities, but the least liquid was instantly rejected.

Drinking very hot water, > thirst and vomiting (dog).

No appetite, yet nourishment is freely taken and digested.

Poor appetite for breakfast.

No appetite, as stomach and bowels feel so full.

No appetite for dinner.

Unusual appetite for chocolate.

Stomach—

Belching of sour water after breakfast.

Nausea and vomiting.

Vomiting: persistent; brownish, coffee-ground; offensive, stercoraceous; with impacted or obstructed bowels.

Vomiting and purging.

Vomits water when it becomes warm in stomach; vomiting >.

Urging to vomit; with cold feet.

Stomach feels too full; < after eating and > by frequent sour eructations.

Nausea > by drinking very hot water and by vomiting.

Vomiting is not infrequent.

Nausea on first rising.

Dyspepsia.

Belching some water after breakfast.

Stomach and bowels feel too full to eat.

Abdomen—

Full feeling and bloating of abdomen.

When lying on left side bubbling or gurgling sensation in hypochondria, extending back to left of spine.

Pain in umbilical region with passage of sticky, yellow, offensive stool.

While riding in a buggy aching in left of umbilicus; < drinking water; > passing flatus.

Soreness of abdomen so severe she can breathe with difficulty, and hardly bear any pressure over right side.

Very severe cutting pains right side going through back, < by every motion, talking, coughing, breathing deep; > lying on right (affected) side; groaning with every breath.

Great distension of the abdomen, with high temperature—lochial discharge, intensely offensive, as if rotten. Peritonitis.

Irregular action of the bowels.

Sensation of cold in abdomen.

Sensation of heaviness in abdomen.

Ascites (Bright's disease).

Stool and Anus—

Feculent and thin mucus, and finally bloody diarrhea and tenesmus (dog).

Two soft, sticky stools, 8 to 9 A.M.

Involuntary escape of stool when passing flatus.

Profuse watery, painless stools, with vomiting.

Stool, horribly offensive, carrion-like.

Stool very much constipated, large, difficult, requires much effort; first part balls, last part natural, with streaks of blood; anus sore after.

Constipation: hard, dry accumulated feces; stool large, black, carrion-like; small black balls like olives.

Congestion and capillary stasis of gastro-intestinal mucous membrane, shedding of epithelium, bloody fluid distending intestines (dog).

(Sweat about anus removed; fistula relieved.)

Usually diarrhea.

Irregular action of the bowels.

No stool today, very unusual.

Sticky yellow stool.

Passing flatus, sometimes involuntary.

Urinary Organs—

Urine scanty; only passed twice in twenty-four hours.

Urine: yellow when first voided; after standing, cloudy with substance looking like orange peel; red deposit on vessel hard to remove; deposits sediment like red pepper with reddish cloud on vessel.

Got up three times in night to urinate.

(Bright's disease.)

Urine contains albumin and casts; horribly offensive, carrion-like.

Frequent calls to urinate as fever comes on.

Intolerable tenesmus of bladder; spasmodic contractions, involving rectum, ovaries, and broad ligaments; [cured in a case of Yingling's with Pyrogen cm. (and higher); patient's next period came on naturally and painlessly, whereas before menses had been painful and extremely offensive].

Irregular urination.

Action of the kidneys irregular.

Aching in region of the kidneys.

Urinated only twice to-day. Very unusual; usually several times a day, normal in quantity.

Urine loaded with albumen.

Red lime inside of vessel, hard to remove.

Sediment like red pepper that floats at the bottom.

Male Sexual Organs—

Testes hang down relaxed; scrotum looks and feels thin.

Female Sexual Organs—

Puerperal fever, with offensive lochia (cured).

Puerperal peritonitis with extreme fetor; a rotten odor.

Parts greatly swollen (Bright's disease).

Menses horribly offensive; carrion-like.

Menses last but one day. then a bloody acrid leucorrhea, horribly offensive.

Hemorrhage of bright red blood with dark clots.

Septicemia following abortion; fetus or secundines retained, decomposed and horribly offensive.

(Has cured prolapsus uteri, with bearing down > by holding the head and straining as in the act of labor.)

Abscess of left ovary, acute throbbing pain, great distress, with fever and rigors (Pyrogen cm. (Swan) produced an enormous flow of white creamy pus with general >).

Lochia: thin, acrid, brown, or fetid; suppressed, followed by chills, fever, and profuse fetid perspiration.

It has cured prolapsus uteri, with bearing down, > by holding the breath and straining, as in the act of labor. Pain starting in the uterine region and passing upward to the umbilicus. It was the reverse (a cork-screw pain); this was momentarily > by holding the breath and bearing down, as in labor; momentarily > by pressing the hands against the vulva, then she said she would have to turn loose, as it made her worse. Lillium had previously failed in this case. Pain starting in the umbilicus or a little above, and passing down towards the uterus, but at midway of abdomen it would be intercepted by the same kind of a pain starting from the uterus and passing upward till they would meet midway between the umbilicus and uterus, then gradually die out till another would come as before; > momentarily by drawing her knees up to her chin and grasping her arms around them, and holding them tight. Intolerable tenesmus of the bladder; it was more of a spasmodic contraction than anything else; at: the same time this condition would be reflected to the rectum-and this strong desire to defecate without ability to do so> would also involve the ovaries and broad ligaments. Nux vom. and Lillium tig. had no effect whatever.

Severe chill; dull frontal headache; restless, pale, anxious.. Sharp shooting pains through abdomen. Pain in head severe; she clasped it with her hands as if she had received a sudden blow and cried, "Oh! my head;" became very restless, said she was going to die, and did not want the baby, of whom she was very fond, near heright Face pallid, with offensive viscid perspiration; abdomen sensitive to pressure; lochia and milk ceased. Thirsty for frequent small drinks. Pulse 140, weak, small; temperature 103. Pyrogen cm. 6 doses in water one-half hour apart. She made a good, though slow recovery. Puerperal septicemia.

Mrs. T. B., pale, slender, delicate, but in good health; primipara; was successfully delivered April 10th, 1901. On the 20th found her with a temperature of 102; lochia scanty, pale, offensive; but she felt well and had no pain. Fever increased in severity gradually for several days, until temperature reached 105 and 106, with a pulse of 120-130; still she insisted she felt well and would not go to bed. Several remedies, Bapt., Bell., Ech., Taright, were given without effect. Finally a severe shaking chill followed in a few hours by another sent her to bed, and the nurse was recalled. Pyrogen was given. Following day temperature 102; lochia reappeared in natural colour; the abdominal sensitiveness ceased and in two or three days disappeared entirely. She rapidly recovered.

Mrs. W. S. C., a slender woman; primipara; delivered June 10th, instrumental. Severe peritoneal laceration, which was repaired. The morning of the third day had shake; cutting spasmodic pain in uterus, which was swollen and sensitive; lochia dark, profuse, clotted; both iliac regions sensitive to pressure < left side. Belladonna gave no relief. Fever continued to rise; lochia darker, more offensive, containing threads and clots. The odor and other symptoms indicating approaching sepsis she received Pyrogen with very gratifying results, and a rapid recovery.

Carrie, aged 16 years, been sick two or three months under allopathic care. Breath, perspiration, expectoration, menses, urine and feces horribly offensive, carrion-like; disgust up to nausea about an effluvia that arises from her own body; soreness of the chest and abdomen, menses last but one day and a sanguineous leucorrhea that is of the same odor; pulse 106, with a bad cough, worse coming into a warm room; large, fleshy, pale, greenish or chlorotic face, mother having just died of consumption. Pyrogen cm., one dose, and better in ten hours, and on November 12th cough, odor and soreness nearly all gone, pulse 80, tongue clean. Sac. lac., and she remains well to this writing.— *Wakeman.*

Respiratory Organs—

Wheezing when expiring.

Cough: expectorating large masses of phlegm from larynx; < by motion; < in warm room; cough, burning in larynx and bronchi; pain in occiput; stitching in small of back, only noticed in the chair; coughs up yellow sputa through night.

Cough > sitting up, < lying down.

Expectoration: rusty mucus; horribly offensive; bloody sputa.

Chest—

Pain in right lung and shoulder, < talking or coughing.

Neglected pneumonia: cough, night-sweats, frequent pulse, abscess had burst discharging much pus of mattery taste (rapid recovery under Pyrogen, three doses).

Chest sore, purple spots on it.

Severe contracting pain within lower sternum, sometimes extending to rib-joints and up to throat, as if esophagus were being cramped.

Ecchymoses on pleura (dog).

J. A. W., aged 61. An old soldier full of rheumatic aches and pains; complaining much.

April 7, 1895. Rode twenty-two miles in a big wind storm, chilling and disagreeable, on the 5th. Taken to bed at once. Hot and cold flashes, < moving about. *Aching and sore all over. Bones ache. Very restless and nervous*. Impatient. *Head feels big,* full and aches all through head and down neck; < coughing. Nasal discharge fluent and thin. *Lungs sore and painful;* < coughing. Coughs considerably, some little expectoration, < at night.

Pulse 84. Bowels not moved since the 4th. Urine scant. Chilly when moving. When first taken sick, and when riding in the storm, his *toe nails felt as if they were flying off,* first one, then anotheright This feeling was very marked and disagreeable.

Pyrogen cmm., three doses, two hours apart.

Within twelve hours the pains were all gone and he had a

good night's rest. Sat up next morning feeling "better and freer from pain than in four months." A very rapid and prompt cure. — *Yingling.*

Respirations are rapid and shallow.

Pain in the chest, and perhaps orthopnea, from pleuritic affections.

Pain in the region of *the left nipple,* as if in the fieart *which* was going to ache.

Heart—

Pain in region of left nipple, as if in heart; increased action; pulse 120.

Heart tired as after a long run; increased action < least motion.

Never free from weary sensation about the heart.

Every pulsation felt in head and ears; a painless throbbing. Sensation as if heart were enlarged; distinct consciousness of a heart.

Sensation as if heart were too full of blood.

Sensation as if the heart were pumping cold water.

Violent, so persistent that it became very tiresome.

Palpitation or increased action without corresponding increase of temperature.

Palpitation < by motion; < lying on affected (left) side. Loud heart-beats, audible to herself and others.

Could not sleep for whizzing and purring of heart; when she did sleep was delirious.

Cardiac asthenia from septic conditions.

Ecchymoses on heart and pericardium (dog).

Palpitation < from motion > remaining quiet; pulse 160-170 per minute.

Tired feeling about the heart, as after a long run, feel as if I would like to take it out and let it rest; it would be such a relief if it would stop its throbbing; temperature not raised.

Back and Neck—

Pains in back in lumbar region.

Bubbling sensation or gurgling in the left hypochondrium, extending back to the left side of the spine, felt when lying on the left side.

Pain in small of back.

Weak feeling in the back.

Stitching pain in the back on coughing.

Throbbing of vessels of neck running up in waves from clavicles.

Limbs—

Aching: in bones; all over body as from a severe cold; with soreness of flesh, head feels hard; > motion (S).

Cold extremities.

Numbness of hands, arms, and feet, extending over whole body.

Automatic movement of right arm and right leg, turned the child round from right to left till feet reached the pillow; repeated as often as she was put right (cerebro-spinal meningitis).

Upper Limbs—

Pain in shoulder-joint; in front, passing three inches down arm (S).

Hands and arms numb.

Hands cold and clammy.

Dry eczema of hands.

Profuse exudation in axillary region.

Pain in left shoulder-joint, in front, passing down the arm from two to three inches, lasting till going to bed.

Lower Limbs—

Aching about knees, deep in bones, while sitting by a hot fire; > by walking.

On going to bed aching in patella; > flexing leg.

Aching above left knee as though bone broken (S).

Aching above knees in bones, > stretching out limbs.

Tingling in right little toe as though frost-bitten.

Feet and legs swollen (Bright's disease). Numbness of feet.

Aching: in bones; all over body as from a severe cold; with lameness and soreness of muscles; bed feels hard; > motion. < from motion.

Cold extremities; feet bathed in cold sweat.

Numbness of hands, arms, and feet, extending over whole body.

Edema of legs, in case of Bright's disease.

Aching pains in legs, as if in the bones.

Skin—

Mrs. I., aged 35, mother of two children, swelling of calf of leg; vesication formed on top of left foot, followed by a large ulcer, which eventually covered the whole foot. As the diseased process extended up the leg, several abscesses formed in succession, the swelling continuing to spread to the hip. About three inches below the trochanter a large abscess burrowed in the soft tissues, discharging great quantities of pus when opened.

Restless, unable to lie in one position; motion caused great pain, but moving gave >; must be continually moved, every hour or two every night, which a dose of Rhus failed to >. The feet, ankles and abdomen very much swollen; urine scanty, with red sandy sediment; constant sensation of repletion; is very thirsty yet unable to drink; hungry, yet the least food causes repletion; very peevish, whines like a child. Swelling and pain still increasing; face and neck yellow, emaciated and wrinkled; temperature 103, pulse 120. After Ars., Rhus, Lye. and Nux v. failed to give any >, Pyrogen cmm., one dose, followed by placebo every hour; improvement began and continued for four days, when a copious, painless, watery, offensive diarrhea began; another dose of Pyrogen was given and the patient went on to a rapid recovery.

Skin and conjunctiva becomes jaundiced.

Soon after the rigor, sometimes a subcutaneous abscess forms, or discolourations and pustules are seen on the skin. Jaundice appears.

Bed sores easily form and skin shows a tendency to slough on very slight pressure.

Patches of superficial gangrene frequently occur, without provocation.

Erysipelas.

Skin pale, cold, of earthy ashy hue.

Obstinate, varicose, offensive ulcers of old people.

Nerves—

Great nervousness and restlessness.

Could not lie long in one place without moving; yet moving gives no relief.

Great debility in the morning. He staggered when attempting to walk.

Nervous weakness attending convalescence from septic fever.

Sleep—

Dreamed he had nosebleed, and on waking the nose had bled all over the pillow.

Restless sleep, with moaning.

Unrefreshing sleep.

Disturbed sleep.

Slept awhile; woke to roll and tumble in every conceivable position.

Unable to sleep from brain activity and crowding of ideas.

Restlessness > after sleep.

Cries out in sleep that a weight is lying on her.

Whispers in sleep.

Kept awake by purring of heart.

Dreams: of various things; of business; of his patients and the remedy which cured them.

Dreamed all night of the business of the day.

Can lie but a few minutes in any position.

Could not sleep till dawn—brain too active—could not keep my eyes shut.

Cries out in sleep as if in pain.

Fever—

"In all cases of fever commencing with pains in the limbs" (Swan).

Shivers and begins to move about restlessly; temperature rises gradually and as gradually subsides (dog).

Chills running up and down the spine in successive waves; heat gives no relief.

Temperature rises rapidly to 104° F., and sinks rapidly from heart failure (dog, fatal dose).

Constant terrible aching all over the body; bed feels hard, must move frequently in search of a soft place.

Chilly at times and a little aching; a little feverish.

After dinner, ache all over, chilly all night, bed feels hard.

After getting into bed, chilly, teeth chatter; woke 10 P.M. in perspiration on upper part of body; > motion (S).

Feels hot as if he had a fever, but temperature was only 99° F., feels like 105°.

Frequent calls to urinate as soon as fever came on; urine clear as water.

Every other day dumb ague.

Perspiration horribly offensive, carrion-like; disgust up to nausea about any effluvia arising from her own body.

Cold sweat over body.

Fevers caused by: sewer gas poisoning; surgical infection; dissecting wounds, blood poisoning, or absorption of pus by medicated topical application.

Delirium when closing the eyes; sees a man at the foot of the bed or in the farther part of the room; hands cold and clammy; abdomen so sore that she can scarcely breathe; bowels so sore cannot bear any pressure over the right side; < from sitting up in bed; vertigo on rising up in bed.

N. B., child 4 years old, resided in a house in which plumbing was being repaired. A few days after was attacked at 2 A.M. with: Vomiting and purging; stools profuse and watery.

Cold extremities, ears and nose; forehead bathed in cold perspiration. Tongue heavily coated, yellowish-gray; edges of tip very red. Great prostration. Great restlessness mental and physical; pulse 140, small and wiry; temperature 99. Great thirst for small quantities, but the smallest quantity was instantly rejected. Later in day stool was horribly offensive, of a carrion-like odor; face pale, sunken, bathed in cold perspiration. Tongue dark red and free from the heavy coating of early morning, intense thirst, but water < both vomiting and purging. After Ver., Ars., Carbo v. and Bap. had been given, with no improvement, the patient evidently sinking, impossible to count the pulse, thinking perhaps sewer-gas poison may have been the factor, and the clean, fiery red tongue called my attention to Dright Burnett's cures in the Homeopathic World with Pyrogen. I gave two doses dry on the tongue with prompt and permanent relief.

Miss K. B., aged 14, complained of feeling weary, unable to go to school. Applying thermometer, found temperature 102, pulse 108, and her father sent for me. I found tongue abnormally red, thin, white fur at base. Had a slight epistaxis in the morning which Bryonia >, but failed to affect the fever. As there was absolutely no pain and very few symptoms, she was allowed to wait a few days on placebo. Sewer-gas was now discovered as the cause; Pyrogen, one dose, was given with rapid recovery.

Inclined to talk all the time at night during the fever; cold sweat over the body; pain in the small of the back; desires to urinate; it is scant; talks to herself; urging to vomit, with cold feet; restlessness > after sleeping; purple spots on the chest; cries out in her sleep that some one or a weight is lying on her; heart beats hard, has a laborious action; sensation as if the heart was too full of blood; it beats very loud, heart sounds can be heard some distance from the thorax, always can hear her heart beat; could not sleep last night for whizzing and purring of heart, when she did fall asleep was delirious. Sensation as if a cap were on her head. When she awakens and finds it there she knows that she is all right, that she is not delirious; > after vomiting; whispers in her sleep; whispers to herself, if you ask her what she said does not answer; sensation as if she covered the whole bed; she knew that her head was on the pillow, but she could not tell where the rest of her body was.

She feels when lying on one side that she is one person and that when she turns to the other side she is another person; sensation as though the fever would not run in each alike, that is to say, she felt as though she was existing in a second person, or that there were two of her.

Coldness and chilliness all day that no fire would warm; sits by the fire and breathes the heat from the stove; chilly whenever leaving the fire; at night when the fever came on he had a sensation as if his lungs were on fire and that he must have fresh air, which soon brought relief.

Sensation as though he was crowded by his arms and legs; When turning over in bed they were still crowding him; as soon as the fever came on he commenced to urinate; he can tell every time when the fever is coming on because of this urgency to urinate. The urine is clear as spring-water. Very severe pain in the right side; knife-like pains going through to the back; < from every motion, from coughing or talking or taking a long breath; > from lying on the affected side; groaning with every breath; redness of the face and also of the ears, it looked as if the blood would burst out of them. After the fever leaves he still has the hallucination that he is very wealthy and he has a very large sum of money in the bank, and this was the last to leave him—this idea that he had the money.

I can hardly mention Pyrogen without becoming enthusiastic, on account of the wonderful results that I have had from it in blood poisoning. In any kind of septic infection, either puerperal or traumatic, Pyrogen will do wonders, when the symptoms correspond. It is similar to Anthracinum in some respects.

An old woman dying with gangrene inoculated one of her nurses; the nurse had chills, high fever and red streaks running up the arm following the course of the lymphatics. Pyrogen rapidly removed the whole process.—*Boger.*

The palmar surface of the left forearm was torn to the bone by a buzz-saw. It was dressed by adhesive plaster, which was put on so tightly that it had to be removed in 24 hours, replaced by another and a few stitches taken; but the whole hand began to swell, became very painful, gradually grew worse for eighteen days, during which patient had but few hours sleep. Whole hand and forearm were enormously swollen, almost black in colour and mortification threatened. Amputation was now decided.

At this stage a homeopathic physician found in addition to the symptoms above the patient delirious and excited; he could not lie down, for the bed was too hard, nor could he rest the arm on anything, for everything on which it lay also seemed too hard. Pyrogen 50m. In a few hours he was sleeping quietly, temperature reduced and pain lessened. Improvement was rapid and steady to complete recovery.

Slight elevation of temperature, severe rigor, followed by sweating. The rigors are usually severe, and they occasionally occur with the regularity of ague.

Pulse becomes weak and rapid.

Pulse felt in head and ears, painless throbbing.

Fever of the intermittent type, with the usual accompaniments of loss of appetite, restlessness, thirst.

Rigors cease after the first few days, but the temperature usually maintains a remittent character.

Puerperal fevers.

Typhoid fever.

Feverishness.

Pyemia.

Septicemia.

Burning in the face.

Blood was throbbing all through every part of head and body—could feel it even in my fingers.

Chilly all night.

Generalities—

Cannot lie more than few minutes in one position, > change.

Debility in morning, staggered on trying to walk (S).

Aching all over, bed feels hard.

Great muscular debility; rapid recovery in a few hours (dog).

Restlessness, turning in bed, groaning.

Pains in limbs and general uneasiness.

Soon after the initial rigor, pain and swelling of one or more joints occurs.

Peculiar sweet smell about the patient, as in diabetes.

A sudden attack of pleurisy occurring in any one with otorrhea. Pyemia may be suspected.

General lassitude.

Nervousness.

Feebleness.

Malaria, pains in limbs, especially in legs and back, with headache, distress in stomach, like a heavy wad.

Restlessness, when beginning to move and during motion.

Restless and moaning, in persons dying, especially from scarlet fever or diphtheria, often enables them to recover.

Great nervousness and restlessness, wants to be covered or rocked.

Great aversion to being washed. Cries when washed.

Will not sleep in bed, but wants to be held in lap and kept in slight motion; wakes when the motion is stopped or on attempting to lay her down.

Aggravation—

Restlessness > when first commencing to move (Rhus < when first commencing to move).

Amelioration—

From hard rocking in a chair.

SECALE CORNUTUM

Synonyms—

Ergota (Ergot or Argot, Fr,, a cock's spur); Ergot of rye; Spurred rye; Secale clavatum; Mater secalis; Seigle ergote (Fright); Mutterkorn; Kornmutter (G).

Characteristics—

Adapted to women of *thin, scrawny, feeble, cachectic appearance;* irritable, nervous temperament; pale, sunken countenance.

Very old, decrepit, feeble persons.

Women of very lax muscular fibre; everything *seems loose and open; no action, vessels flabby;* passive hemorrhages, copious flow of thin, black, watery blood; the corpuscles are destroyed.

Hemorrhagic diathesis; the slightest wound causes bleeding for weeks (Lach., Phos.); discharge of sanious liquid blood with a strong tendency to putrescence; tingling in the limbs and great debility, especially when the weakness is not caused by previous loss of fluids.

Leucorrhea: green, brown, offensive.

Boils: *small, painful with green contents,* mature very slowly and heal in the same manner; very debilitating.

Face: pale, pinched, ashy, sunken, hippocratic; drawn, with sunken eyes; blue rings around eyes.

Unnatural, ravenous appetite; even with exhausting diarrhea; craves acids, lemonade.

Diarrhea: profuse, watery, putrid, brown; discharged with

great force (Gamb., Crot.); very exhausting; painless, involuntary; anus wide open (Apis, Phos.).

Enuresis: of old people; urine pale, watery, or bloody; urine suppressed.

Burning, in all parts of the body, as if sparks of fire were falling on the patient (Ars.).

Gangrene; dry, senile, < from external heat.

Large ecchymoses; blood blisters; often commencement of gangrene.

Collapse in cholera diseases; skin cold, yet cannot bear to be covered (Camph.).

The skin feels cold to the touch, yet the patient cannot tolerate covering; icy coldness of extremities.

Menses: irregular; copious, dark fluid; with pressing, labor-like pains in abdomen; continuous discharge of watery blood until next period.

Threatened abortion especially at third month (Sab.); prolonged, bearing down, forcing pains.

During labor: pains irregular; too weak; feeble or ceasing; everything seems *loose and open but no expulsive action;* fainting.

After pains: too long; too painful; hour-glass contraction.

Suppression of milk: in thin, scrawny, exhausted women; the breasts do not properly fill.

Pulse small, rapid, contracted and often intermittent.

PROVERS.

1 Mrs. L. M. Hayes, with the 200th. This prover knew the potency but not the drug. She was perfectly convinced that in the 200th potency no drug was capable of producing medicinal symptoms on the healthy, and persisted in repeating her experiments to verify or disprove former results. Took November 4th, six drops every other day for a week. November 17th, took six drops twice a day for a week. January 5th, took fifteen drops every day for a week. March 1st, took fifteen drops every morning for three days.

2. Miss R. C. Wilder, took six drops, 30th potency, in morning of November 5th, 8th, 12th, 15th.

3. H. B. Reynolds, took one drachm of 2d potency, in repeated doses.

4. J. S. Campbell, took several doses of 2 potency.

5. F. W. Rogers, took one drachm of 200th potency, a dose twice a day for two weeks.

6. Mrs. M. T. Hathaway, repeated doses of 200th potency.

7. D. M. Finley, 100th potency; repeated the proving four times with same results each time.

8. Miss H. M. Swathel, took 200th potency, from March 1st to April 23, two or three times a day. Took 100th potency from May 2 to May 15th, once or twice daily.

9. G. D. Green, took 2 potency for two weeks.

10. C. S. Erswell, took 100th potency, one drachm, in daily doses for two weeks.

1 E. H. Pond, took 30th potency.

12. E. C. Watts, took 30th potency daily for a week.

Since March, 1880, the drug was given out to seventy-two volunteers, as follows:

Second potency to 16 provers.

Third potency to 4 provers.

Sixth potency to 17 provers.

Thirtieth potency to 13 provers.

Sixtieth potency to 5 provers.

One hundredth potency to 6 provers.

Two hundredth potency to 8 provers.

Blanks potency to 3 provers.

The blanks were given to those whose health, on examination, was not deemed sufficiently good to warrant a reliable proving, only one of whom (a young man who afterwards died of albuminuria) obtained or returned any results.

RULES OBSERVED

So far as possible, every prover was examined as to health

and personal qualifications; and questioned or cross-questioned on the recorded results.

Provers were directed to follow the rules laid down by Dun-ham for proving a drug.

No person knew what she or he was taking.

BOTANY.

Adam Lonicer, of Frankfort, about the middle of the 16th century, is the first botanical writer to notice Ergot, and soon after Thalius speaks of it as used "*ad sistendum sanguinem.*"

In 1623, Caspar Bauhin mentions it under the name of *Secale luxurians,* and in 1693 the English botanist Ray alludes to its medicinal properties.

The true nature of Ergot, whether a product of diseased vegetable life or a true vegetable itself, has long been a source of a great diversity of opinion. But according to the latest authorities, Secale cornutum belongs to the order Thallophyta—cellular or non-vascular plants. This is the lowest order of the vegetable kingdom and is divided into two classes, Algae and Fungi, which is based upon the presence in the former of Chlorophyll, and its absence in the latteright They produce no differentiation of root, stem or leaf. In the lowest members of the group there is no sexual reproduction; in the higher the sexual union may be by a single spore, or a mass of spores, or a fructification within which spores are found. De Candolle and Fries in 1816, and Leveille, in 1827, added, by their researches, much to our knowledge of the intimate structure of Secale, but it remained to L. R. Tulsane, in 1853, by his admirable monograph "Memoire sur 1' Ergot des Glumacees," to clear up many disputed points in the formation, growth and development of this fungus, and this monograph is still referred to by nearly every author as the best work on the subject. Yet Fluckiger and Hanbury maintain that *the true nature of Ergot has not been settled* even by Tulsane's long continued and admirable researches.

FORMATION

Hamilton sums up the conflicting views entertained by various writers as follows:

a. "Some regard Ergot as a fungus growing between the glumes of grasses, in the place of the ovary (hence Leveille calls it *Spacelia segetum).*

b. "Some regard Ergot as a diseased condition of the ovary or seed.

c. ' Some have supposed that ordinary morbific causes (such as moisture combined 'with warmth) were sufficient to give rise to this diseased condition of the grain.

d. "Some have ascribed the disease to the attack of insects or other animals.

e. "Some, dissatisfied with the previously assigned causes of the disease, have been content with declaring Ergot to be a disease, but without specifying the circumstances which induce it."

Fluckiger and Hanbury state, "That the tissue of the seed of the rye, in the process of development, does not undergo a *transformation,* but is simply *destroyed."*

Neither in external form, nor in anatomical structure, does Ergot exhibit any resemblance to a seed, although its development takes place between the flowering time and that at which the rye begins to ripen. It has been regarded as a complete fungus, and as such was named by De Candolle *Sclerotium Clavus,* and by Fries *Spermoëdia Clavius.* No further change occurs in the Ergot while it remains in the ear; but laid on damp earth, interesting phenomena take place.

At certain points small, orbicular patches of the rind fold themselves back, and gradually throw out little white heads. These increase in size whilst the outer layers of the neighbouring tissue gradually lose their firmness and become soft and rather granular, at the same time that the cells, of which they are made up, become empty and extended. In the interior of Ergot, the cells retain their oil drops unaltered. The heads assume a grayish-yellow colour, changing to purple, and finally after some weeks stretch themselves towards the light on slender, shining stalks, of a pale, violet colour. The stalks often attain an inch in length with a thickness of about half a line. Fluckiger further says: "Ergot of rye collected by myself in August, placed upon earth in a garden-pot and left in the open air unprotected through the winter, began to develop the *Claviceps* on the 20th of March."

Hering calls it an undetermined fungus, and from the doubtful position it has so long held in the world of science classes it, not without some reason, as a 'Nosode;' and when a doubtful point in Materia Medica is to be solved, the opinion of the venerated and scientific Hering is deserving of some consideration.

Nosode, he says: "Is the general term given to the alcoholic extracts of morbid productions, foolishly called isopathic remedies. The most useful and fully proved are Hydrophobinum and Psorinum. To these ' Nosodes' belong the Ustilago maidis, the Secale cornutum, the fungus of the potato, the ambra of the pot-fish, anthracin, vaccinin, variolin, etc., etc. The sneering remarks of Trinks and others in 1826 against Sepia and the ignorant opposition to Lachesis have sunken into oblivion during the succeeding score of years. All the condemning remarks against the Hydrophobinum, Psorinum and other ' Nosodes' will meet the same fate. We can afford to wait."

PREPARATION.

For homeopathic use the Ergot of rye should always be prepared fresh, as it is fed on by a small acarus which destroys the interior of the grain, leaving it a mere shell. Ergot kept in stock longer than a year should always be rejected on this account.

MEDICAL HISTORY.

Among the writings of the ancients there is no distinct notice to be found of Ergot. In 1089 the French historian, Sigebert, refers to an epidemic in the following passage:

"A pestilent year, especially in the western parts of Lorraine, where many persons became putrid, in consequence of their inward parts being consumed by St. Anthony's fire. Their limbs were rotten and became black like coal. They either perished miserably or, deprived of their putrid hands and feet, were reserved for a more miserable life. Moreover, many cripples were afflicted with contraction of the sinews."

An epidemic disease in Hessia in 1596 first attracted the attention of the medical profession to Ergot as a cause. Rathlaw, a Dutch accoucher, employed it in 1747, but it was not until thirty years later, 1777, that the essays of Desgranges, and especially those of Stearns and Prescott in the United States, that its medicinal properties became known.

To the use of rye flour, more or less adulterated with Ergot, is attributed the formidable disease known in modern medicine as *Ergotism,* but in early times by a number of names: *Morbus spasmodicus, Convulsivus Malignus, Epidemicus vel Cerealis, Convulsion Rapkania, Ignus Sancti Antonia.* There is now little doubt that the terrible epidemics which occurred in France in the tenth century and in Spain in the twelfth century were due to Ergot. Fluckiger and Hanbury says:

"In the year 1596 Hessia and the adjoining regions were ravaged by a frightful pestilence, which the medical faculty of Marburg attributed to the presence of Ergot in the cereals consumed by the population. The same disease appeared in France in 1630; in Voightland, Saxony, in the years 1648, 1649 and 1675; again in various parts of France in 1650, 1670 and 1674. Freiburg and vicinity were visited by the same malady in 1702; other parts of Switzerland in 1715-16; Saxony and Lusatia in 1716; many other districts of Germany in 1717, 1722, 1736 and 1741-42. The last European epidemic occurred after the rainy season of 1816 in Lorraine and Burgundy, and proved very fatal among the poorer classes."

From time to time a number of monographs giving a more or less accurate description of the various epidemics supposed to have been caused chiefly by Ergot and other adulterations in

France, Germany and Switzerland have appeared. In 1825, the year previous to his departure for South America,. Hering made a collection of these monographs which he left with Trinks, who had it completed by one of his assistants and published. These comprise the first 80 of the 170 authorities of the *encyclopdaeia,* taken from Hartlaub and Trinks. The later additions are chiefly toxicological and clinical.

Dr. R. B. Johnstone, of Pittsford, N. Y., writes:

"In 1883-84, during the building of the West Shore Railroad, I was called upon to treat many of the Italian employes for an eruption which appeared upon the body in many places, but usually on the shoulders, neck and inner surface of the upper arms. In the majority of cases it was on the right side alone, but if on both sides was always worse on the right. The eruption would begin in a small point, like the prick of a pin, which would soon assume a pimple-like form and finally become pustular and as large as a small pea. At other times they would appear as large as a small boil (half an inch across the base), of a dark bluish hue, shading off to the healthy colour of the skin an inch or more from centre of boil. They were *intensely painful to touch, aching, burning and itching, better from light rubbing, worse from scratching, worse from heat.* The small ones would dry up leaving no cicatrix, but the large ones would fill slowly with a bright yellow pus-like material, or at times a bloody, watery serum, remaining open for days, having extremely painful edges and base, and discharging towards its close a thick, dirty, offensive serum. They were decidedly indolent in character, and left a prominent cicatrix. Cool air blowing over the eruption would relieve the itching and burning, but not the pain. Secale, Lachesis, Causticum were the remedies chiefly indicated. Having learned that the Italians ate largely of rye bread made of a very poor and cheap quality of flour, while other nationalities (not eating the rye bread) did not suffer from it at all, I attributed the eruption to poisoning by *Ergot* in the bread; and if a patient presented without an interpreter I usually gave Secale, which would cure about seven cases in ten."

"H. G. K.—A miller of Pittsford, N. Y., informs me that he is unable to grind rye even for a short time. Upon entering a rye mill, had a sensation of constriction in the throat, great difficulty in breathing; difficult inspiration; expiration accompanied by soreness all over the chest; oppression of the chest; soreness of the chest; intercostal pains; pricking of the tongue.

"The foregoing symptoms are distinctively of rye grinding; when grinding wheat no symptoms follow. He also informs me that in two rye mills in Rochester he knows a number of individuals engaged therein who suffer as above with the addition of an eruption particularly on the neck, chest, behind the ears and around the waist. The eruption is pustular, itching violently, and discharges a yellow matter. One man he knew who was compelled to give up rye grinding because of the many *boils* and *carbuncles.* He recovered entirely after changing his occupation. Nearly all rye grinders have enlarged finger joints and poor teeth."

DAY BOOK OF MRS. M. F. HATHAWAY.

March 6, 1885.—Took a powder (Secale 200) every morning and at night on retiring, for three days, then at night only, for a week.

March 9th—A sore spot felt on back part of base of tongue, left side, as though a 'canker sore' were making its appearance; it was not felt in day time and passed away after a few days.

March 10th and 11th—A slight frontal headache and some mental confusion, but not very troublesome. Sore spot on base of tongue, right side.

March 13th—Spots with a sore bruised feeling appeared about and below the left knee. On looking found a swollen patch about the size of a silver half dollar, of a purple red colour. Towards evening three or four similar spots appeared further down the leg, about the top of the shoe, so sore could scarcely bear the touch of the shoe, and attended with violent itching, but were so extremely sore could not scratch them, and when touched gave me a faint, sick feeling.

March 14th—Headache and confusion more pronounced, and chiefly in frontal region. Three or four spots appeared on right leg below the knee, with violent itching and the same sore bruised feeling.

March 15th—An eruption in the form of a rash or small pustules appeared on the face, left side chiefly, very sore and sensitive to touch. It would begin in fine points like the prick of a pin or the sting of an insect and gradually increasing in size to a small pustule as large as a pea. Felt like the spots on the legs, with the same sore, bruised feeling in the skin of face and neck. There were twenty-eight small pustules on left side of face and neck.

March 18th—The eruption appeared on the left shoulder, several small pustules in a cluster, with the same characteristic soreness. Ceased taking drug. Dull, heavy headache in forehead and eyes; much throbbing.

Before the menses (four or five days) a dark coloured leucor-rhea was observed, not very profuse, but attended with a tired and uneasy feeling in the pelvis.

April 5th—The eruption on face, neck and shoulders gradually disappeared, but left discoloured, ecchymosed spots and patches like the remains of an old bruise for several weeks, especially on lower leg.

April 18th—Menses appeared on time, *very profuse* for the first three or four days, accompanied by a good deal of pain and an uneasy sore feeling through the pelvis (much more than usual), but an unusual amount of pain for a week before the menses. Flow darker, much more profuse (formerly profuse for one day) for four days. Considerable clotting. The flow continued for ten days, a circumstance which never occurred before. Vertigo during entire menstrual period, with inclination to fall forwards.

Was attacked while at lectures with palpitation which continued nearly all the afternoon. Could feel the heart flutter and remit. Pulse 108 and 110. Violent throbbing of the carotids, faint for several hours. Never had palpitation before in her life. Headache; full, throbbing, bursting, like a Glonoine headache (has proved Glonoine), only not so sore on shaking the head.

Mind—

Stupid, half-sleepy state.

Impaired power of thinking.

Delirium: quiet; wandering.

Mania: with inclination to bite; with inclination to drown.

Uncomfortableness and depression.

Fear of death.

Anxiety, sadness, melancholy.

Great anguish; wild with anxiety.

Apathy, indifference.

Constant moaning and fear of death.

Great anxiety and difficult respiration.

Excessive sadness, gradually changes to cheerfulness; talks and acts foolishly; rage, followed by continuously deep sleep.

Paralytic mental diseases; treats his relations contemptuously and sarcastically; wandering talk and hallucinations; apathy and complete disappearance of the senses.

|| Laughs, claps her hands over her head, seems beside herself.

After miscarriage.

Memory failed. Forgot names of friends whom I met daily.

Confusion of mind. Unpleasant forebodings.

Anticipated misfortunes, as though about to lose something of great value.

|| Sensation of intoxication while undressing, to retire (third day and for several successive evenings).

During entire proving I experienced an elevation of spirits, felt buoyant and exhilarated.

Sensorium—

Unconsciousness, with heavy sleep, preceded by tingling in head and limbs.

Diminution and loss of senses, sight, hearing, etc.

All the senses benumbed.

Consciousness seems to continue until the last breath, and just before death it seems as if patient would improve.

Stupefaction; stupor.

Vertigo: constantly increasing; with stupefaction and heaviness of head; reeling, inability to stand erect; peculiar feeling of lightness of head, particularly in occiput; as from intoxication; unsteady gait.

Heaviness of head and tingling in legs.

|| Sensation of intoxication while undressing.

Inner Head—

Pulsations in head with giddiness, she cannot walk.

Pain and confusion most in occiput.

Congestion to head and chest.

Headache; hemicrania on left side.

Vertigo during entire last menstrual period; inclination to fall forwards.

Head heavy. Sharp stinging pain running upwards through the left eye into forehead and left side of head; coming in paroxysms.

A dull, heavy, at times pressing headache, most severe on right side; aggravated in warm room, but not ameliorated in open air.

Dull pain on each side of the head, above and before the ears, worse in warm room. At times it was throbbing, and continued with more or less severity for three weeks after leaving off the drug. It was semi-lateral at times, and seemed to prefer the right side and forehead.

Feels oppressed; stupid, heavy; aches every night; would waken me at night; ameliorated by eating breakfast and exercise.

Could not sleep on account of the fearful oppressive headache, extending from occiput up over head to the eyes.

Severe pain in occiput, forehead, temples, back of eyes aggravated by pressure on nape of neck.

Headache aggravated in open air, and first entering warm room; as after riding in cold north wind in winter, when entering warm room the head aches so fearfully.

More or less, a dull headache during the entire proving, especially in the forehead and eyes.

Head full, throbbing, bursting, like a Glonoine headache, though not so sore on shaking the head.

Continuous, supra-orbital headache (developed after proving the remedy a week).

Pain from forehead to the eyes; burning sensation in the eyes; no inflammation; pain shoots through the eyeball backward.

Outer Head—

Hair falls out.

Twisting of head to and fro.

|| Scalp sore.

Scalp sore; so painful, cannot bear to move the hair.

Felt as though the hair had been parted in a new place, or pressed by hair pin.

Hair looked at roots as though bulbs were enlarged.

Scalp slightly pink in irregular spots; pimples appeared over scalp; small, very sore to touch, with slight burning sensation.

Eyes and Sight—

Photophobia.

Dimness of vision; mistiness before eyes. Cataract.

Double or triple vision.

Blue and fiery dots flying before eyes.

Pain in eyes with feeling as if they were spasmodically rotated.

Stitching pain in eyes; pressure on balls.

After an epidemic of the rye disease an unusually large

number of cataracts occurred in young people, twenty-three of whom gradually became blind (fifteen men and eight women), associated with headache, vertigo and roaring in ears; of the cataracts two were hard, twelve soft, and nine mixed.

| Cataracta senilis.

|| Suppuration of cornea; < from warm applications.

|| Retinitis diabetica.

Dilation of pupils.

Suppressed secretion of tears.

Injection of conjunctiva.

Eyes sunken, surrounded by a blue margin.

Paralysis of the upper lids, from coal gas.

Immovable state of eyelids after facial erysipelas.

Eyes look fixed, wild, glazed; staring look.

|| Pustulous conjunctivitis and blepharitis.

|| Exophthalmos with struma.

Exophthalmic goitre.

Ears and Hearing—

Undue sensitiveness of hearing, even slightest sound re-echoed in her head and made her shudder.

Confused hearing; deafness. After chorea.

Singing in ears and difficult hearing.

Humming and roaring in ears, with occasional deafness.

Nose and Smell—

Sneezing.

Nose feels stopped up, yet watery discharge runs from it.

|| Nose stopped up on left side as with a solid plug.

|| Nosebleed: blood dark, runs continuously, with great prostration, small, threadlike pulse; in old people or drunkards; of young women; from debility.

Passive morning epistaxis from left side, bright red.

Morning nose-bleed, something very unusual; left side only, passive, but bright red.

Nose stopped up on left side as with a solid plug, but not much discharge.

Nose sore to touch externally and internally.

Nose-bleed not very profuse, recurring for several successive days.

Bleeding at the nose on every attempt to wipe it.

Face—

Face: pinched, pale, earthy-looking; sunken, hip-pocratic, ashy; swollen; contracted, discoloured, with sunken eyes, blue rings around eyes; risus sardonicus; distorted; wan, anxious.

Tingling in face.

Muscular twitchings usually commence in face and then spread all over body, sometimes increasing to dancing and jumping.

Spasmodic distortion of mouth and lips.

Forehead hot.

Lockjaw.

Lips deathly pale or bluish.

Oppressed, full of blood during fever.

Face and neck feel hot, as if full of blood and ready to burst.

Teeth and Gums—

Looseness of teeth.

Grinding of teeth.

Bleeding from gums.

|| Difficult dentition; great weakness; vomiting of everything taken; great thirst; pale face; eyes dim, sunken; dry heat, with rapid pulse; restlessness and sleeplessness.

Taste and Tongue—

Tongue: thickly coated with yellowish-white, dry, tenacious substance; discoloured, brown or blackish; deathly pale; cold and livid; clean, with dry, red tip; red tip and edges, centre coated.

Slight but unpleasant warmth on tongue, during day.

Spasm of tongue, projecting it from mouth, forcing it between teeth and rendering speech indistinct.

Feeble, stuttering, indistinct speech, as if tongue were paralyzed.

Coated yellowish brown through middle, sides clean.

In the evening (second day) a sore spot felt on the back of the tongue, left side, as though a 'canker sore' were making its appearance.

In the evening of the third day the same sore feeling on the tongue, but on right side. This is not felt at all during the day time.

Mouth—

Bloody or yellowish green foam at mouth.

Increased secretion of saliva; ptyalism.

Much acid fluid in mouth.

Spitting of blood.

Fetid breath.

Speech difficult, slow and weak, with a feeling at every motion as if there was some resistance to be overcome.

Dryness of mouth.

Dry, but seldom thirsty. Burning, dry sensation, not relieved by drinking. Brackish taste.

Stammers unintelligible words between teeth; speech, difficult and stammering; speech, slow and weak, with a feeling on every motion as if there were always some resistance to be overcome.

Throat—

Dryness of soft palate, throat and esophagus, with thirst.

Burning in throat with violent thirst.

Painful tingling in throat and on tongue.

| | Throat sore on left side running up into ear.

| Follicular pharyngitis; hawking up of little follicular exudates.

Diphtheria: loss of strength; rapid loss of sensibility;

numbness of extremities; painful tingling and crawling on tongue; dry gangrene; apathy; dilated pupils; burning pains of affected parts; stammering speech; absence of all reaction.

|| Severely paralyzed both in swallowing and in speaking; could scarcely take food without great danger of choking; speech reduced to a whisper; could not bear heat or covering and would throw all covering off. Post-diphtheritic paralysis.

Soreness with dryness and sensation of constriction, better by swallowing; symptoms worse mornings.

Rawness, dryness and constriction of throat, without any pain.

Throat sore on left side running up into ear.

Throat on right side red, sore, with a feeling as if it were constructed of tense and hard fibres, very slightly hoarse.

Later throat felt constricted, chiefly on right side; right side and back of throat inflamed, red and 'stiff,' some pain on swallowing. (I am not inclined to right sided sore throat, almost all my attacks of the kind being confined to the left side.)

Appetite, Thirst, Desires, Aversions—

Ravenous, insatiable appetite, even when dying from exhausting discharges from bowels.

Hunger as from long fasting.

Disgust for food, especially for meat and fatty things.

Thirst: during all stages of fever; unquenchable; for acids.

Great thirst and dryness of mouth and throat, with burning and tingling of tongue.

Desire for: sour things; lemonade.

Hiccough, Belching, Nausea and Vomiting—

Eructations: with disagreeable taste; sour, tasteless, but with subjective, disagreeable, empyreumatic odor; empty.

Nausea: inclination to vomit; painful retchings; constant, < after eating.

Excessive nausea and debility, with very little vomiting of a dark brown coffee-grounds fluid.

Vomiting: of food; of bile; of mucus; of green, offensive, watery fluid, painless and without effort, with great weakness; immediately after eating; of lumbrici; of blood; black vomit.

Hematemesis, patient lies still; great weakness but no pain; abdomen soft.

Scrobiculum and Stomach—

Tenderness of epigastrium.

Anxiety and pressure in pit of stomach, with great sensitiveness to touch.

| Severe anxiety and burning at pit of stomach.

Pain in pit of stomach.

Violent pressure in stomach, as from a heavy weight.

Warmth and feeling of repletion.

Burning in stomach.

Painful constriction of epigastrium.

Great distress and oppression of stomach.

|| Bilious vomiting, with cramping pains in stomach; burning in stomach extending up esophagus; head sunk upon breast, face pale, yellowish, voice weak, pulse small. Cardialgia.

|| Attacks of severe pressure and constriction in region of stomach extending through to spine, extremely painful and followed in half an hour by vomiting of tasteless fluid or of contents of stomach, thereupon an intermission of several hours occurred; during attack region of stomach felt as if contracted, and on percussion gave a tympanitic note; has three to four attacks daily.

| Hemorrhage from stomach; lies still with great weakness but no pain; face, lips, tongue and hands deadly pale; skin covered with cold sweat, pulse frequent, threadlike; oppression; abdomen soft, without pain. Hematemesis.

|| Hematemesis; attacks preceded by pains in epigastrium and nausea, pain going to left side when pressure is made in epigastrium; marked protrusion in left hypochondrium, with

pain; blood red, never containing particles of food, and when collected in basin appears more like bloody serum than pure blood and is of offensive odor, quantity vomited not very large; frequent chilliness at night, followed by profuse sweat; strength not much impaired; appetite and sleep good.

Eructations: having the odor of burnt horn.

Appetite much increased; was very hungry, ashamed to eat as much as desired.

Felt as though I had dined on chopped cabbage.

Nausea after leaving table.

Felt too full, fermented; much flatulence.

Flatulence rumbling through stomach and bowels.

A tired sensation—one of distress and oppression—over region below the stomach, was present much of the time during the proving.

Hypochondria—

Enlargement of the liver.

Inflammation and gangrene of liver; acute pains in hepatic region; tongue thickly coated with a brown tenacious substance, burning in throat, unquenchable thirst; great weakness, but no pain; limbs cold and covered with cold sweat.

Burning in spleen; thrombosis of abdominal vessels.

Abdomen—

Distension of abdomen; tympanites; meteorism.

Flatulence with rumbling.

Painful sensitiveness and rumbling, with continual nausea and confusion of head.

Inclination to colic, diarrhea, and bloatedness of abdomen.

Pain in lower belly, preventing an upright position, even forcing him to lie doubled up in bed.

Colic with convulsions.

| Pain in abdomen with burning in stomach.

| Pains in hypogastric region.

Pain in loins as from false labor pains.

Continual bearing down in lower abdomen.

Burning in abdomen.

Cold feeling in abdomen and back.

Strong pulsation in umbilical region.

Lumps and welts in abdomen; in affections of uterus.

|| Aneurism of mesenteric artery, in women.

Abdomen much distended.

Distension of abdomen; much flatulence as though soon to suffer from diarrhea.

Spasmodic jerking of small intestines near sigmoid flexure as though tied about with strings, which were interruptedly pulled. Worse evening, and better by pressure and lying on affected side. This lasted for about three weeks.

Bowels felt weak, sick, faint, as in summer from eating too much fruit; no pain but hot and dry internally.

Bowels did not pain, and seemingly would have been relieved of heat, dryness and uncomfortable feeling if I could have drunk water enough to reach them, which I was unable to do. Neither drinking water nor an enema gave relief.

Stool and Rectum—

|| Diarrhea: very exhausting; pernicious; very offensive; involuntary, profuse, watery, putrid, brown; discharged with great force; very exhausting; urine suppressed; painful with great prostration; painless with tingling and numbness in limbs; putrid, fetid, colliquative, patient does not want to be covered or to be near the heat, but prefers to be in the air or wishes to be fanned; sudden attacks; of children, discharges whitish, watery; chronic in overfed children, great prostration; during August; great stools undigested, or watery, at times yellowish, also greenish, with forcible expulsion, accompanied by discharge of flatus; paralytic weakness of sphincter ani with involuntary discharges.

Stools: yellowish; greenish; brownish; watery and flocculent; colourless, watery; profuse; frequent; putrid; gushing;

involuntary; watery, slimy; thin, olive green; offensive, watery; fetid, dark coloured; thin, involuntary; watery, yellowish or greenish, discharged rapidly with great force and even involuntarily; painless, without effort and with great weakness.

Before stool: cutting and rumbling in abdomen.

During stool: cutting; great exhaustion; coldness.

After stool: exhaustion.

|| Five to ten minutes after taking least quantity of food, severe colic which made her bend double and cry out; pain begins between region of stomach and navel, extends thence to sides and rest of abdomen and down to sacral region, accompanied by severe urging and tenesmus, followed by a thin, slimy, yellowish stool with some relief of pain; four to five such attacks follow each other; then relief until she eats again; four to five evacuations during night; she compares pains to labor pains; great thirst; thick mucous coating on tongue; sleep disturbed; prostration. Diarrhea.

|| Uncomfortable fullness of abdomen, with transient pinching pains in upper abdomen as from flatus; at night severe cutting pains throughout whole abdomen; restless anxious tossing about, with short and unrefreshing naps; during night anus firmly closed, "as if locked up;" in morning frequent short watery evacuations, in gushes, preceded by cutting pains in abdomen.

|| Stools yellowish-white, slimy, undigested, escaping involuntarily, < at break of day. Diarrhea.

| Interminable diarrhea in summer, which resists everything, especially in scrofulous children; putrid, fetid and colliquative; choleraic symptoms, with cold, clammy perspiration; sinking spells at 3 A.M. (not the restless anguish of Arsenicum).

|| Colliquative diarrhea.

Cholerine with more retching than vomiting.

| Cholera infantum; profuse undigested stools, watery and very offensive, discharged by fits and starts and followed by

intense prostration; pale face, sunken eyes, dry heat, quick pulse, restlessness and sleeplessness; great aversion to heat and to being covered. Cholera infantum.

|| Vertigo, cramps or drawing in calves of legs, rumbling in abdomen, nausea, stools in rapid succession, brownish or colourless, rapid prostration, coldness of limbs, tongue but slightly coated.

|| Profuse prostrating evacuations, severe painful cramps in feet, toes, hands and fingers which are spread apart or extended toward back of hands; cramping pressure in stomach; dry, wrinkled, cold skin; cyanotic colour Cholera.

| Cholera infantum; cholera morbus; cholera Asiatica.

|| Patient cold, almost pulseless, with spasmodic twitching of muscles in various parts of body; spreads fingers asunder; eyes sunken, features pinched; much spasmodic retching although not much vomiting; skin harsh, shrivelled, dry, as if there were no moisture left in system; urine suppressed; tingling or formication all over body; stools profuse, watery, ejected with great violence; is cold but cannot bear to be covered. Cholera.

|| Aversion to heat or being covered, with icy coldness of extremities.

| Diarrhea after cholera.

| Cholera Asiatica, with collapse, sunken, distorted face, particularly mouth; crawling sensation as from ants.

Paralysis of rectum; anus wide open.

| Hemorrhage from bowels.

| Constipation.

Constipated; dry, dark, detached, yet difficult to expel.

No desire for days; feels as though rectum was full.

Frequent stools; light coloured, soft.

Diarrhea: stool small, scanty. Almost every time urine was passed during the day, a small stool.

Constant desire for stool.

Urinary Organs—

Retention of urine; urine pale or bloody; discharge of thick black blood from kidneys; obscuration of sight. Scarlatina.

Diabetes; great general lassitude; heaviness of limbs; loss of strength; emaciation; gangrene; skin dry and withered; furuncles; petechias; fever, with unquenchable thirst; diminished power of senses; dryness of mouth; morbidly great appetite; cardialgia; costiveness; diarrhea; watery urine; increased quantity of urine.

| | Hematuria in a boy suffering from suppuration of the glands of neck after scarlet fever; urine also very albuminous; anasarca; great thirst.

| Passive hemorrhage; blood thin; blood corpuscles wanting in consequence or dissolution; or painless discharge of thick black blood in consequence of kidney disease; coldness of body; cold perspiration on forehead; great weakness. Hematuria.

Urine suppressed; on introducing catheter a gill of dark, prune-coloured urine passed, which appeared to be full of gritty sediment emitting a very disagreeable odor.

Unsuccessful urging to urinate.

Ischuria paralytica.

| Paralysis of bladder.

|Enuresis: old people; pale, watery or bloody urine.

Urinary deposit looking like white cheese.

| Bloody, albuminous urine.

| Discharge of thick black blood from bladder; kidney affections.

Urine increased in quantity, lighter colour, passed more frequently, especially at night. Milky on standing a short time.

Pressure in bladder at night.

Male Sexual Organs—

After lightness in occiput, violent dragging in spermatic cord causing sensation as if testicle were being drawn up to inguinal ring.

After sexual excess palpitation of heart.

| Weak memory after exhausting coition; impotence.

Clonic spasmodic stricture of urethra.

Female Sexual Organs—

Uterus and right ovary much congested, very sensitive to touch.

|| Pain in ovaries and uterus.

Pains of an expulsive character in uterus.

Prolonged bearing down and forcing pains in uterus; thin and scrawny subjects.

Burning pains in greatly distended uterus, which felt hard and was painful to touch.

|| Putrescence of uterus; abdomen distended, not very painful; discharge from vagina, brownish, offensive; ulcers on external genitals discoloured and rapidly spreading; burning hot fever, interrupted by shaking chills; small, sometimes intermittent pulse; great anguish, pain in pit of stomach, vomiting decomposed matter; offensive diarrhea; suppressed secretion of urine; skin covered with petechial and miliary eruptions or shows discoloured, inflamed places, with a tendency to mortification; the patient lies either in quiet delirium or grows wild with great anxiety and a constant desire to get out of bed. Metritis.

||Metritis; tendency to putrescence; inflammation caused by suppression of lochia or menses; discharge of thin black blood, a kind of sanies, with tingling in legs and great debility. Metritis.

| Cancer and gangrene of uterus.

| Uterine ulcers feel as if burnt, discharge putrid, bloody fluid.

The uterus that had previously been in a normal condition descended so that it almost protruded, was hot and painful; os open as large as middle finger; excessive desire to urinate; labor pains only relieved by wet bandages or pressure upon abdomen; lasted three days, did not miscarry though os remained open during this period; afterward uterus gradually ascended, pains diminished, and after five or six days os contracted; went on to eighth month, when she miscarried.

|| Uterus about an inch from labia inferiora, membrane around it felt hard, while rest of mucous membrane of vagina was very much relaxed and gathered into a fold at lower part.

| Partial prolapsus of uterus for eight months after a forceps delivery; dysuria; sense of weight over pubes as if contents of abdomen would fall forward.

| Prolapsus of three months' standing; frequent severe cutting pains in abdomen; occasional nausea.

| Dreadful bearing down, dragging out feeling in lower abdomen, so that her life is almost unbearable; every four or five days profuse, thick, yellow discharge from vagina; hesitation in urinating; rheumatism. Hysteralgia.

Hemorrhage from uterus; apparent death of newborn child. Incessant metrorrhagia.

Uterine hemorrhage: when uterus is engorged; with pains in sacrum, extending down thighs and pressing into lower abdomen of a pregnant woman; profuse protracted flow; tearing, cutting colic, cold extremities and cold sweat, weak, hemorrhage < from slightest motion, blood thin and black, black, lumpy or brown fluid, of disgusting smell; black liquid blood.

|| A woman, aet. 45, passed through a normal confinement seven years ago; miscarried about two years ago, hemorrhage kept up for five months under allopathic treatment, with exacerbation during time of menstruation; after ceasing for seven months, hemorrhage set in again with slight intermission of one or two weeks; excessive anemia; sunken features; skin cold and dry; pulse small and quick; heavily coated tongue; loss of appetite; headache; since five days, daily ten or twelve painless stools, of mucous, watery, sometimes foul-smelling masses; thin, black, foul-smelling bloody discharges.

|| Feeble and extremely emaciated, skin flaccid, face very

pale and sunken, with an expression of suffering, mucous membranes pale and cool, hands and feet deficient of natural warmth, action of heart quickened, breathing short and oppressed, pulse very small, 120; abdomen distended; os uteri very open, with indented and puffy edges, flaccid and soft, vagina tender and cool; manual examination caused much uneasiness and flooding; violent headache limited to one spot, throbbing in temples, roaring in ears, giddiness on slightest movement; enfeebled nervous system showed extraordinary excitability; many times in day, and especially at night, cramps in calves and spasmodic twitching of limbs, causing exhaustion, remains several hours in bed as if paralyzed; digestion and sleep disturbed to some extent; hemorrhage still continued, even in horizontal position, and elevation of pelvis caused no diminution in large quantity of blackened coagula which were constantly passing, while least movement increased discharge in a very great degree. Chronic passive hemorrhage.

| Uterine hemorrhage, flow passive, dark and may be offensive; tingling or formication all over body, holds her fingers spread asunder, asks to have her limbs rubbed; finally lies unconscious and cold.

|| Metrorrhagia; relaxed condition of body; depressed, anxious state of mind; unusual drowsiness by day; gush of thin black blood on least movement of body; general feeling of prostration; diminished temperature of body; wooden, numb feeling in lower extremities.

Uterine hemorrhage; did not wish to be covered, desired windows to be open, though room was very cold and surface of body like a corpse.

| Painless flooding in feeble, cachectic, dyscratic women, or such as have long resided in tropical climates.

|| Since last delivery menses too seldom and very irregular, last time rather copious in consequence of unusual exertion; at night dreamed she was ascending the stairs with a heavy load, and suddenly a clot of blood came away and the blood seemed to gush forth; the alarm awakened her and she

found that she was bleeding fast; on following morning strength greatly reduced; lips and whole body, even tongue, deathly pale; pulse could not be distinguished; frequent fainting fits; periodic pains with expulsion of clots of blood and between these attacks constant oozing of thin bright blood.

|| An excessive menstrual flow every two weeks, lasting seven to nine days; for last four weeks flow is continuous; very weak and thin; has severe pains in loins and uterine region; bearing down pains as if in labor.

(Menses: too profuse and lasting too long; with tearing and cutting colic, cold extremities, cold sweat, great weakness and small pulse; or with violent spasms.

Menstrual blood: thin and black; black, lumpy or brown fluid and of disgusting smell.

|| Menstrual colic; pains so severe as to frequently cause spasms; uterine region very sensitive to touch; high fever; pains > when flow appears.

|| Menstrual colic; pale face; coldness of limbs; cold sweat; small, suppressed pulse; tearing, cutting pains in abdomen.

|| Menses irregular; every four weeks for three to four days, copious dark-red fluid discharge of blood, with pressing, labor-like pains in abdomen; constipation; pressure in occiput; afterward continuous discharge of watery blood, until next period.

Suppression of menses with pain.

|| Gangrene of whole vaginal mucous membrane; on holding apart the labise this membrane was found of a dark slate, colour, emitting the characteristic odor.

Vagina hot or cool.

| Discharge from vagina almost black, fluid and very fetid.

| Leucorrhea: in thin, scrawny women, with prolapsus uteri; green, brown, offensive; like cream, from weakness and venous congestion.

Ulcers on outer genitals, discoloured and rapidly spreading.

Sharp pains in left ovarian region, week before menses.

Menses a week too soon (always regular before to a day).

Flow bright red and coagulable; many clots.

Offensive in odor; *a cold cadaverous smell.*

Before the menses (four or five days) a dark coloured leucor-rhea was observed, not very profuse, but with a very uneasy feeling about the pelvis.

Menses appeared very profuse, lasting for ten days, but only profuse for the first three or four days, accompanied by a great deal of pain and an uneasy sore feeling (more than usual), and a dull headache during entire proving, especially in fore-head and eyes.

Catamenia occurred on time. Flow easy, abundant, pain-less and entirely without clot.

Passed a membrane. Period ceased (fifth day), having been entirely free from discomfort.

At second period the flow was of good colour, rather fluid, a few clots.

Continuous exercise stopped it on the second day, but no backache, headache or other disagreeable symptoms appeared in consequence.

Next period appeared at proper time "with few premoni-tory symptoms," but with a feeling all day as if I *must keep still* or have the flow checked. Passed a membrane. In four days menses ceased. (During the spring months of the past two years have passed membranes at the monthly period, but never be-fore in *consecutive* months.) The flow is usually attended with uneasy feelings and is always *greatly clotted.*

Leucorrhea the week before, discharge like white of egg (many times daily), changed just before menses to a yellowish offensive discharge; irritating; relieved by bathing parts in cold water.

After menses sharp pains in uterus and pelvic region,

with dragging, bearing down sensation, and aching across small of back.

Genital organs feel as if full of hot blood, pressed to their utmost capacity. The surface did not burn, but felt as though blood-vessels were filled with hot blood.

Uterus prolapsed; region sore to touch. This condition continued for weeks.

Menses one week too soon, too profuse, and what is very unusual, attended with much bearing, pressing down pain.

Second month, four days too soon, flow darker than custernary and offensive, but not clotted; lasts two days longer and is too profuse but not weakening.

Vertigo at the time of the menses with pain and heaviness in the pelvis for a week before the menses.

Unusual amount of pain and heaviness in pelvis for a week before menses.

Flow darker, much more profuse (formerly profuse for one day only) but this lasted four days.

Considerable clotting.

Pregnancy. Parturition. Lactation—

Arrested development of fetus.

Discharge of blood during pregnancy.

| Threatened abortion: more especially at third month; with copious flow of black, liquid blood; false labor pains, with bloody discharge; in feeble, cachectic women, having a wan, anxious countenance, pulse almost extinct, fear of death; convulsive movements.

|| Extremely violent pains, almost without intermission, she seemed to be in the last stage of labor, but on examination os was found about the size of a half dollar, thick and somewhat rigid.

|| Extremely violent pressing labor pains, os, however, being only about as large as a ten cent piece; hysterical convulsions.

|| When advanced about seven and a half months in pregnancy was taken with labor pains, wriggling and not distinctly

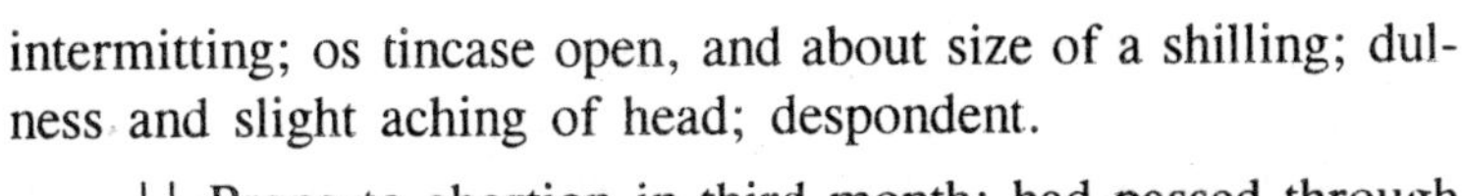
intermitting; os tincase open, and about size of a shilling; dulness and slight aching of head; despondent.

| | Prone to abortion in third month; had passed through five, although she kept her bed as soon as pregnant; some labor pains with bloody discharge; was able to attend to her household duties and went to full term.

| | After lifting a heavy weight during sixth month of pregnancy severe pains in stomach, abdomen and small of back and a pushing-down sensation; violent movements of fetus; cold feet; numbness and tingling in feet; small, weak pulse.

After abortus: difficult contraction of uterus; thin, black, foul-smelling discharge.

| Retained placenta, after miscarriage, especially when occurring during early months of pregnancy; offensive discharges; patient cold and often almost pulseless from loss of blood; uterine contractions very imperfect, or else prolonged tonic contraction.

| | During eighth month of pregnancy violent convulsions with frothing at mouth, etc., followed by variable spasms; insensibility and clonic spasms, < at every pain; on return of consciousness complained of dull frontal and occipital headache and incessant uterine pains. Premature labor.

| | During pregnancy: frequent and prolonged forcing pains, particularly in thin, ill-conditioned women; cramps in calves.

| Uterine pains prolonged but ineffectual.

A sensation of constant tonic pressure in uterine region; causes great distress; desires fresh air; does not like to be covered.

| Hour-glass contraction.

| | During labor: prolonged bearing-down and forcing pain in uterus; pains irregular; pains too weak; pains feeble, or ceasing; everything seems loose and open, no action; fainting fits.

| Strength of uterus weakened by too early or perverted efforts.

| Thin, scrawny women, skin shrivelled, dry and harsh, sallow face, weak in labor; pains seem to be entirely wanting; uterus flabby; bearing down in sacral region, a sort of prolonged urging feeling in abdomen.

|| While the head was passing in lower strait, she was suddenly seized with violent convulsions lasting about three or four minutes, followed by a stupid state with stertorous breathing and uneasy moaning as if from pain.

| Labor ceases, and twitchings or convulsions begin.

| Puerperal convulsions with opisthotonos.

| Retained placenta, with constant, strong bearing-down in abdomen, or with relaxed feeling of parts.

|| After labor, pale, weak; uterus distended, burning pains therein, hard, painful to least touch; discharge of black, coagulated or brown, watery offensive-smelling blood; throbbing, tearing pains in thighs extending down to toes; pain < from motion; strong pulsations in umbilical region, which could be felt by the hand; pulse at wrist weak and rapid; frequent yawning.

|| Post-partum hemorrhage, with relaxation of uterus, only temporarily relieved by compression: after-pains excessive, < when child nursed.

|| After-pains: too long and too painful.

|| Violent after-pains with hemorrhage arising from irregular contractions; the longitudinal fibres alone contracting in such a manner as to leave a sulcus in middle, making it appear as if uterus were split open from top to bottom.

|| Cessation of lochia, with fever; inflammation of uterus, subsequently an abscess opened through vagina.

||| Lochia: dark, very offensive; scanty or profuse; painless or accompanied by prolonged bearing-down pain; suppressed, followed by metritis; suddenly changes character and

becomes of a dirty brown or chocolate colour, with fetid odor, grows sad and melancholy and fears death; of too long duration.

| Fever with frequent watery stools. Puerperal fever.

| Strong tendency to putrescence; discharge of sanious blood, with tingling in legs and great prostration; urine suppressed; offensive diarrhea; voice hollow with difficult breathing, feeble and inaudible; burning fever interrupted by shaking chills, does not care to be covered; cold limbs; cold sweat over whole body; gangrene.

| Suppression of milk; the milk will not flow from the breast.

| Lack of milk with much stinging in mammae.

| In women who are much exhausted from venous hemorrhage; thin, scrawny women; the breasts do not properly fill with milk.

Thin, scrawny children with shrivelled skin; spasmodic twitchings, sudden cries, feverishness.

Pendulous abdomen.

Promotes expulsion of foreign bodies from uterus.

Married woman, aged 25, had severe pain in the pelvic region; great bearing-down, excruciating rectal and vesical tenesmus; restless sleep, high fever, and heavily-coated tongue. Subperitoneal hematocele was diagnosed in consultation. Tumor increased rapidly, and increased fever; pulse 130 to 150; tongue dry, dark-brown; sordes on the teeth; vaginal secretions fetid; frequent urgent micturition; mucous dysentery, with increased tenesmus; countenance expressive of great suffering. Under Secale, tumor discharged through the rectum, large quantity of dark, thick blood; patient gradually recovered.

Voice and Larynx, Trachea and Bronchia—

| Voice: hollow, hoarse, with difficult breathing; feeble and inaudible; weak, unintelligible, stammering.

Thickening of mucous membrane of air passages.

Lungs during chill felt as though respiration fanned air.

Respiration—

Respiration: slow; labored and anxious; oppressed; moaning; constant sighing; hiccough.

Blood is sometimes expectorated during violent efforts to breathe.

Lungs during chill felt as though respiration fanned air on a perfectly dry surface; only during chills.

Sharp pains through left chest, especially when walking.

COUGH—

Hard, hoarse cough, with but little expectoration.

|| Concussive cough; profuse perspiration; sleepless nights; inclination to colic; diarrhea; bloatedness of abdomen; emphysema. Bronchitis.

| Spitting of blood, with or without cough;

Inner Chest and Lungs—

Cramp in chest.

Pains over nearly whole front part of chest, < from coughing and motion.

|| Expectoration of dark, frothy, rather viscid blood, brought up by a slight cough and amounting to a teacupful in four hours; a spot as large as a crown piece on right side of chest to right of nipple, dull on percussion, with bronchial respiration and mucous rale over that part.

Heart, Pulse and Circulation—

Palpitation; hot fore-head; inclination to sleep; spasmodic shocks from right half of chest into right arm and leg; in paroxysms every two or three hours; oftener in night, after each meal; less in open air; coldness and numbness of right hand, with tingling in fourth and fifth fingers; loss of muscular power and feeling in hand; after sexual excess.

Palpitation of heart: with contracted and frequently intermitting pulse.

| Pulse: often unchanged even during violent attacks; generally slow and contracted, at times intermittent or suppressed;

somewhat accelerated during heat; small; empty, weak; thread-like, in hemorrhages.

During the entire proving palpitation of the heart (something I never had before in my life); could feel the heart flutter and remit.

Palpitation nearly all the afternoon.

Violent throbbing of the carotids; faint for several hours.

Was attacked while at lectures with palpitation which continued about eight hours.

Pulse 108 and 110.

Neck and Back—

Tumors on neck discharging yellow pus.

Gentle, creeping sensation in back, as if a soft air were blowing through it.

Tingling in back, extending to fingers and toes.

Pain in small of back.

Stitch in back.

Sudden 'catch' or 'kink' in back.

Pains in sacrum with bearing down as if parts would be forced out, < when moving.

|| Hard, hoarse cough, with but little expectoration; pains nearly all over front part of chest, < from coughing and motion; for several years tenderness of lower cervical and upper dorsal spinous processes, with stiffness of neck; < from every exertion or strain upon spine; pressure upon diseased portion of spine produces pain there, as well as all through chest, with irritation to cough.

|| Stitches in upper dorsal vertebral (between shoulders), constant when sitting, intermittent when standing, at times extending into hands, < by pressure upon vertebrae; frequent formication through all limbs; at times rigidity and spasmodic stretching of fingers so that for several minutes he cannot sew; frequent pressure and swelling beneath epigastrium; pain in back < when sewing.

Violent pain in back, especially in sacral region;

anesthesia and paralysis of limbs, convulsive jerks and shocks in paralyzed limbs; painful contraction of flexor muscles; paralysis of bladder and rectum. Myelitis.

| Myelitis diffusa.

Paraplegia preceded by cramps and muscular pains.

Difficult, staggering gait; complete inability to walk, not for want of power but on account of a peculiar unfitness to perform light movements with limbs and hands: contraction of lower limbs on account of which patient staggers; trembling of limbs, sometimes attended with pains; formication of hands and feet; excessive sensation of heat, with aversion to heat or being covered.

Spine disease with gressus vaccinus.

Muscles of neck stiff, sore.

Shoulder-blades and clavicle lame, as though wrenched or twisted.

Back aches; feels weak, especially in sacrum.

Sharp, shifting pains in all parts of body.

Upper Limbs—

Arms fall asleep.

Rough rash all over arm.

Spasmodic jerks of hand, with flexion of hand at wrist or of forearm.

Numbness and insensibility of hands and arms.

Burning in hands.

Hands deathly pale.

Coldness and numbness of right hand with tingling of ring and little fingers.

Loss of feeling in backs of fingers.

Loss of muscular power and of feeling in hand.

Fingers convulsively drawn in toward palm, clasping thumb.

| Contraction of fingers.

Fingers bent backward or spasmodically abducted.

|| Left thumb spasmodically drawn toward dorsum of hand, followed in a few minutes by cramping and flexure of rest of fingers toward palmar surface; hands feel numb like velvet; next day both hands became affected and after several days felt a tingling and stitches in legs, followed by heaviness of same, < after walking, generally appearing while sitting, while cramps in hands always appear after using them.

Loss of sensation in tips of fingers.

Numbness of tips of fingers.

Crawling in tips of fingers as if something alive were creeping under skin or as if fingers were asleep, as from pressure upon arm.

Peculiar prickling feeling in tips of fingers; they are sensitive to cold.

Painful swelling of fingers.

Violent pains in finger tips.

| Gangrene of fingers; senile gangrene.

Shifting pains first through my hands from one finger to another, then through the wrist joint.

Wrist weakened so it was painful to lift weights.

Sensation of burning on left hand as though irritated with Cayenne; warm after rubbing.

Dull, spasmodic pain from shoulder to elbow along median nerve, worse on right side and in morning.

Lower Limbs—

Hammering, tearing pain in both thighs increased by motion.

Legs heavy and tired.

Tingling in legs.

Creeping feeling in anterior femoral and posterior tibial regions.

Shuffling gait as if feet were dragged along.

Rheumatic pains of joints.

| Cramps in calves of legs and soles of feet, disturbing sleep at night and hindering walking in pregnant women.

| | After an attack of cholera cramps in calves and sensation of numbness and formication in toes.

| | Cramp in calves.

| Burning in feet.

| The feet seem asleep and stiff.

Toes of right foot spasmodically drawn upwards, continuously during day and occasionally at night, causing a peculiar limping gait; this cramp was accompanied by no pain, but by a very tiresome sensation rendering walking, particularly going up and down stairs, very difficult; tendons running along dorsum of foot to toes were tense as wires and the corresponding muscles of leg larger and harder than normal; now and then slight sensation of coldness in back and also a peculiar buzzing (formication) in spine.

Swelling of feet with black spots.

| | Beginning senile gangrene; swelling and livid colouring of right foot extending to malleoli; foot cold; severe indescribable pains.

| | Senile gangrene commenced in great toe of right foot and slowly extended; foot was livid and swollen; all the symptoms pointed to its complete loss,

| | Dry gangrene of foot with constant severe, burning tearing pains.

Severe pains in sole of foot and toes: black spot on plantar surface of heel; toes livid, blue, cold; burning pains; foot swollen; walking impossible. Senile gangrene.

| |Profuse, stinking and corrosive perspiration of feet, softening and bleaching soles and destroying quickly stockings and shoes; existing two months in a girl eighteen years old.

Tingling in toes.

| | Gangrene of toes.

Shifting pains through ankles and knees.

Legs so weak gave out while walking.

Knees so weak could hardly reach top of stairs.

Legs would 'give out' suddenly.

Lassitude, weakness, heaviness, trembling of limbs.

Limbs cold; covered with cold sweat.

Formication; pricking; tingling; numbness; insensibility of limbs.

Spasmodic pains; drawing and crawling in limbs.

Burning in hands and feet.

| Fuzzy feeling in limbs.

Cramps in hand and toes.

Painful jerkings in limbs at night.

Most violent convulsive movements of limbs occur several times a day; during intervals ringers are numb and often contracted.

Sudden periodic contraction of limbs, with tensive pain.

Contractions of hands, feet, fingers and toes.

Gangrene of limbs, limbs suddenly became cold, leaden coloured and lost all sensation.

| Paraplegia.

Internal pain greatly < by heat, whether of bed or atmosphere; somewhat > when exposed to a cooler atmosphere, though even then it was scarcely tolerable; the pain extended by degrees from toes to legs and thighs, and from fingers to arms and shoulders, gangrene supervened.

Not the slightest pain in gangrenous limb when pricked or cut, though frequently motion is not entirely lost.

Absolute insensibility of tips of fingers and toes.

|| Cold gangrene of limbs.

True anthrax, rapidly changing into gangrene.

Hands and feet swollen with a gangrenous black and suppurating eruption.

Pain with some swelling without inflammation, followed by coldness, blue colour, cold gangrene and death of limb.

The limbs become cold, pale and wrinkled as if they had been a long time in hot water.

Have pained me much.

No strength in limbs or between shoulders.

Glad to sit down; too weak to talk; tired.

Rest. Position. Motion—

Must lie doubled up in bed; pain in belly.

Sitting: stitches in vertebra, constant; cannot bend forward or backward without losing his equilibrium.

Holds hands with fingers spread widely apart.

Standing: stitches in vertebra intermittent.

Inability to stand erect: vertigo.

Every exertion: tenderness of cervical process <.

Motion: hemorrhage <; giddiness; after labor pains <; pains over chest<; pains in sacrum <; tearing in thighs <.

Walking: heaviness of legs >; impossible from gangrene.

Every attempt to walk knees sink from under him.

Cannot walk: giddiness.

Nerves—

| Hyperesthesia of cutaneous nerves, especially of spine.

|| Sensation of soreness in abdomen; formation of large lumps and swellings in abdomen; right hand very weak, particularly fingers, so that she could hold nothing, nor sew with that hand; when placing open hand to side and taking it away a spasm of hand occurs, the fingers are spread apart and she cannot close the hand; rapid alternations of heat and cold in hands and feet; cramps in legs; icy coldness of knees; trembling of right arm and hand while eating, must use the left; sensation of coldness in stomach, > for a short time by warm drinks; habitual constipation.

|| Burning: in all parts of the body as if sparks of fire were falling on them.

Neuralgia, caused by pressure of distended veins upon a nerve trunk.

Spasmodic twitchings.

Irregular movements of the whole body.

Spasmodic distortion of limbs, relieved by stretching them out.

|| Expression of countenance varied every moment from a constant play of the muscles; eyes rolled about, pupils dilated, tongue jerked out, head moved about from side to side; arms in constant action with most diverse movements; snatched objects rather than took hold of them, could hold nothing securely; trunk also in constant motion; urine could not be retained; pulse small, weak, quick; heart beat tumultuously; appetite poor; bowels torpid; aching in occiput; sensation of formication in extremities; memory impaired; speech difficult, hurried; no relief at night; staggered about the house almost all night.

| Chorea associated with menstrual irregularities.

|| The muscular twitchings usually commence in face and spread thence all over body, sometimes increase to dancing and jumping.

Spasms with fingers spread apart.

Convulsive jerks and starts in paralyzed limbs.

Painful contractions in flexor muscles.

Tetanic spasms, with full consciousness, followed by great exhaustion.

| Convulsions.

Tonic spasms.

Epileptiform spasms; epilepsy.

|| Complains of great weakness, constipation, heaviness in epigastrium, formication in legs and cramps; at night while asleep gets epileptiform attacks of which she knows nothing next morning except that she feels greatly prostrated and has a constant heaviness in head.

|| After abortus, spasms with full consciousness, afterward great exhaustion; heaviness in head and tingling in legs.

|| Convulsions first occurring after a fright when a little girl, returned after each confinement.

|| Twitching of single muscles; twisting of head to and fro; contortions of hands and feet; labored and anxious respiration.

|| Numbness of extremities; paralysis of some parts; painful tingling (like crawling of ants) on tongue.

| Paralysis after spasm, and apoplexy, with rapid emaciation of affected parts and involuntary discharges from bowels and bladder.

|| Suddenly fell to ground, but without loss of consciousness; on every attempt to walk the knees would sink from under him; especially right; while sitting cannot bend forward or backward without losing his equilibrium; arms slightly weak, sensation of touch not affected; general dulness; difficult speech; inclination to weep; complains of headache and pain in lumbar region; sleep poor; urine and feces escape involuntarily; no stool for several days; at times oppression of breathing.

|| Paralysis of lower extremities, in a woman past climacteric; a hard, sensitive tumor in one of her breasts had been developing for several years, but for the last year or two had rapidly increased in size and become very painful; by continued application for several months of a yellowish salve the tumor was enucleated; in about a month after ceasing to use the salve, a peculiar torpor or deadness was felt in great toes, which extended to whole foot and ankle joint; feet seemed large and heavy and could be moved only by moving whole limb; gait shuffling as if feet were dragged along by lifting legs; slight numbness in hands.

| Paralysis with rapid emaciation, with relaxation of sphincters.

Myelitis and softening of cord.

Trembling; unsteadiness of whole body.

|| Restlessness; extreme debility and prostration.

Loss of power of voluntary motion.

|| Sinking spells from diarrhea, at 3 A.M.

|| Collapse from choleroid diseases, etc., with cold skin, yet unable to bear warmth.

Sleep—

Frequent yawning.

Inclination to sleep; drowsiness; deep, heavy sleep, stupor.

Sleep at night disturbed by frightful dreams.

Restless and sleepless.

Disturbed by distressing dreams. Surrounded by danger, constantly trying to escape evils. Sometimes my family were sick unto death, or the house on fire; again I was pouring water from one bucket into another to free it from lizards and reptiles, that would crawl over the sides of the vessel and endanger my children.

Night after night my dreams would continue of this character I would waken, my head would be in such distress, not from pain but oppression. I would turn my pillow and change my position to endeavor to forget my dreams, and after some time would again fall asleep, to be awakened by another equally unpleasant dream.

This condition of head and sleep lasted six or seven weeks. (November 17th to January 5th.)

Time—

At 3 A.M.: sinking spells.

At break of day: diarrhea.

In morning: frequent short evacuations.

During day: warmth on tongue; unusual drowsiness; toes drawn up continuously.

During night: anus firmly closed; cramps in calves and twitching of limbs; dreamed she was ascending stairs; palpitation; toes drawn up occasionally.

Jerking in limbs; staggered about house with chorea; ulcers <.

Temperature and Weather—

Open air: palpitation less.

Wants to be in air or be fanned: with diarrhea.

Warm applications: suppuration of cornea <; ulcers <.

Warm drinks: coldness of stomach <.

Does not wish to be covered; diarrhea; uterine hemorrhage.

Heat: could not bear it and would throw off all covering, in post-diphtheritic paralysis; with diarrhea, did not wish to be near; aversion to, with cholera; internal pain much <; gangrene <.

Wet bandages: > labor pains.

Cold: ulcers >; gangrene >.

Fever—

Disagreeable sensation of coldness in back, abdomen and limbs.

Skin cold, with shivering.

Coldness of surface of body, particularly extremities.

| Violent chill of but short duration; followed soon after by internal burning heat, with great thirst.

Chill with thirst.

|| Violent shaking followed by violent heat, with anxiety, delirium and almost unquenchable thirst.

|| Intense, icy coldness of skin, with shivering; pale, sunken face.

| Cold limbs, cold sweat, great weakness.

Cold stage preceded by vomiting, succeeded by moderate sweating.

| Severe and long-lasting dry heat, with great restlessness and violent thirst.

|| Heat with thirst and hot skin.

| Burning heat, interrupted by shaking chills, then internal burning heat, with great thirst.

| Sweat: all over body, except face; profuse cold, cold

limbs; from head to pit of stomach; especially on upper body; cold, clammy over whole body; colliquative.

|| Exhausting perspiration, accompanied by evening fever and alarming cough.

Cold surface; sunken pale face and blue lips; will not be covered; tingling in limbs; holds hands with fingers widely spread apart; cold, clammy sweat; speech feeble, stuttering. Ague.

|| Aversion to heat or to being covered; may feel cold but does not wish to be covered.

| Great tendency to typhoid. Intermittent.

Chilly sensation from least motion in bed at night, not ameliorated by covering up.

Chilly all over, especially shoulders and back, but do not shiver or shake.

Kept limbs drawn up close to body, are too cold to lie straightened out; they ache but are too cold to straighten out.

Limbs and whole body ache as though tired and lame, particularly hips and knees.

Get warm about 5 A.M., then hands, chest and back moist with perspiration.

Chill at 11 A.M., lasting three hours.

Chills would creep up and down the back between the shoulders, spreading down and out into the limbs.

Chills in back up and down the spine.

Fever followed with great *oppression* of face and head.

Desired fresh air constantly, though walking any distance would aggravate the headache, especially over eyes and through the forehead.

Slight in the morning.

Hands, back and chest moist with perspiration about 5 o'clock in the morning.

Severe chill, from 4 A.M. to 10 A.M., in small of back, along spine; during chill, shooting pains chiefly in legs and arms; very thirsty during chill, little thirst during or after the fever; slight sweat; mouth dry; wants to drink continually; violent nausea; vomiting great quantity of bile; superficial congestion; veins of extremities very full.

A man, 67, has suffered from emphysema and asthma; cardiac complications with hypertrophy and weak, rapid, irregular pulse; < by ascending stairs and walking. For two or three years been subject to attacks of severe coldness that came on irregularly, followed by great weariness for two days. The hands and feet became pale and cold with an intense feeling of weariness; some throbbing of head which seemed warm; after some hours limbs became warm again leaving only weariness. Temperature, normal during attacks; arteriosclerosis was no doubt due to tension of arteries and its consequent anemia. Aconite, Arsenic, Cedron, Chin. sulf. gave only temporary relief; Secale cured.— *Tessier.*

Attacks, Periodicity—

Sudden attacks: diarrhea.

Alternation: of heat and cold, in hands and feet.

Five to ten minutes after taking least quantity of food severe colic.

Every two or three hours: paroxyms of palpitation.

Several times a day: convulsive movements of limbs.

For several weeks: formication in tips of fingers.

Every two weeks: excessive menstrual flow; lasting seven to nine days.

For two weeks: profuse corrosive foot sweat.

For four weeks: flow is continuous.

During August: diarrhea.

In Summer: interminable diarrhea.

For several years: tenderness of cervical process.

Locality and Direction—

Right: ovary congested; a spot on side of chest dull on percussion; spasmodic shocks from half of chest into arm and leg; coldness of hand; toes drawn up; swelling and livid colouring of foot; gangrene in great toe of foot; hand very weak; trembling of hand and arm.

Left: hemicrania; nose stopped up; throat sore; protrusion in hypochondrium; thumb spasmodically drawn toward dorsum of hand.

Sensations—

As if intoxicated while undressing; as if eyes were spasmodically rotated; as of a solid plug in nose; as if tongue were paralyzed; as if there were some resistance to overcome in speech; as of a heavy weight in stomach; region of stomach as if contracted; anus as if locked up; as if testicles were being drawn up to inguinal ring; uterus as if burnt; as if contents of uterus would fall forward; as if soft air were creeping through back; as if sacrum would be forced out; as if something alive were creeping under skin; as if fingers were asleep; as if limbs had been a long time in hot water; as if sparks of fire were falling upon different parts of body; in lumbar region; as if mice were creeping under skin.

Pain: in occiput; in eyes; in pit of stomach; in epigastrium; in lower belly; in abdomen; in hypogastric region; in loins; in ovaries and uterus; in sacrum, down thighs and into lower abdomen; over front part of chest; in small of back; in sacrum.

Excruciating pains: in spine.

Violent pains: in back; in finger tips.

Acute pain: in hepatic region.

Severe pains: in stomach; in abdomen and small of back; in sole of foot and toes.

Cutting: in abdomen.

Tearing pains: in both thighs; in foot.

Throbbing, tearing pains: in thighs.

Tearing, stinging pains: in extremities.

Pinching pains: in abdomen.

Forcing pain: in uterus.

Stitches: in upper dorsal vertebrae.

Stitching pains: in eyes; in legs.

Stitch: in back.

Sudden catch: in back.

Throbbing: in temples.

Cramps: in calves of legs; in feet, toes, hands and fingers; in chest.

Cramping pains: in stomach.

Cramping pressure: in stomach.

Rheumatic pains: in joints.

Tensive pain: in limbs.

Drawing pains: in calves of legs.

Drawing: in limbs.

Dragging: violent in spermatic cord; in abdomen.

Stinging: on mamma.

Burning: in throat; of tongue; at pit of stomach; in spleen; in abdomen; in uterus; in hands; in feet.

Soreness: of throat; in abdomen.

Tenderness: of epigastrium; of lower cervical and upper dorsal spinous processes.

Distress: of stomach.

Painful constriction: of epigastrium.

Painful jerkings: in limbs.

Jerking: under skin.

Pulsations: in head.

Pressure: in eyeballs; in pit of stomach; in occiput; in uterine region.

Heaviness: of head; in epigastrium.

Lightness: of head.

Peculiar prickling feeling: in tips of fingers.

Tingling: in face; in throat and tongue; of legs; on tongue; in limbs; all over body; in fourth and fifth fingers; in back; in toes.

Crawling: on tongue; in tips of fingers; in limbs; all over body; between skin and flesh; in upper lip; all about mouth.

Formication: in face; in gums; in extremities; in tips of fingers; over whole body.

Gentle creeping sensation: in back.

Fuzzy feeling: in limbs.

Dryness: of soft palate, throat and esophagus; of mouth.

Numbness: in limbs; of feet; of right hand; of tips of fingers.

Cold feeling: in abdomen and back; in limbs; of body; of right hand; in stomach.

Tissues—

It destroys the activity of the cord; convulsive twitchings and shocks, painful contractions, tetanic manifestations; perfect paralysis, with increased reflex activity; most excruciating spinal pains, especially in sacral region; paralysis of bladder and rectum; tendency to gangrene; rapid emaciation.

Dissolution of blood corpuscles; blood thin; passive hemorrhages.

Anemic state, either from exhaustive diseases or artificial depletion; the blood is thin and does not coagulate.

Thrombosis of abdominal vessels.

| Neuralgia caused by pressure on nerves by a distended vein.

Tumefaction of glands.

| Lymphatic tumors.

|| Collapse from choleroid diseases.

| Rapid emaciation of paralyzed parts.

Malignant pustule.

Emphysematous swellings.

Passive hemorrhage; blood dark and red, in feeble and cachectic persons, accompanied by tingling in limbs and prostration; desire for air; does not like to be covered; wishes to have limbs extended; skin cold.

Rheumatism (peliosis rheumatica of Schoenlein) generally is found in cachectic individuals, with purpura; affects joints, especially of lower extremities; thrombosis of abdominal vessels.

| Ulcers: bleeding; becoming black; feeling as if burnt; painless; pricking, producing a prurient sensation; pus putrid; < at night, touch, from external warmth; > from cold.

|| Gangrene: from anemia; external injuries, application of leeches or mustard; > from cold, < from heat; dry, of old people.

| Dry gangrene of extremities, parts are dry, cold, hard and insensible, of a uniform black colour and free from fetor; large ecchymoses, blood blisters on extremities, becoming gangrenous, black suppurating blisters; limbs become pale, cold, shrivelled or lead-coloured, losing all sensibility.

Touch, Passive Motion, Injuries—

Touch: pit of stomach very sensitive to; right ovary sensitive to; uterus painful; ulcers <.

Pressure: upon abdomen > labor pains; upon vertebra stitches <.

After lifting heavy weight: during sixth month of pregnancy; severe pain in stomach, abdomen and small of back.

External injuries: gangrene.

Skin—

Skin dry and cool.

Cold and dry; dingy, wrinkled, dry and insensible; desquamation.

|| Formication: with a sense as if mice were creeping under skin; on face, gums and other parts of body; in extremities with tearing, stinging pains; in tips of fingers, lasting several weeks, with a partial loss of sensibility; over whole body.

| Crawling: all over body; between skin and flesh; and jerking under skin.

Violent crawling and prickling over whole body, especially in upper lip and at times all about the mouth.

| Bloody blisters on extremities, becoming gangrenous.

|| Boils, small, painful, with green contents, mature very slowly and heal in same manner; very debilitating.

| Carbuncles; extensive ecchymoses.

| Petechia and miliary eruptions.

|| Purpura hemorrhagica.

| Cachectic females, with rough skin; pustules showing tendency to gangrene.

| Varicose ulcers and enlarged veins in old people.

| Ulcers turn black, copious vomiting of a mixture of a thick, black, pitchy, bilious or shiny matter.

| Indolent ulcer, ichorous, offensive pus, > from cold.

General desquamation in scarlatina.

| Variola pustules of abnormal appearance, either fill with a bloody serum or dry up too soon.

Several sore pimples, the size of a pin's head, gradually increasing to the size of a pea or larger, appeared on face, worse on right side; lastly, boil, very red, sore, swollen, painful, on right cheek near insertion of masseter muscle.

Made me sick in bed, so fearfully painful; whole face congested and swollen. Discharged much *green pus,* finally a *green core* (bright green), and leaving a deep scar, which was long in healing.

On the seventh day several spots with a sore, bruised feeling appeared about and below the knee, the size of a half dollar, of a purple red colour; then three or four similar spots appeared further down the leg, about the shoe top, which were so sore could hardly bear the pressure of the shoe. They itched violently, but were so sore could not scratch them, and when touched gave me a sick faint feeling.

These first appeared on the left side, then three or four appeared on the right leg.

With them a rash appeared on the face which was very sore and felt like the spots on the legs, only they were smaller, but there was the same sore, bruised feeling in them. It would begin in fine points like the prick of a pin or the sting of an insect, and gradually increased in size to a small pustule as large as a pea.

When spots disappeared they left a blue (ecchyrnosed) mark for several weeks especially on the legs.

Immediately after the same kind of spots appeared on the shoulders, three or four in a cluster, with the same sore, bruised feeling.

The same characteristic spots appeared six weeks later in another proving, twenty-eight of them in all, which were peculiarly sensitive to touch, accompanied by faintness and nausea. Some result in pustules.

Generalities—

Many sharp, shifting pains in different parts of body, and stiffness of back and neck as though muscles were swollen close to occiput.

SYPHILINUM

Authorities—

Drs. Sam'l Swan, I. C. Boardman, Thomas Wildes, E. A. Ballard, Wm. Eggert, Laura Morgan, H. I. Ostrom, Wm. Bradshaw, Thomas Skinner, R. M. Theobald, S. Morrison, D. W. Clauson, C. F. Nichols, E. W. Berridge, Francis Burritt, S. W. Jackson, R. N. Foster, E. B. Nash, Julius Schmidt, C. W. Boyce, W. A. Hawley, D. B. Morrow, J. R. Haynes, H. H. Carr, H. C. Alien, J. T. Kent.

Dr. Swan's provers: Miss Eva Spalding, Miss Hays, Mrs. Mary B. Pitts, Mrs. S. S., Mr. Brown, a lady, a woman, five provers (names and sex unknown). Dr. Morrison's prover: Mrs. ———. Dr. Berridge's prover: Mrs. W. Heitts. Dr. H. B. Carr's provers: Dr. ——, Mrs. Henry Hake, Mrs. Kelt. Copland's Dictionary.

Dr. Fellger said it was absurd to claim that any disease could be cured by its nosode, for after potentizing the nosode, we cannot be satisfied that it is in the same condition as when first taken from the diseased individual. Thus the syphilitic poison is composed of molecules: the molecules of atoms. When the poison is potentized the essential character of the molecules is undoubtedly lost, and hence it is not the same substance any longeright Therefore, there can be no certainty that the potentized preparation is the same poison. But if, for argument, we allow that the molecules of the poison can be potentized without change of character, we still are not relieved of the dilemma, for primary syphilis in any one person will make a different set of symptoms from syphilis in another person. The variations are endless. Hence, we must then have a potentization of each one of these different kinds of syphilis, which would be impossible. Mercury is a staple substance, always unchanged; it might then be expected to produce identical sets of symptoms on any number of the most different people. Yet its action is different upon every person to whom it is given. How much more, then, must be the individual variations in the case of the poison of syphilis, and if Mercury requires so many different remedies to antidote it, how much more, then, must syphilis need a variety of remedies to treat it. It is folly, then, to expect to treat symptoms with its nosode, and the folly is the more apparent when we realize that the character of this nosode is essentially changed in the process of potentizing. The only way, therefore, to use a nosode is to *prove* it on the healthy, like any other drug, and note its symptoms in the regular way.

Characteristics—

Pains from darkness to daylight; begins with twilight and ends with daylight (Merc., Phyt.).

Pains increase and decrease gradually (Stan.); shifting and require frequent change of position.

All symptoms are worse at night (Merc.); from sundown to sunrise.

Eruptions: dull, red, copper-coloured spots, becoming blue when getting cold.

Extreme emaciation of entire body (Abrot., Iod.).

Heart: lancinating pains from base to apex, at night (from apex to base, Med.); from base to clavicle, or shoulder, (Spig.).

Loss of memory: cannot remember names of books, persons or places; arithmetical calculations difficult.

Sensations: as if going insane; as if about to be paralyzed; of apathy and indifference.

Terrible dread of night on account of mental and physical exhaustion on awakening; it is intolerable, death is preferable.

Fears the terrible suffering from exhaustion on awakening (Lach.).

Leucorrhea: profuse, *soaking through the napkins* and running down to the heels (Alum.).

Headache, neuralgic in character, causing sleeplessness and delirium at night; commencing at 4 P.M.; worse from 10 to 11 and ceasing at daylight (ceases at 11 or 12 P.M., Lye.); falling of the hair.

Acute ophthalmia neonatorum; lids swollen, adhere during sleep; pain intense at night < from 2 to 5 A.M.; pus profuse; > by cold bathing.

Ptosis: paralysis of superior oblique; sleepy look from drooping lids (Caust., Graph.).

Diplopia, one image seen below the other.

Teeth: decay at edge of gum and break off; are cupped, edges serrated; dwarfed in size, converge at their tips (Staph.).

Craving alcohol, *in any form.* Hereditary tendency to alcoholism (Sar., Psor., Tuber., Sulph., Sulph. ac.).

Obstinate constipation for years; rectum seems tied up with strictures; when enemata were used the agony of passage was like labor (Lac d., Tub.).

Fissures in anus and rectum (Thuja); prolapse of rectum; obstinate cases with a syphilitic history.

Rheumatism of the shoulder joint, or at insertion of deltoid, < from raising arm laterally (Rhus—right shoulder, Sang.; left, Fer.).

When the best selected remedy fails to relieve or permanently improve in syphilitic affections.

Syphilitics, or patients who have had chancre treated by local means, and as a result have suffered from throat and skin troubles for years, are nearly always benefited by this remedy at commencement of treatment unless some other remedy is clearly indicated.

Relations: antidote; Nux vomica, for over-action or excess of action in sensitive organisations, or too frequent repetition of the remedy, especially in the higher potencies.

Compare: Aur., Asaf., Kali iod., Mer., Phyt., Nit. ac. in

diseases of bone and syphilitic affections. Ech., Lac can., Med. in dysmenorrhea. Calc., Tub., headache deep in the brain. Plat., Stan., pains increase and decrease slowly. Alum., Kali bi., Puls., Psor., Sep., Teuc., post-nasal catarrh, or ozena, with offensive plugs or clinkers. Hepar, Sil., Psor., tendency to successive abscesses (succession of boils, Anthr.). Auright, Lac can., Lach., Mer. iod., syphilitic stomatitis. Calc. fl., Fluor, ac., Kali bi., Kali iod., Mang., Mer., syphilitic nodes. Abrot., Iod., Tub., progressive emaciation. Med., lancinating pains in heart (from apex to base). Spig. (from base to clavicle or shoulder). Syph. (from base to apex). Lach., fear of exhaustion on awakening. Caust., Gels., Graph., paralysis of upper lids. Asaright, Med., Psor., Sul., Tub., hereditary tendency to alcoholism. Lac d., Tub., paralytic weakness of rectum with labor-like pains. Nat. mur., Sanic., Thuja, fissure ani. Kreos., Mer., troubles during detention, especially if hereditary syphilis be suspected. Phos., X-ray, bad effects of thunder-storms.

Aggravation: motion, touch, hot or cold things, warm or damp weather, seaside, electric storms, winter, raising arms laterally, at night (in common with all anti-syphilitics).

Amelioration: cold bathing, in the mountains, warmth, walking.

Mind–

Loss of memory.

Loses remembrance of passing occurrences, names, dates, etc., while all occurrences previous to inception of disease are remembered as distinctly as ever, almost without effort.

Very nervous, weeping without cause.

|| Cross, irritable, peevish.

Irritable, excited, walking much of the time, does not want to be soothed, violent on being opposed, has tremors, seems on the verge of convulsions, dazed, absent-minded, always washing her hands.

Periodical neuralgia in head.

|| Very despondent, does not think he will ever get better.

Feeling as if going insane, or about to be paralyzed.

A far-away feeling, with apathy and indifference to future.

Crying infants, who begin immediately after birth.

Difficulty in making arithmetical calculations.

|| Terrible dread of night, not on account of cough so much as on account of mental and physical exhaustion when she awakes; it is intolerable, death is preferable; she fears to prepare for night and is positively in abject fear of suffering, in form of exhaustion on awaking; it is < by cough, but it is quite independent of cough as she wakes in this awful state; always < as night approaches; leaves her about daylight, which she prays foright Spring cough. Had had a dose of Syphilinum cm., twenty-four hours before; on third night her anxiety and cough returned, though very much less. Another dose of Syphilinum cm., next morning, removed all symptoms, including aphonia, and exhaustion requiring brandy.

Great difficulty, and sometimes impossibility, of concentrating the thoughts on particular subjects; yet at the same time can recollect consecutive events and details which occurred 25 or 30 years previously in the order of occurrence, almost without effort.

Cannot remember names of persons, books or places.

Head.—Vertigo on looking up, seems to be caused by heat.

| Headache: linear, from or near one eye backward; lateral; frontal; from temple to temple; deep into brain from vertex; as from pressure on vertex; in either temple, extending into or from eye > by warmth; in bones of head; < by heat of sun; after sunstroke.

Sick headache, pains intolerable, arteries of head full and pulsating violently; high fever, frequent retching on trying to vomit; menses regular, but very scanty.

| | Lancinating pain in occiput, < invariably at night, and causing sleeplessness, but always ceasing with the coming light of morning.

Headache and great debility.

| Neuralgic headache causing sleeplessness or delirium at night, always commencing about 4 P.M.; < at from 10 to 11 P.M., and ceasing at daylight.

Bursting sensation in vertex as from severe cold.

Pain from eyes through to occiput, with sensation of weight in occiput drawing head back; or as if it were pulled back; eyes ache and smart.

Constant linear headache, commencing at both angles of forehead and extending in parallel lines backward—a precursor of epileptic attack.

Heavy, crushing, cutting pain across base of cerebellum.

Heavy, clouded, dull feeling in base of brain.

| Headache through temples, thence vertically like an inverted letterT.

| | Coronal headache.

| Headaches accompanied by great restlessness, sleeplessness and general nervous erethism.

| | Syphilitic headache for many months, piercing, pressing excruciating over right eye; extending deep into brain; losing continuity of thought and memory; makes repeated mistakes in figures.

Suffusion and full feeling in face, throat and head, with innumerable small enlarged cervical glands.

Sore, one and a half inches in diameter, on occipital bone, covered with a thick, yellow-white scab.

| | Dirty eruption on scalp.

Great loss of hair.

| | Nervous chills preceded by aching pains in head, especially in occipital and integuments thereof, head feeling heavy, sore, congested; also frontal headache about one-half or two-

thirds inches wide across forehead under eyebrows; aching pains below waist, in pelvis and extremities, especially in tibia, which is sensitive to touch; pains commence about 4 P.M., culminate about midnight in delirium, and cease entirely at daylight.

|| Syphilitic cephalalgia in occiput, intolerable, extending to nervous ganglia of neck, causing hardening of cords; attacks at irregular intervals, especially after excitement.

Cephalalgia in nerves of scalp, invariably worse at night and better after daybreak.

Eyes—

|| Red papulous eruption round left inner canthus, with isolated pimples on side of nose, cheek and eyebrow; these pimples were red, with depressed centre, circumscribed areola, became confluent where they were most dense; pimples bleed when scabs come off; agglutination of lids.

Sensation of heat with a little pain in outer half of left lids.

Myopia.

Sharp, pulsating pain, occasionally at outer end of superior border of right orbit, apparently in periosteum.

| Upper lids swollen.

| Ptosis: paralytica; eyes look sleepy from lowering of upper lid.

Diplopia, one image seen lower than the other.

Strabismus paralytica, eye turning inward, and pupil can only be turned outward as far as median line.

| Chronic recurrent phlyctenular inflammation of cornea; successive crops of phlyctenules and abrasion of epithelial layer of cornea; intense photophobia; profuse lachrymation; redness and pain well marked; delicate, scrofulous children, especially if any trace of hereditary syphilis remains.

||eyeball covered with fungus-like growth, pain intense < at night.

| Acute ophthalmia neonatorum.

|| Redness and swelling of outer half of both lower tarsal edges.

|| Syphilitic iritis, intense pain steadily increasing night after night; < between 2 and 5 A.M., coming almost at the minute and ceasing same way.

|| Pain in right inner canthus as if blood went there and could go no farther, also in right temple.

|| Both eyes glued in morning; conjunctiva injected; photophobia, constantly wears a shade.

|| Eyes dull.

Infantile syphilis.

|| Ophthalmic pains, < at night, > by cold water.

|| R. eye alone affected, congestion of conjunctiva and sclerotica, with some chemosis; lids inflamed, especially at outer canthus; sensation of sand in eyes; lids agglutinated in morning; great photophobia (hereditary syphilis).

|| Neuralgia every night, beginning about 8 or 9 P.M., gradually increasing in severity until it reached its height about 3 or 4 A.M., and after continuing thus for two or three hours, gradually decreased and finally ceased about 10 A.M.; attacks gradually get more severe and last longer; first feels cold all over, almost a shiver; then soreness as if beaten in right half of head, extending a little beyond middle line on vertex; in about thirty minutes scalding lachrymation from right eye, with shooting backward therein; eye is very red and closes, with photophobia; gnawing pains extend down right side of face and whole of nose; head is worst when eye is bad; during paroxysm right eye feels as if lids were open wide, and cold air blowing on exposed eye; she perceives a horizontal band across pupil of right eye hindering sight; this came on soon after paroxysms commenced; eye > by placing handkerchief on head and letting it hang over eyes, also by gentle pressure, though she cannot bear much pressure; it is more painful when lying on right (affected) side when also right side of head feels sore; right eye red, and red vessels run all over it, converging towards iris; right pupil horizontally oval; right iris looks dull and there is a slight brown hue around pupil; left eye normal; attacks

seem to have originated from sitting at a window in a cold draft, right eye being next window.

| During sleep lids adhere; in infantile syphilis.

| Paralysis of superior oblique.

| Chronic recurrent phlyctenular inflammation of cornea; successive crops of phlyctenules and abrasion of epithelial layer of cornea; intense photophobia; profuse lachrymation; redness and pain well marked; delicate scrofulous children, especially if any trace of hereditary syphilis remains.

Interstitial keratitis.

Photophobia, black spots, shreds or veils before sight.

Itching of left inner canthus.

|| Eyes very red and inflamed. Acute ophthalmia neonatorum.

|| Eyes swollen and closed with syphilitic ophthalmia, pus running out of them.

|| Acute left conjunctivitis, with considerable pain in eyeball, photophobia and lachrymation, followed by iritis; nocturnal aching in eyeball, pain extremely violent from 2 to 5 A.M.; sight impaired.

Iritis with photophobia, congestion of conjunctiva and sclerotica, with puffiness of conjunctival mucous membrane; chemosis, pupil immovable, diminution of sight; supraorbital pain.

|| Pain in right inner canthus as if blood went there and could go no further, also in right temple.

|| At 1 P.M. scalding lachrymation of right eye with shooting therein, followed by shooting from around eye into eye; eye red and closed; this lasted about an hour, then decreased, ceasing about 3 P.M.; recurred for two successive days and again four days afterwards in a slighter degree, but at same hour.

|| On turning eye to left feels momentary coldness in inner half of right eye.

|| On waking, gum in right canthus.

|| On walking across room, right eye sensitive to air, aches on using it.

|| Left eye closed, upper lid swollen as large as half an English walnut; deep red, not much pain, with oozing of purulent matter from between lids.

Strabismus paralyticus, the rectus internus being involved, and the eye turning outward.

Left eyeball covered with a fungus-like growth, pain intense, worse at night.

Ears–

|| Intense earache in right ear, incisive pains thrusting into ear; purulent watery discharge from ear with pain.

|| Gathering in left ear which discharges a great quantity of pus (hereditary syphilis in a child).

|| Deafness gradually increasing until she could scarcely hear at all.

|| Complete deafness; nothing abnormal to be seen.

|| Catarrhal or nerve deafness with marked cachexia.

| Calcareous deposit on tympanum.

|| Small, acrid, watery discharge occasionally from ears, no deafness (ozasna).

Nose–

Left side of nose, inside ala, itching.

Nose stuffed up and burning.

| Attacks of fluent coryza.

|| Offensive, thick yellow-green nasal discharge; during sleep dry scabs form in both nostrils; following an application of salve for sore eyes; left submaxillary gland, which had been swollen and indurated, softens, discharges, and, after forty-five days, begins to heal slowly.

|| Ozaena syphilitica. (Syph. brought out an eruption of sores with a fiery-red base on nose over frontal sinuses.)

||Left side of nose inside and out very sore, likewise lips and chin; sores itching and scabbing over; after Syphilinum 1m.

much better in twelve hours, many drying up and scabs falling off, leaving skin beneath of a dull-reddish copper colour.

| Itching in nostrils.

Face—

Face drawn to one side, difficulty of speaking, masticating, blowing.

|| Spasmodic twitching of many muscles, especially in face (paralysis agitans), with great melancholy and depression of spirits.

|| Facial paralysis right side, thick speech, hemicrania, jactitation of right eye and lid.

An old gentleman has had for some years cancer on right malar bone; no rest, his agony excruciating in extreme (relieved).

|| Face pale.

| Itching, scabby, eczematous eruptions singly or in clusters, looking like herpes.

|| Nose and cheeks covered with eruptions and scabs in layers rising to a point.

| Dark purple lines between alae nasi and cheeks.

|| Lips and teeth covered with bloody mucus.

Sores on lips and chin, especially left side, scabbing over.

|| A boy, aged 20 months, fretful, peevish, cross and crying, tossing in his sleep, grinding his teeth, face dotted with papules filled with a watery yellowish matter, most on edges of lids; teeth irregular, arms and legs emaciated, very tottery on his feet, very nervous.

Left submaxillary gland which had been swollen and indurated, softens and discharges, and after forty-five days begins to heal slowly.

Teeth—

Single small lunae cleft in upper incisors, permanent set, which incisors are dwarfed in their general dimensions, and converge at their tips; inherited syphilis.

Children's teeth are cupped.

Teeth decaying at edge of gum and breaking off.

| | Felt like a worm in tooth, could not tell which tooth.

Singular feeling as if teeth had all got out of place, and on closing jaws teeth do not come well together.

First central upper incisors serrated, permanent teeth point towards each other, inner side concave; edges serrated. Medorrhinum.

Pain in right upper jaw, as if from teeth, with swelling of face.

Painless fluttering occasionally in teeth, very peculiar, as if something alive, cannot detect which tooth it is.

Mouth—

Tongue red and thick; two deep cracks running lengthwise in it; one on each side of median line.

| | Aphasia, difficulty of finding words; debility.

Tongue feels as if paralyzed.

| | Fetid breath.

| Tongue coated white, edges indented by teeth.

Tongue turns to one side when protruded; difficulty in mastication, cannot turn food with tongue so readily from right to left as in other direction.

| | Putrid taste in mouth before epileptic fit.

| | Tongue very red and thick; covered with herpetic eruption, two deep cracks running lengthwise on each side of median line, making it difficult to swallow.

Tongue thickly coated, dirty, edges indented or serrated by teeth.

| |Twenty ulcers in mouth, every part involved, top and under side of tongue, lips, buccal cavity, fauces and nose. Two large ulcers, one on eaeh side near apex of tongue, were very much swollen, and the one on right side had a gangrenous center, the rest lardaceous bottoms with bright fiery red edges, and were cut down as with a knife, and felt hard like an in-

durated chancre. Septum of nose threatened, both alae nasi very painful, smarting with burning as if on fire; pains and burning prevented sleep; hungry but could eat nothing but fluids, as mastication was impossible; tongue heavily coated white, large quantities of stringy, viscid saliva running from mouth, of a sweetish taste; a putrid sickening odor filled whole house; all symptoms < toward night. This attack excited by exposure to rain.

Herpetic eruption in mouth, tonsils, hard palate and fauces, completely covering inside of mouth and throat, making it difficult to swallow even liquids.

| | Syphilitic destruction of hard and soft palates.

Chancre on hard palate exposing the bones of roof of mouth.

Throat—

| | Chronic hypertrophy of tonsils.

| | Chancrous ulcer extending across velum palati to left pillar of pharynx, which was congested and thickened, interfering very much with his speech; voice husky.

| Acute pharyngitis.

Sore throat.

Deglutition painful, especially with liquids.

Excoriation of throat when swallowing.

Sore throat with granulations.

Chancrous ulcers in pharynx.

Herpetic eruption in mouth, tonsils, hard palate and fauces, completely covering inside of mouth and throat, making it very difficult to swallow even liquids.

Appetite—

| | Appetite indifferent and capricious.

| | Total loss of appetite for months, little or nothing satisfies him; formerly was generally ravenous.

| | Loss of appetite.

Thirst.

Appetite good again; ravenous desire for food even after a meal.

| Tendency to heavy drinking; alcoholism.

| Aversion to meat.

| Dyspepsia; flatulence, belching of wind; nervous dyspepsia.

Stomach—

Nausea.

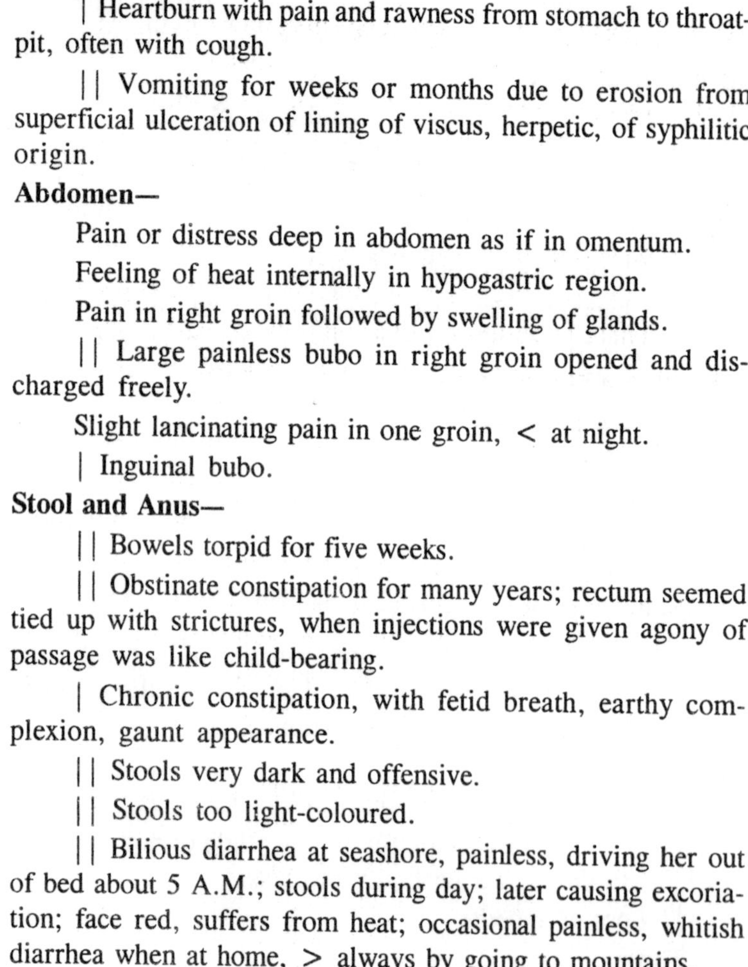

| Heartburn with pain and rawness from stomach to throat-pit, often with cough.

|| Vomiting for weeks or months due to erosion from superficial ulceration of lining of viscus, herpetic, of syphilitic origin.

Abdomen—

Pain or distress deep in abdomen as if in omentum.

Feeling of heat internally in hypogastric region.

Pain in right groin followed by swelling of glands.

|| Large painless bubo in right groin opened and discharged freely.

Slight lancinating pain in one groin, < at night.

| Inguinal bubo.

Stool and Anus—

|| Bowels torpid for five weeks.

|| Obstinate constipation for many years; rectum seemed tied up with strictures, when injections were given agony of passage was like child-bearing.

| Chronic constipation, with fetid breath, earthy complexion, gaunt appearance.

|| Stools very dark and offensive.

|| Stools too light-coloured.

|| Bilious diarrhea at seashore, painless, driving her out of bed about 5 A.M.; stools during day; later causing excoriation; face red, suffers from heat; occasional painless, whitish diarrhea when at home, > always by going to mountains.

| Obstinate cases of cholera infantum.

| | Fissures in anus and rectum.

| | Two indurated ulcers at mouth of anus somewhat sore; slight itching of anus.

| | Lower portion of rectum hanging out like a ruffle, looking like a full-blown rose fully three inches in diameter, and sensitive; constant weak dragging sensation in rectum, extending as far as sacrum.

Urinary Organs—

Itching in orifice of urethra.

A sensation, in morning on going to urinte, as if male urethra were stuffed up or clogged, about an inch from orifice.

Scalding urine.

| | Urination difficult and very slow; no pain, but a want of power, so that he has to strain.

Urine infrequent, not oftener than once in twenty-four hours, scanty, of a golden-yellow colour; after Syphilinum 1m., woke next morning with great distention of abdomen and pain in region of kidneys; rising she passed a large quantity of normal coloured urine, after which the distention and pain were relieved; next day regular urination, watery.

| |Profuse urination after chill; passed during night nearly a chamberful.

| | Rich lemon-yellow scanty urine.

| | Frequent urging to urinate all night, at least from 7 P.M. until 5 A.M., or sunset to sunrise.

Male Sexual Organs—

Chancre on prepuce.

| Buboes.

Burning in chancre; ulcer size of a split pea, on prepuce above corona glandis; edges raised, bottom covered with lardaceous deposit; no pain or sensation in it. Glans purple, on left side covered by an exudation.

| Chancre on penis, third in two years, all on same spot.

Aching of genitals, could not sit still for over a month.

|| After suppressed chancre, disease attacked testes and scrotum, which became painful and swollen; this was supposed to be cured, but ever since, every few weeks, if exposed to damp weather would be seized with pain as if in kidneys, seemingly traversing ureters, but instead of passing into bladder followed spermatic cord, down groins and into testes; pain agonizing, chiefly in cord, in present attack in right; pricking in chancre, as though punctured by pins.

|| Chancroid, phagedenic, spreading rapidly; buboes commencing in each groin.

| Inflammation and induration of spermatic cord.

|| Constant pain in anterior part of right thigh, < while standing, painful all night, preventing sleep; bubo in left inguinal region size of a pigeon's egg, purple, fluctuating; night sweats.

Bubo, purple, pointing in left groin, size of pigeon's egg; accompanied with night sweats, and constant pain in anterior portion of right thigh, < at night.

Female Sexual Organs—

|| Uterine and all surrounding parts loose, soft and flabby; profuse, thick, yellow leucorrhea; constant pain across small of back.

Slight whitish leucorrhea.

| Yellow offensive leucorrhea, watery or not, so profuse it daily soaks through napkins and runs to heels of stockings if much on her feet.

| Profuse yellow leucorrhea < at night; in sickly, nervous children.

|| Soreness of genitals, and muco-purulent discharge, in a child.

||Acrid discharge causing violent itching and inflammation of external organs < at night from warmth of bed, parts very tender; itching and inflammation > during menses.

| | Nocturnal < of right ovarian pain, preventing sleep.

| | Sore on right labium majus, extending to left

Intense itching of vulva on rising in morning, continuing until 10 o'clock.

Menstruation painful, two weeks too soon; pink-red, bright, profuse, running free for some days; napkins wash easily. Menses returned in 28 days, painless.

| | Painful menstruation.

The usually painful menstruation with all its concomitants, was very easy and the best for years.

Sensitiveness of os uteri, < to intolerable pain at menses, or on introduction of finger or penis; frequently causes abortion.

Sharp zigzag shooting pains in region of uterus.

Ovaries congested and inflamed; tendency to ovarian tumors.

Sore aching in left ovarian region, extending to right with darting pains.

Left ovary swollen, during coitus, at moment of organism, a sharp cutting pain like a knife, and twice there was smarting as of a sore; ovary swelled so much that its size and shape could easily be felt through abdominal walls (caused by *Buboin).*

| Uterine and ovarian diseases with pronounced nervous disorders, especially in married women.

Mamma sensitive to touch, feeling sore; during menses, and at other times.

Respiratory Organs—

Hoarse, almost complete aphonia, day before menses.

| Diseased cartilages of larynx.

Pain and oppression at bifurcation of bronchia and in larynx, it hurts her to breathe.

| |Attacks of spasmodic bronchial asthma for twenty-five years; they come on only at night after lying down or during a thunder-storm, producing most intense nervous insomnia, entirely preventing sleep for days and nights.

| Violent attacks of dyspnea, wheezing and rattling of mucus, from 1 to 4 A.M.

Cough—

Hard cough < at night, when it is continuous preventing sleep.

Hard, constant cough with thick, yellow, tasteless expectoration.

|| Dry, racking cough, with thick, purulent expectoration, caused by a sensation of rasping or scraping in throat, always < at night.

|| Whooping-cough with terrible vomiting.

|| Cannot lie on right side, as it causes a dry cough.

|| Muco-purulent expectoration, greyish, greenish, greenish-yellow, tasteless.

|| Expectoration without cough, quite clear, white, feels like a round ball and rushes into mouth.

Cough and dyspnea come on after midday dinner, has to fight for breath, feels as if she would be suffocated; symptoms last all night, > at daybreak (improved).

Expectoration of white phlegm.

|| Dry, sharp, hacking cough without expectoration, but with rawness, scraping and burning from fauces to stomach pit; with a whoop in inspiration and a choking sensation from fauces to bifurcation of bronchia, great mental distress.

Hard cough, < at night, when it is continuous, preventing sleep; white phlegm expectorated.

Cough < on lying on right side.

Hoarse, almost complete aphonia, the day before menses; no catarrh or sore throat.

Chest—

|| Chronic asthma; in Summer, especially when weather was warm and damp; most frequently in evening, passing off at daybreak; soreness of chest, with great anguish and inability to retain a recumbent position; in Winter severe bronchial cough succeeded by asthmatic attacks; a regular type of chills

and fever developed; suffered from this many years before. Within 24 hours after taking the 1m. the character of the asthma changed, during the night it disappeared, and the hour which had been that of relief, now became that of aggravation. The attacks only lasted a few minutes, and gradually becoming less severe, did not return for several months.

Oppression of chest to such an extent as to almost arrest breathing; asthma caused by sensation as if sternum were being gradually drawn toward dorsal vertebra; expansion of chest difficult; confusion of mind, as if unconsciousness might follow. Attack lasted about ten minutes, followed by general weariness which passed off in a few hours.

|| Rattling in chest and throat.

Pain in centre of chest as if skin were drawn up, on drawing the head back.

Lack of sleep produces sudden faintness and sinking sensation in chest; three spells succeeded each other during a single night.

Sensation of pressure under upper part of sternum.

| Pain and pressure behind sternum.

| Angina; ptosis left eye; facial paralysis left side, slight asphasia; impotence (relieved).

Eczematous herpetic eruptions on chest.

A lady, 78 years of age, had suffered from attacks of spasmodic bronchial asthma (?) for 25 years. The attack would come on *only at night after lying down or during a thunderstorm,* and produces the most intense insomnia, entirely preventing sleep for days and nights together. Under allopathic treatment full doses of Morphine brought relief for twenty months. Ars., Amb., Bell., Ipecac, Nux, Phos., SuL, Op. high, and other apparently well selected remedies entirely failed. Syphilinum cm. cured.

Heart—

Lancinating pain in heart at night, from base to apex (Medor. has reverse).

Valvular disease of the heart.

Neck and Back–

| Heavy aching and stiffness from base of neck up through muscles and cords into brain.

| | Great pain in back in region of kidneys, < after urinating.

Pain in coccyx at its junction with sacrum, sometimes in lower sacral vertebrae; < on sitting, with a sensation as if swollen, though it is not. Pains commencing in sacral regions internally, and apparently coming around to uterus.

| | Caries of cervical spine with great curvature in same region, directly forward, occiput sinking down to a level with it and resting on protuberance of curvature; often nearly a teaspoonful of calcareous matter would be discharged at a time and on evaporating it a quantity of dry powder, looking like phosphate of lime, would be left; pain in curvature always < at night (no proof of syphilis).

Rigidity of muscles.

A heavy, dragging, dull feeling in lumbar region, with stiffness and want of elasticity.

| | Caries or dorsal vertebras with acute curvature, numerous cloacæ communicating with diseased bone, one much larger than the rest, exuding a sanious, offensive pus, and surrounded with proud flesh; great thickening and induration of surrounding parts from effusion of lymph; percussion or pressure not endurable; two abscesses in groins, left having been opened a year before right about a month ago; least motion gave him great pain by day; and terrific pain by night; for five months, every night most intense neuralgic pains, commencing generally from 5 to 7 P.M. and never terminating till about daylight or about 5 A.M.; pains in muscles of loins, generally in left, sharp, cutting spasms, terrible to bear, preventing sleep and forcing him to cry out; < at least motion, and slightly > by warm poultices.

| | Psoas abscess first left then right, latter discharged more than a quart of offensive greenish pus when opened; se-

vere nocturnal pains, affecting upper sacral, lower dorsal and left cervico-facial regions, steadily increasing: they occurred twice, each time twenty-one days after either psoas abscess had been opened.

|| Enlargement of cervical glands and a number of pedunculated pin-head warts on neck; cured by *syco-syphilinum.*

Enlargement of glands in different parts of the body, particularly abundant about the neck; indurated and slightly painful causing a sensation of uncomfortable fulness and suffusion in face, throat and head.

|| Nocturnal aggravation of pains in back, hips and thighs.

|| Enormous swelling of glands in head and neck; no relief from any remedy. Cured with Buboin syphilitica cm.

Syphilitic sores on back near spine on hip.

Pains commencing in sacral region internally, and apparently coming around to uterus.

Indurated lumps between muscles of the neck.

Aching pains in lirnbs like growing pains.

Upper Limbs—

| Rheumatism of shoulder-joint or at insertion of deltoid, < from raising arm laterally.

Can only raise arms to a right angle with axilla; trying to force them higher causes muscles to suddenly become paralyzed and they drop pendant.

Lameness and pain of arm on motion < on raising arm up in front as if reaching; pain located about insertion deltoid in upper third of humerus, not painful to pressure.

|| Fingers and thumbs have runarounds (infantile syphilis).

Always washing the hands.

|| Hands badly ulcerated on backs.

|| R. second finger is swollen and stiffened.

Lower Limbs—

Swelling of legs from knees down, soles painful when

standing on them; swelling goes down in morning, comes back at night.

Pains in lower extremities, excruciating, completely banish sleep; < from hot fomentations; > pouring cold water on them > for an hour, after which the pains returned.

Cannot sit in a low chair, or squat down, owing to loss of control over knee and hip-joints.

Pains in long bones of lower extremities, also on joints.

Dull pains over back of feet to toes, began soon after getting into bed, lasting until 4 or 5 A.M.

|| For two or three winters intense cold pain in both legs, < in left, came on every night on lying down, lasting all night; > by getting up and walking, and in warm weather.

Pain in three toes of right foot as if disjointed.

|| Slight contraction of tendons beneath right knee.

Tearing pains in hip and thighs, < at night > about daybreak, < by walking, not affected by weather (improved).

|| Redness and rawness with terrible itching between toes.

|| Bubo with pain in spot on middle of right thigh in front, only when standing and on deep pressure, which seemed to touch spot, which was apparently on periosteum.

|| Two ulcers larger than a crown piece, dirty stinking, sloughing, with jagged, elevated edges, one on thigh above patella, another on head of tibia; two large pieces of bone came away from head of tibia.

|| Osteosarcoma in centre of right tibia the size of half an ostrich egg, pains agonizing at night, growth irregular, spongy, partly laminated, very hard.

| Contracted, painful feeling in soles, as if tendons were too short.

Aching pains in limbs, like growing pains.

Bone pains in knees and feet.

Gradual rigidity of all joints after eruption; flexors seem contracted.

|| Rheumatic swelling of left wrist and big toe, bluish red, with pains as if somebody sawed at his bones with a dull saw; > by heat of stove; < from sundown to sunrise; no appetite; has lasted two weeks.

Feeling of numbness in palms and soles, at times a prickly sensation as if numb parts were punctured by a great number of needles.

Excruciating arthritis; swelling, heat, and redness intense. Rheumatism, muscles are caked in hard knots or lumps.

|| Severe attacks of aching in lower limbs.

|| Sharp rheumatic pain, burning like fire, in 1, side of right instep and below inner malleolus, prevents her from moving foot < when toe is pointed inward; < in evening, continuing during night, waking her up suddenly every two or three hours, worst from 1:30 to 3:30 A.M., < toward daybreak (improved).

An old doctor residing here had been troubled for two or three winters with an *intense cold pain* in both legs, left one worse. It came on every night on lying down and lasted all night, only relief was by getting up and walking, and everything had failed to help. Magnetic leggings had afforded most relief. The trouble ceased in warm weatheright He happened to speak of it one day, and I told him I would stop it. As he wanted to try it, I gave him one dose of Syphilinum mm., dry. He lost his pain for six or eight weeks, when it returned in a milder form, and he received one dose of Syphilinum cmm., and he has never had it since. Went all winter without pain. But he said the second powder made his genitals ache so that he couldn't sit still, and this continued for over a month.

Skin—

Pustular eruption on different parts of body; in patches on certain places, particularly on wrists and shins, where bones are nearest cuticle, and isolated other large pustules on other parts, these break, discharging an ichorous fluid for one or two days, then heal, leaving characteristic pockmark cicatrice;

patches take longer to heal, discharging same fluid till healing process commences.

After healing of chancre a fresh pustular eruption appears on different parts of body, which when pustules have discharged an ichorous liquid and healed up, leaves fresh coppery pockmarks; Medor removed it permanently, causing it to turn yellow-brown, dry at edges and scale off, leaving skin permanently clear and free.

|| Biting sensation in different parts of body, as if bitten by bugs, at night only.

|| Syphilitic rash, very prominent on forehead, chin, arms and front of thorax, an abundance of fine scales peeling off; large prominent spot on centre of forehead, filled with fluid, as also are some smaller patches.

|| Syphilitic bulla discharging freely on cheeks, under chin, on back of shoulders, on scalp and other parts of body (infantile syphilis).

|| Macula; copper-coloured; from crown of head to sole of foot.

| Pemphigus, looking like a pock, often confluent and persistently reappears. Skin bluish.

|| Macula over back, chest, abdomen, arms and legs, but not on any uncovered part of body.

|| Several elevated spots on arm, stomach, leg and finge; has them habitually on face, chiefly on left cheek.

|| A blood-boil on arm: face broken out with a lumpy fiery rash.

|| Eruption over whole body not elevated, but could be distinctly felt by passing hand over skin; after Syphilinum 1m. eruption came rapidly to surface; at same time a disagreeable odor began to be developed; eruption reddish-brown like small-pox pustules, without central depression; body covered with it, except scrotum and penis; increased, completely covering inside of mouth and throat, making it difficult to swallow even liquids; eyes also covered, making him completely blind; in-

tolerable smell from body; tips of pimples became filled with pus; < from warmth of bed; fetid breath; eruption developed still more, a great quantity of pus, with intolerable itching, yet could not scratch as it was extremely sore; eruption left skin of entire body covered with dull, reddish, copper-coloured spots, which in cold, looked blue.

Sleep—

Great restlessness at night, impossible to keep long in one position.

| Absolute sleeplessness (vies with Sul. in producing quiet, refreshing sleep).

Wakes soon after midnight and cannot sleep again till 6 A.M.

During the whole 24 hours can only rest from 8 to 10 A.M.

Total loss of sleep for 22 successive days and nights.

Absolute sleeplessness for 11 to 14 days and nights.

Fever—

|| Great pains in head, whole body extremely cold, looked blue; wanted to be covered with blankets or couldn't get warm; no appetite; sleeping almost continually, could not be aroused.

|| Nervous chills preceded by pains in head, especially occiput and scalp of that part; pains below waist, in pelvis, legs, especially tibia, which is sensitive to touch; bowels torpid; cross, irritable, peevish; pains begin every day at 4 P.M., culminate at midnight, disappear at daylight.

After retiring nerve chill beginning in anus, running down legs with spasmodic sensation; desire for stool; > by profuse urination and by eructations.

Fever: dry, hot, shortly after going to bed, parched lips, great thirst; during fever intensely hot, wants to throw off covering, puts feet out of bed and against wall to cool them; high fever in middle of day, heat being intense, with sensation as if burning up; thirst for large quantities often, sensation of burning internal heat very marked; fever preceded by slight chill and followed by sweat and great debility.

|| Sweat: profuse at night, sleepless and restless; especially between scapulae and down to waist, with excessive general debility.

|| Fever from 11 to 1 P.M. daily; perspires when she begins to get over fever; pain in back, < between shoulders, no ambition or desire to move.

| Excessive general debility and continued night sweats, latter being most marked between scapulae and down to waist

Generalities–

Utter prostration and debility in morning.

Epilepsy.

Dwarfed, shrivelled-up, old-looking babies and children.

Epileptic convulsions after menses.

|| Body, extremities and face covered with syphilides; a sticking soreness begins in throat every evening between 6 and 7 o'clock and continues to grow < during night; exceedingly restless until 4 A.M.; then a restless sleep for a few hours; can scarcely swallow; when swallowing a sensation as of throat tearing to pieces; continual throbbing in throat, < from cold and hot drinks, and < lying down; throbbing in temples and ears, boring in ears meeting in centre of brain; sensation as if top of head were coming off; drawing pain in eyes < from lamplight; teeth pain when eating, also when taking anything hot or cold, feel as if they were loose, > pressing teeth together and pressing throat with hands; excessive flow of saliva, it runs out of mouth when sleeping; severe pain in neck; bending back head, > pain in neck; aching pain in shoulders and knees; rending, tearing pains throughout body, > moving about slowly; had his wife hide his revolver lest in a fit of desperation he might kill himself, as was his desire during extreme paroxysms of pain; strikes wall with fist and beats head against wall for relief; stools hard, dry like sheep dung; desire for stool three or four times a day, but only a little scentless

wind passes which gives relief; sitting at stool, > pain in head; is easily offended, gets desperate, cannot bear to be alone, great anxiety about getting well; at night no position suits him, walks floor or goes into street and moves about slowly; sleepy all the time but cannot sleep; dreams about his disease; < in open air; frequent urination with sudden desire; discharges large quantities of muddy urine.

Shifting pains of a rheumatic character obliging a repeated change of position and posture.

Lancinating rheumatic pains, slightly relieved by a change of position at times, and sometimes relieved by motion.

Pains commence at 2 P.M., gradually increasing till they reach their acme at 9 P.M., continuing exceedingly acute till 3 or 4 A.M., subsiding with daybreak.

Pains more particularly < in, or confined to, the muscles and joints of lower limbs, for four or five weeks, then they seemed to go to the periosteum and bone itself, consequently becoming deeper and more profound.

The pains produce two sensations, an external one which seems to lie in muscles and joints, and an internal one which is deeper and much, more unbeartable, so much so that it seems by its profound nature to control the external ones and to cause those pains to disappear, afterward reappearing intensified in the external sensation.

Pains in all the limbs every night after midnight, weary, tired pains, making rest impossible, as he could lie nowhere without suffering in the part on which he rested. Pains worse in lower limbs, much perspiration which partly >.

Rheumatic neuralgic pains in all the muscles, even in cremaster, *not* in joints; darting pains in irregular attacks, sometimes lasting a week or two. The pains gradually increase and decrease; they are worse in damp and especially in frosty weather; they get worse at 4 or 5 P.M., attain their height at 2 or 3 A.M., ceasing about 8 A.M. Never contracted syphilis —very much improved by dm.

Rheumatism with sweating of hands, wrists and legs below the knees, and feet, with great soreness of soles, all < at night.

Extreme emaciation.

Hardly able to lift hand.

Feels < mornings: utter prostration and debility in morning.

Weak, emaciated.

Though 17 looked 12, was so reduced and dwarfed; great attenuation of soft parts throughout, spare and hollow; confined to couch for about three years, and for one year was scarcely ever off back.

After the disappearance of the pustular eruption, a gradual rigidity of all the joints ensues, and all the flexors seem to become contracted and shortened; this causes inability to close the fingers on a knife, fork or spoon, and a partial inability to lift the foot in order to step up-stairs, except with great difficulty by using a cane, and only a step up or down at a time. (NOTE.—This is not the case where the pustular eruption is acurative effect of the Syphilinum high.—*Swan.*

Feeling of numbness in palms and sole, which have also at times a prickly sensation as if the numb parts were punctured by a great number of needles.

Slight rigidity of joints.

Rheumatic swelling of left wrist and left great toe which is bluish-red, with pains like sawing off his bones with a dull saw; better from heat of stove, worse from sundown to sunrise; no appetite.

THYROIDIN

Thyroidin. Thyroid Extract. A Sarcode. Trituration of the fresh thyroid gland of sheep or calf. Attenuation of a liquid extract of the gland.

Mind—

Acute stupor alternating with restless melancholia; at times could not be got to speak, but would lie on floor with limbs rigid; at other times would weep and undress herself; at times dangerous and homicidal, would put her arms round the necks of other patients so tightly as almost to strangle them (in this case the insanity was primary and the myxedema secondary; both conditions were removed). Evinced increased vivacity by quarreling with another patient about a trifling difference of opinion.

Depression.

Fretfulness and moroseness gave way to cheerfulness and animation.

"All progressed cases of myxedema show some mental aberration which tends towards dementia, usually with delusions, the latter taking the form of suspicion and persecution. Occasionally actual insanity is present in the form of mania and insanity."

Delirium of persecution (three cases observed, one fatal, the result of taking Thyro. in tablets to reduce obesity).

Sudden acute mania occurring in myxedema, perfectly restored mentally and bodily under Thyr.

Mental aberration dating three years before onset of myxedema, subject to attacks of great violence, with intervals of depression and moroseness.

State of idiocy; fearful nightmares.

Excited condition, lasting all the rest of the day, grunting continuously and laughing in a way that was peculiar to herself.

Very excited; excited state followed by considerable depression.

For several hours in what can be only termed a hysterical condition.

Profound depression.

Irritable and ill-tempered.

Became a grumbler.

Angry.

Had frights.

Head—

Vertigo.

Feeling of lightness in the brain, scarcely amounting to giddiness.

Much giddiness and headache for twenty-four hours.

Awoke about 4 A.M. with sharp headache and intense aching in back and limbs, which continued for three days and compelled him to keep his bed.

Ever since taking the first thyroid [had had five glands altogether, at intervals] he had a strange feeling in his head, with vertigo and palpitation on stooping.

Headache (with fever symptoms); disappeared on suspending treatment, reappeared seven days after recommencing.

Frontal-coronal headache after taking one tabloid for four successive days.

(Constant headache, pains in occiput and vertex.)

(Headache in case of acromegaly.)

Headache.

Headache and pains in abdomen.

Fresh growth of hair (many cases).

Black hairs growing among the grey.

In one case of scleroderma and in one case of myxedema the hair fell off permanently.

In a case of myxedema the patient lost all the hair of his head and face and had a thick growth over his arms and thorax; under Thyright The hair of the head and face grew again and that of the arms and chest fell off.

Eyes—

(Prominence of eyeballs—exophthalmic goitre.)

Optic neuritis (in five persons, four of them women, under treatment for obesity; no other symptoms of thyroidism).

Accommodative asthenopia.

Ears—

Moist patches behind ears heal up (case of psoriasis). Hyperplastic median otitis with sclerosis and loss of mobility of the ossicles (rapid amelioration—several cases).

Face—

Flushing: with nausea and lumbar pains; loss of consciousness, tonic muscular spasms; immediate; with rise of temperature, and pains all over; suddenly became breathless and livid.

Faintness, with great flushing of upper part of body and pains in back.

Swelling of face and legs.

In lupus of face, tight sensation, heat, and angry redness removed.

Burning sensation of lips with free desquamation.

Mouth—

Tongue became thickly coated.

Feverish and thirsty.

Great thirst.

(Ulcerated patch on buccal aspect on left cheek near angle of mouth.)

Throat—

(Full sensation.)

Goitre, exophthalmic, cured.

Goitre reduced.

Stomach—

Loss of appetite.

Increased appetite with improved digestion.

Eructations.

Dyspeptic troubles.

Nausea, with flushing and lumbar pains.

Nausea, slight vomiting.

Slight nausea recurring on thinking of it.

Nausea soon after taking the gland.

On five occasions the patient (a woman) vomited the thyroid.

Always felt a sensation of sickness after the injections.

Sensation of faintness and nausea (after a few injections).

Feels tired and sick.

Gastro-intestinal disturbance and diarrhea.

Abdomen—

Flatulence increased, followed later in the case by amelioration.

Headache and pain in abdomen.

Stool—

Diarrhea, with gastro-intestinal disturbance.

Relief of constipation with more natural actions.

Constipation.

Urinary Organs—

Increased flow of urine.

Increased urination, usually with clear, pale yellow secretion.

Slight trace of albumin found in urine.

Albuminuria.

Diabetes mellitus; caused and cured.

Female Sexual Organs—

Increased sexual desire.

Six days after commencement of treatment menstruation, which has been absent over a year, reappeared and continued profusely (in several cases of myxedema with or without insanity).

Menses profuse, prolonged, more frequent; early amenorrhea.

(Painful and irregular menstruation.)

(Constant left ovarian pain, and great tenderness).

Looks pale and feels ill.

Pain in lower part of abdomen, headache and sickness (in 33 girl of sixteen, probably menstrual effort provoked by Thyright;no catamenial flow appeared).

Acts as a galactagogue when milk is deficient; when a deficiency is associated with a return of the menses it will suppress the latter.

(Puerperal insanity with fever.)

(Puerperal eclampsia.)

Respiratory Organs—

Slight attack of hemoptysis, followed by cough and signs of phthisis at apex of left lung.

(Voice became clear.)

Dormant phthisis; lighted up the disease in five cases.

Heart and Pulse—

Death, with all the symptoms of angina pectoris.

On trying to walk uphill died suddenly from cardiac failure.

While stooping to put on her shoes she 'fainted' and died in half an hour.

On one occasion, after exerting herself more than she had done for a long time previously, "suddenly became extremely breathless and livid, and felt as if she was dying;" < by rest in recumbent position and stimulants.

Two fainting attacks.

Frequent fainting fits.

Complained occasionally of a feeling of faintness, not occurring particularly after the injections.

One patient showed extraordinary symptoms after the injection; the skin became so livid as to be almost blue-black.

Degeneration of heart muscle in animals.

A systolic cardiac murmur was less loud after the treatment than before.

Sensations of faintness and nausea.

Palpitation on stooping.

Weakness of heart's action.

Tachycardia and ready excitability of the heart persisting for several days after the feeding was stopped.

Pulse rose to 112.

Relaxation of arterioles.

(Rapid pulsation, with inability to lie down in bed.)

(Jumping sensation at heart.)

Back—

Flushing, nausea, and lumbar pains, lasting a few minutes.

Stabbing pains in lumbar region.

Intense aching in back and limbs, which continued for three days.

Flushing of upper part of body and pains in back.

(Backache.)

Upper Limbs—

After injection, to a great extent lost the use of her hands for two days; recurred later, lasting a few hours.

Felt queer and unable to raise her arms (after injection, another case).

Arms less stiff and painful (psoriasis).

Lower Limbs—

Tingling sensation in legs.

Edema of legs appeared, and subsequently subsided and continued to reappear and subside for a month.

Pain in legs.

Incomplete paraplegia.

Swelling of face and legs.

Feet frequently peel in large flakes, leaving a tender surface.

Profuse flow of fluid from feet (in case of dropsy cured by Thyr.).

Quivering of limbs; tremors.

Intense aching in back and limbs, lasting three days.

Pains in arms and legs, with malaise.

Skin of hands and feet desquamated.

(Acromegaly, subjective symptoms.)

Generalities—

Malaise > by lying in bed.

Stooping = palpitation.

Rest in recumbent position > extreme breathlessness with lividity, felt as if dying.

Myxedematous patients are always chilly; the effect of the treatment is to make them less so.

Loss of consciousness and general tonic muscular spasm for a few seconds.

Fainting attacks (many cases).

Tremors, quivering of limbs, complete unconsciousness.

(Tetany.)

Epileptiform fit, after which he was unconscious for an hour; next day felt better and warmer.

Malaise so great she refused to continue the treatment.

Agitation.

Incomplete paraplegia.

Hysterical attack.

(Hystero-epilepsy with amenorrhea.)

Nervous and hysterical, had to have nurse to watch her.

Feels tired and sick.

Stabbing pains.

Aching pains (many cases).

Aching pains all over.

Diffused pains.

Aching pains in various parts of body.

Pains over whole body.

Brawny swelling at point of injection, followed by abscess of slow development.

Myxedema removed (many cases).

A series of abscesses resulting from the injections, but probably originating from an accidental abscess quite independent of them."

A small abscess formed.

Increased suppuration in case of lupus.

Gained a stone in weight.

Lost weight enormously (may cases of myxedema).

Rapid gain of flesh and strength.

Anemia and debility.

Infiltration rapidly absorbed (psoriasis).

Persons suffering from skin disease can bear much larger doses than those suffering from myxedema.

(Acromegaly, headache, and subjective symptoms.)

(Fractures refuse to unite.)

A peculiar cachexia more dangerous than myxedema itself.

Syphilis, secondary, tertiary.

Skin—

Flushing of skin.

Skin became so livid as to be almost blue-black.

Skin has desquamated freely, but there has been no perspiration or diuresis.

Psoriasis: eruption extended and increased.

(Psoriasis: redness and itching reduced; eruption separating and being shed in great scales, angry, inflamed appearance completely gone.)

Moist patches behind ears heal up.

Arms less stiff and painful; swelling diminished.

Crusts separated, leaving faint red skin; eruption not nearly so painful.

(Symmetrical serpiginous eruption; dark red; edges raised and thickened.)

Lupus: tight feeling, heat, angry redness removed; suppuration increased.

Eczema: irritation of skin markedly allayed.

Scattered pustules of eczema mature quickly or abort.

(Teething eczema.)

(Syphilitic psoriasis.)

(Rupia.)

Scleroderma.

Peeling of skin beginning on legs and extending over whole surface; skin has since become comparatively soft and smooth.

Peeling of skin of lower limbs, with gradual clearing (eczema).

Skin of hands and feet desquamated.

Sleep—

Continual tendency to sleep.

Awoke about 4 A.M. with sharp headache.

Fearful nightmares disappeared.

Insomnia.

Excited condition; could not sleep.

Fever—

Flushing: with nausea; with loss of consciousness.

Always felt hot, and had a sensation of sickness after the injections.

Felt better and warmer.

Flushing of upper part of body and pains in back.

Temperature never rose above 99° but she felt feverish and thirsty.

Temperature rose to 100° F., and remained there several days; pulse 112.

Rise of temperature; diaphoresis.

Profuse perspiration on least exertion.

TUBERCULINUM

Mind—

Anxiety, gloomy, melancholy humor.

Has lost melancholy expression she formerly had.

Is disposed to whine and complain; dejected mind, anxiety.

She is very sad.

Nervous irritation; aversion to labor.

Indifferent.

Forgetful.

Aversion to all labor, espcially mental work.

Sensibility to music.

Does not like to be disturbed by people; trembling of hands.

Felt positively ugly; personal aversions became almost a mania.

Trifles produced intense irritation and I could not shake them off.

Very irritable, want to fight; no hesitancy in throwing anything at any one, even without cause.

Memory weak, unable to think.

Comprehension and concentration almost impossible.

Great anxiety for future, otherwise marked indifference.

Great sleepiness and weariness; entire muscular system relaxed; desire to lie down all the time.

Nervous; Weak Irritable.

Melancholy, despondent, morose, irritable, fretful, peevish.

Dejected, taciturn, sulky; weeps, but knows not why; naturally of a sweet disposition, now on the borderland of insanity.

Fretful, snappish, morose, depressed and melancholic, even to insanity.

Ill-mannered, quarrelsome; lies in bed and complains; lachrymose, weeps without any provocation, cannot help it.

Irritable on waking; nothing can please him; nothing satisfies.

Melancholy with marked hypochondriacal delirium.

Everything in the room seems strange, as though in a strange place.

Intense restlessness; and inward restlessness.

||With every little ailment whines and complains; easily frightened, particularly by dogs; screams in terror when approached by a dog.

Anxiety, gloomy, melancholic humor.

Very restless in the evening when aroused.

Periodical anxiety and terror.

She is very sad, dejected, and complains continually.

Nervous irritation; averse to physical or mental labor.

Indifferent; forgetful; averse to all labor, especially mental work.

Extremely sensitive to music.

Sensibilities dulled; with chill and aching in the head, back and limbs.

Somnolence; loss of vital power; great physical weakness.

Does not like to be disturbed; trembling of hands and feet.

Soporous, dazed condition; unable to find the right way; is confused; surroundings appear strange.

Memory weak or lost; unable to think or comprehend.

Comprehension difficult; must read a paragraph several times before he can understand it.

Sopor; somnolence; with dyspnea.

Coma: profound, lasting three days, with temperature 106.

Delirium and serious meningeal symptoms, following an injection of Tuberculinum.

Complete unconsciousness; stupor and stertorous breathing.

Insanity; acute or chronic, with a family history of tubercular affections.

When the best selected remedy fails to relieve or permanently cure in a marked tubercular diathesis, with a tubercular family history.

Despondent, discouraged, feel as if I would rather die than live.

|| Although naturally of a sweet disposition, became taciturn, sulky, snappish, fretty, irritable, morose, depressed and melancholic, even to insanity.—*Burnett.*

Head—

Vertigo, especially in morning; heavy with obscuration of eyes; is obliged to lean on something; by bending down, especially by rising after bending down; with palpitation; with nausea; with backache in morning; after dinner.

Great heat in head; flushes of heat after dinner; sensation of heat in head in evening.

Headache: deep in forehead; deep in temples; on vertex, with sensation of heat; from neck to forehead; in morning, passing away in afternoon.

Sensation of heaviness on vertex.

Headache with obscuration of sight.

Headache with vertigo.

Piercing headache.

Piercing pain in forehead from 10 A.M. to 3 P.M.

Headache in evening; in afternoon.

Frontal headache in morning.

Headache with rushing in ears.

Headache in morning with bleeding of nose.

Headache from neck to forehead; burning, piercing.

Colossal hyperemia of pia mater and brain substance; extreme engorgement of vessels on the surface, internally dusky red; tubercles presented no retrogressive changes (arachnitis).

(Sensation as if brain were squeezed with iron band.—Bac.)

Headache < by motion.

Sick-headache commencing about 8 A.M., increasing in severity through the day; very changeable, leaning the head to one side would increase the pain on that side.

Brain seems loose and rolling around from side to side.

Darting pain in occiput, extending down the spine.

Headache commencing about 10 A.M., increasing until 3 or 4 P.M. Pains erratic, changing place rapidly; first in one place then in another, not > in any position.

Headache in evening 8 P.M., neurotic, first in one place then in another, over one eye then the other, then the occiput and down the spine.

Headache in afternoon, worse from going up stairs, better in open air.

Severe headache and vertigo in afternoon; a dizzy, sick at stomach sensation, like sea-sickness.

Dull headache on waking.

A strange sensation in head on first lying down as if some light substance was rolling from above eyes to vertex.

Severe headache beginning upon mastoid process on left side and extending over head to opposite side.

Complete physical exhaustion without any apparent cause.

Chilly all day, although room was warm; muscles of the whole body sore to touch or pressure.

In morning so weary and muscles ache so severely it is difficult to arise.

Great heaviness in head and pain in occiput and neck.

Severe headache, < on second day, lasting until the third, recurring from time to time for many weeks and compelling quiet fixedness.—*Burnett.*

Headache, *with frequent sharp, cutting pains passing from above right eye through head to back of left ear.—Rose.*

|| Headache of great intensity preceded by a shuddering chill passing from brain down spine, with attack a feeling as if head above eyes were swollen; became unconscious with screaming, tearing her hair, beating her head with her fists or trying to dash it against wall or flooright—*Swan.*

|| Headache of forty-five years' standing, *pain passing from right frontal protuberance to right occipital region.—Swan.*

|| Terrible pain in head, as if he had a tight hoop of iron around it; trembling of hands; distressing sensation of damp clothes on his spine; almost absolute sleeplessness; profound adynamia; was thought by his friends to be on verge of insanity; most of his brothers and sisters had died of water on brain; right lung solid, probably from healed-up cavities, as he at one time suffered from pulmonary phthisis.—*Burnett.*

|| Sullen, taciturn, irritable, screams in his sleep, is very restless at night, constipated; sister died of tubercular meningtis.—*Btirnett.*

|| Fretful and ailing, whines and complains, indurated glands can be felt everywhere, child hot, drowsy, urine red and sandy, much given to be frightened, particularly by dogs; was vaccinated and had a very bad arm for four months thereafter; would not smile, whimpers when spoken to, skin dingy, skull hydrocephalic.—*Burnett.*

|| Boy, aged 20 months, ill for days with head, high fever, restlessness and constant screaming; finally no sleep for forty hurs, followed by a condition of collapse; peculiar smell of body; family history of tuberculosis.—*Burnett.*

| Tubercular meningitis, with effusion; head gradually enlarged; alternately wakeful and delirious at night, talked non-

sense by day, at intervals; nocturnal hallucinations and fright, delirium; pyrexia; had eczema which almost disappeared after two unsuccessful vaccinations, and which were soon followed by above condition; after administration of remedy there occurred a severe pustular eruption, then patches of a lepra and eczema appeared.—*Burnett.*

|| Basilar meningitis—*Sinker.*

Tubercular meningitis— *Sinkeright*

|| Acute cerebral meningitis, with intense strabismus.—*Biegler.*

Plica polonica: several bad cases permanently cured with Tuberculinum.—*Jackson.*

Eyes—

Swollen lids; headache with swollen lids in morning.

Right eye much swollen, conjunctiva inflamed.

Dulness and heaviness of eyes; darkness before eyes.

Obscuration of vision with vertigo.

Opens right eye (which had been closed).

Breaking down of cicatrices of old corneal ulcers (Stoker).

Clearing of corneal opacity the result of old tuberculous corneitis (Stoker).

Tuberculosis of eyelids, small grey and yellow nodules, existing in conjunctiva of outer sections of lids, increased in size, ran together, then suddenly disappeared.

Phlyctenulae appeared where none existed before (Maschke).

Conjunctivitis; herpes on lids.

Amblyopia with irregularity and complete paralysis of pupils (in an alcoholic).

Stye appeared on upper lid of right eye. Lid swollen, intensely painful; four days later opened discharging green pus.

Stye on lower lid of right eye, appeared suddenly, began to swell like a bee sting. Opened within 48 hours discharging green pus.

Ears—

Tinnitus.

Rushing in ears with heavy head.

Sticking pain from pharynx to ears.

Headache with rushing in ears and pressure on vertex.

Great aching in ears and teeth.

Discharge of yellowish matter from the ears.

Swelling of the glands around the ear and on the neck, worse below the ear and behind.

Slight discharge of yellowish matter from right ear.

No pain.

Earl, aged 2 years. Light complexion.

January 25, 1895. Consumption on the father's side. Since last February has had a discharge from the ears of a yellowish matter without special indications. Was relieved by some medication until within the last two or three weeks.

Now there is considerable swelling of the glands around the ear and on the neck, worse below the ear and behind, with a slight discharge of yellowish matter from the right ear. No pain. No appetite; will only take milk when it has tea in it. Not in poor flesh, but thinner than usual. Desires fresh air and wants to be out of doors. Fretful at night; seems to be better during the day. Was very feverish a day or so before the ear commenced to run. Tuberculinum 50m., one dose.

February 7. The swelling about the ear increased till Sunday night (three days) and looked as though it would break on the outside. Since then it has been going down; his ear quit running yesterday. The discharge became thick and would not run; they kept it syringed out with warm water and soap; it gradually grew less. Hardly any odor about the discharge. Stool once or twice a day. Appetite better. A little more restless at night. Anxious to get out of doors, but cried to get back into the house again. Head seems to hurt when he cries. Disposition better; he is not so cross. The swelling about the glands almost gone. Seems to be gradually improving. Placebo.

February 26. Better in every way. No swelling or running at the earight The family consider him well. The only thing noticeable is that he seems somewhat pale and nervous when first getting up in the morning, but this soon wears off. Is in better flesh. Sac. lac. The case required no more medicine and rapidly went on to a cure.

Nose—

Coryza.

Secretion of mucus from nose, viscid, yellow-green.

Increased secretion of mucus, with frontal headache.

Aching of ears and teeth with coryza in evening, with headache.

Bleeding of nose.

Comedones on nose, surrounded with minute pustules.

The nose, which used to feel 'hot and burning,' has lost this sensation.

Profuse discharge of blood mixed with mucus from nares.

Seem to have a fresh cold with each change of weatheright Blowing blood from nose constantly. Profuse discharge of bloody mucus.

Small boil at end of nose; at upper nasal commissure, and one on upper lip. The boils were small, dark-red in colour and contained green pus. Very slow in healing.

Sneezing, burning, watery coryza. Seemed to have fresh cold all the time.

Fluent coryza.

Discharge of thick tenacious, gray-coloured mucus.

Awakened every morning at 5 A.M. to clear nose and throat.

Rattling of mucus in throat immediately after eating, which must be expectorated.

Soreness inside of nose, commencing as watery pimples, which, suppurating, form scabs; nose and lips somewhat swollen; itching slightly.—*Rose*.

Face—

Edematous, pale face.

Clonic convulsions of musculus orbicularis inferior, acute.

Convulsions in region of facial muscle, especially buccinator.

In one case the inflammation of the lupus (on face) presented unquestionable erysipelas of a rather severe type, and the patient was for some time in danger.

Flushing of cheek of same side as lung affected, during the reaction (Borgherini).

Upper lip and nose became swollen during the first two or three reactions, the lip becoming cracked on inner surface.

Herpes on lips and eyelids (Heilferich).

After the tenth injection his left moustache, which was kept cut to prevent scabs from gathering, ceased to grow, every hair fell out, and for a month the left upper lip was perfectly denuded of hair, and had all the appearance when seen under a lens of being depilated; however,-the hairs began to grow well before he left the Home. (Hine).

Slight swelling and itching of lips.—*Rose.*

Teeth—

Vague toothache.

Teeth felt loose.

"Feeling as if the teeth were all jammed together and too many for his head."

Sordes on teeth.

Inflammation of gums, scurvy-like.

Gums turgescent, felt swollen.

Mouth—

Tongue foul, furred.

Tongue much coated.

Coating on soft palate and tongue.

Taste: salty, purulent.

Aphthae on tongue and buccal mucosa.

Tongue dry.

Dryness of lips.

On lips black blisters.

Palate: granulations enormously swollen and vascular.

Breath offensive.

Spit up blood streaked mucus from mouth and throat.

A bitter, disagreeable taste; nothing tasted natural. This continued for more than a month.

Tongue coated white at back and through the center.

Scalded sensation on tongue and in mouth as though burned; tongue sore at tip.

Lips dry, chapped; entire mouth very dry, but no thirst, worse in morning on rising.

Thirst for small quantities of water.

Wakened several times in the night on account of dryness of mouth.

Throat—

Aching in pharynx and larynx.

Scratching in pharynx.

Tickling in throat exciting cough.

Sensation of mucus in throat.

Sensation of a tumor in throat.

Dryness in throat; tonsilitis; general inflammatory condition of pharyngeal mucous membrane.

Retropharyngeal abscess.

Burning pain in throat.

Sensation of constriction in throat; in larynx.

Heaviness and sensation of rattling in throat.

Aching extending from throat to ears.

Dysphagia increased; later diminished (in laryngeal phthisis).

Intense pain in naso-pharynx on swallowing.

Sensation as if throat was swollen on the right side; expectorating a great deal of mucus from posterior nares, worse immediately after eating.

Needle-like pains in left side of throat < by swallowing.

Pains shooting to the left ear when swallowing; unable to eat solids.

Dryness of the throat and posterior nares, with a dry, tickling cough at night.

Appetite—

Appetite good; enjoy food. It is all right until it reaches lower bowel, then urging begins. Stool mostly undigested; lienteria; weight 112; previous to proving, weighed 134.

Loss of appetite, especially in morning.

Thirst: extreme, day and night; burning in morning.

Always drank coffee, but now cannot bear even the odor of it, which < the headache.

Great thirst.

Mouth, lips and tongue dry and parched.

Craving for food, for something to eat, but not relieved by eating.

Stomach—

Eructations and sensation of fulness over stomach.

Nausea, vomiting.

Vomited severely with decreasing to headache.

Nausea and vomiting, nausea with efforts to vomit with colic and diarrhea.

Transitory sickness and vomiting after dinner.

Vomiting after every meal.

Nausea and sickness in morning with heaviness in stomach region.

Pressure in stomach, going to throat, as if the clothes were too tight.

Cramping pain in stomach.

Nausea with pains in umbilical region with diarrhea.

Nausea with racking and stirring in stomach and increased thirst.

Sickness in stomach and pressing.

Nausea in morning.

Sticking pains in stomach region.

Belching of tasteless gas.

Constant nausea, but could not vomit.

Belching, with burning sensation in esophagus from stomach to mouth.

Tasteless eructations with much belching.

Nausea and repugnance at sight or odor of food.

Empty, twisted sensation in epigastrium, followed by another stool.

Much pressing, continuous pain in epigastrium.

Feels as if stomach was gripped by a hand.

Great thirst for hot water, which does not relieve.

Empty sensation after eating as if not satisfied.

|| Windy dyspepsia, with pinching and pains under ribs of right side in mammary line.—*Burnett.*

Abdomen—

Cramping pains in stomach and abdomen.

Sensation of constriction in abdomen.

Colic with diarrhea and heaviness in stomach.

Colic with great thirst.

Fatigue and sickness in region of stomach and abdomen; sticking pain's deep in spleen; severe pain in region of liver.

Aching (sticking) in region of liver, spleen, ovaries, spermatic cord, testicles (especially left), in hip-joints, in rectum.

Pains in region of appendix vermiformis.

Mass of enlarged glands, in right iliac fossa much smaller.

Six pustufes at different parts of skin of back and abaomen, and after discharging have healed.

Discrete papular rash over chest and abdomen.

Perforating ulcer in intestines.

Bloated sensation in abdomen all day.

Borborygmus, much rattling and rumbling.

Seems as though something would start in left groin and crawl upward, with persistent rumbling.

Dull pain and rumbling in abdomen, constantly changing from one side to the other.

Great exhaustion and weakness.

Sensation in abdomen as if greatly distended; clothing very oppressive, particularly about the waist; obliged to remove corset immediately for fear of suffocation.

Bursting sensation in abdomen.

Empty sensation in abdomen followed by burning from waist through lower extremities.

|| Fever, emaciation, abdominal pains and discomfort, restless at night, glands of both groins enlarged and indurated; cries out in sleep; strawberry tongue.—*Burnett.*

|| Tabes mesenterica; swelling on left side, also on right; complains of a stitch in side after running; languid and indisposed to talk; nervous and irritable; talks in his sleep; grinds his teeth; appetite poor; hands blue; indurated and palpable glands everywhere; a drum belly; spleen region bulging out. —*Burnett.*

|| Inguinal glands indurated and visible; excessive sweats; chronic diarrhea.

Stool and Anus—

Obstipation; stool hard, dry, with wind and colic.

Diarrhea with pinching and burning pains.

Pressure and constriction in rectum.

Pain in rectum.

Itching sensation in anus.

Constant urging to stool; often ineffectual.

Tenesmus, painful, constant; not so severe when lying down, but not > by lying.

Ineffectual urging; no reference to stool; seems to be the sphincter muscles.

Stool seems to drop for some distance above, coming chiefly in small diarrheic dribbles without pain, until sphincter is touched. Tenesmus begins as soon as feces pass over lower portion of rectum.

Tenesmus and ineffectual urging day and night; no rest; disturbed, unrefreshing sleep.

Pain dull, more or less severe; about hips, sacrum and entire pelvic region.

When I cough seems as if the rectum was being torn out.

Get very weary sitting, but dread to move, as motions < the tenesmus.

Early morning diarrhea: urgent, watery, dark-brown and offensive, passing with great force, 5 A.M. This early morning stool continued for eight days, invariably from 5 to 6 A.M.

Early morning, urgent, ineffectual with tenesmus.

Early morning diarrhea; watery, painless, bright yellow, but little or no exhaustion followed.

Mrs. S——, aged 27, Denver, catarrh of nose, throat and larynx; cough severe < by lying down; for ten or fifteen minutes after retiring coughs severely, loosens some tough mucus which can neither be raised nor swallowed. Night-sweats if warmly covered. Morning diarrhea: watery, profuse, gushing, at 6:30 A.M.; a slight motion, turning in bed, necessitates getting up in a hurry, with a rush. Rumbling, gurgling in abdomen as if quarts of water were in stomach and bowels. By careful eating can go rest of day without. Going without noon-day meal stool is natural, but it would not affect morning diarrhea. In morning, weak; exhausted. In afternoon, feels fairly well. Excessively nervous during menses. Last three periods have been ten or fifteen days late and more scanty than usual. Under the care of one of our best homeopathic prescribers has had Aloe, Sulphur, Podophyllum, Gamboge and Rumex.

Profuse, watery stool two or three times a day.

Constant urging for stool. Formication.

Loose stool; slight tenesmus.

Constant, ineffectual desire.

Loose, yellow coloured stool, with considerable straining; three stools since 5 P.M., attended with much thirst and borborygmus.

Griping pain with bearing down in lower part of abdomen; some relief after stool.

Stool pale yellow colour.

Sensation of drawing and constricting of sphincter.

Profuse, watery, ill-smelling, like old cheese, at 5 P.M.

Sudden diarrhea before breakfast, with nausea.

Diarrhea, furious fever, burning hot skin, great heat in head, red, flushed face, eyes turned upward, quivering and rolling; peculiar fetid smell of body.—*Burnett.*

|| Cholera infanturn.—*Swan.*

|| Severe hemorrhage from bowels, cough; emaciation; family history of phthisis.

Urinary Organs—

Urine intermits, stops and starts; flows slowly; must strain at stool to pass urine.

Unabla to pass urine no matter how hard he strains or how full the bladder until after spasm of anus; then it flows and stops and flows again for several times.

Diminished quantity of urine.

Is obliged to urinate very often, especially during changes of weather.

One-tenth albumin in height of reaction; disappeared afterwards.

Specific gravity of urine increases from 1016 to 1023, with an excess of urates and ropy mucus.

Peptonuria in man, 33 (Maregliano).

Hematuria with renal pain.

Excess of urates.

Abundant viscid mucous discharge.

Urine frequent, copious; deposits yellow, reddish cloud on standing, loaded with urates.

Urine: odor of boiling beans.

Male Sexual Organs—

Pains in testicles, and cord of left side.

Mr. G. A. T., 28, dry goods salesman, light complexion, mental, motive temperament, active, wirey, well nourished. Father and three uncles died of pulmonary tuberculosis, leaving him the only living male representative of the family; is strictly temperate, uses no coffee, tea, beer, or tobacco. Has suffered for nine years from involuntary emissions, with or without erections, and with and without dreams; weak and exhausted for two days following emissions; has six or eight per month. Has had some of the best men of both schools in the city caring for him, and the last six years under homeopathic treatment, and for three years under one of the ablest members of this association.

Female Sexual Organs—

Severe pains in breast in evening at beginning of menstruation.

Menstruation with pains in lumbo-sacral and ovarian region.

Sticking pain in lower abdomen; pains in lumbo-sacral region < when walking.

Weakness in genital region; painful menstruation.

Blood lumpy, menstruation lasting more days than usual; menstruation antepones eight days.

Burning pains in external genitals; sharp leucorrhea; pains in sacral and ovarian region to hip-joints.

Sensation of heat in genitalia externa, with increased leucorrhea.

Cramps in uterine region with pains in sacral and ovarian region.

Burning pain in ovarian region.

Menstruation returns fourteen days after parturition.

Menses five days early, offensive, scanty, dark flow only two days; ceased one day, returned on the fourth. The function was wholly unnatural in appearance.

Menses usually one or two days late and four days in duration.

Miss Mary K. A., 29, University student, one brother living in poor health. Mother, several aunts and rest of family died before thirty of tuberculosis. In July, when 11 years old, was severely poisoned with ivy, and has annual attacks in summer ever since. Menstruated at 13; early, full, scanty, dark, clotted, exhausting, dribbles for a week; omits in June, July and August every year.Stomach and abdomen bloated < in summeright Perspires easily on single parts. Hands and feet edematous. Nape and occiput heavy; painful. Mental labor; her college work can only be done with great effort. Restless, dreamful sleep, unrefreshing. Feet and hands cold and damp. Summer heat exhausts her. Leucorrhea: acrid, profuse, brownish-yellow, offensive, running down to the heels in large quantities. Not relieved by bathing.

Case of cancer of the breast, so diagnosed by best allopathic authority in Boston; no history of grief or traumatism. The most peculiar symptoms about it were its tubercular—small hard nodules in the gland, a superficial string extending to the axilla. Previously had suffered from severe headaches; since the growths appeared, headaches ceased. The nipple was retracted. On account of tubercular character of growths, the history of former headaches, which were similar to those of Tuberculinum, I gave the patient one dose. In 48 hours burning, lancinating pains began in the growths; had previously suffered from burning pain which was palliated by sedatives. The burning, lancinating pains continuted two or three days, then gradually disappeared. The retraction of nipple was less marked, the tubercles softened, the pains disappeared and general health promptly improved.

Respiratory Organs—Decided effect in laryngeal cases, mostly beneficial.

After ten injections, larynx markedly affected, inflammatory swelling and ulceration.

Central infiltration of mucous membrane of larynx, high red colour, brighter than normal.

Enormous swelling of arytenoids appeared.

Tuberculous outgrowth.

Exfoliation at right vocal cord, appearance extravasated below its posterior part.

Hyperemia of cords intensified and covered with minute ulcerating points.

Cough and expectoration lasting four months, from a wetting (removed, no bacilli found).

Sensation of pressure on chest.

Cough and sputa.

Irritating cough, < in night.

Little cough in night with aching in side and blood-tinged sputa.

Severe cough in evening with pains below mamma on right side.

Inclination to cough.

Severe cough with muco-purulent secretion in morning.

Cough prevents him sleeping in evening.

Cough, secretion of phlegm, especially by walking, with sticking pains in lungs and palpitation.

A sort of whooping-cough.

Dry cough; in night.

Cough with viscid mucus.

After much cough sensation of mucus in pharynx, mucous secretion being easily ejected.

Expectoration diminished.—*Heron.*

Palpitation and pains in back with cough.

Crackling rales at right shoulder, behind.

Copious watery expectoration usually seen during the reaction.— *Wilson.*

With every increase of dose he suffered with asthmatic fits, lasting from three to seven hours.

Extreme rapidity of respirations, without dyspnea, 60 to 90 in the minute; if the patient is spoken to, the rapid breathing ceases at once (as with a dog panting in the sun).—*Heron.*

Is obliged to take deep inspirations; dyspnea.

Difficulty in breathing speedily increased.

Marked feeling of suffocation.

|| Slight tedious hacking cough, which had lasted for months in a girl of a distinctly phthisic habit.—*Burnett.*

|| Hard, dry cough, sometimes slight, but generally no expectoration, slightly feverish.—*Boardman.*

|| Hard, dry cough, shaking patient, more during sleep, but did not waken him.—*Boardman.*

|| Expectoration of non-viscid, very easily detached, thick phlegm from air passages, followed after a day or two by a very clear ring of voice.—*Burnett.*

Chest—

Sensation of pressure in chest.

Heat in chest.

Sticking pain in chest, especially at the apex of left lung.

Sensation of constriction in the precordial region.

Pains in both sides of chest going to back.

Pains in left side.

Sticking in side.

Nightly pains on chest.

Sticking pains: in lungs; in left side, pains between scapulae.

Aching in side in night.

Sticking pain in chest on right and 1, side.

Sticking pain in left side in morning and afternoon.

Sticking pain in lungs when laughing.

Pain in axilla, especially when elevating arm.

Sticking pain: in lungs with cough and palpitation.

Pressure in chest, sticking pain on both sides of chest, in back.

Palpitation caused by deep inspirations, aching in back with pains under ribs.

Pains in subclavicular region with cough.

Sticking pain in left lung.

Pain from clavicles to throat.

Pain in apex pulmonis radiating to axilla and arm.

Sticking pain in chest and in back < from every movement.

Pain in left lung to axilla.

Pain on left side going back.

Pain in left apex and in region of spleen.

Severe pain in back, in axilla and arms.

Pains in left side, must take deep inspiration.

Bronchitic sounds in both lungs.

Dulness right apex.

Sudden, profuse hemoptysis, ends fatally.

Developed a cavity on side opposite to that first affected.

New deposits of tubercles on pleura.

Surface of old pulmonary cavities showed unusually intense redness of granulation layers.

Hemorrhagic infiltration of walls.

Recent hemorrhage observed in the cavities.

In fatal cases of ulcerative phthisis the lungs especially, and also the pleura, showed extensive and severe recent changes— pleurisy, for the most part very severe, simple and tuberculous, frequently hemorrhagic, and not infrequently bilateral.

Caseous pneumonia or caseous hepatization—the lung appearing like blood-pudding studded with pieces of lard (the patient an architect, 33, had six injections, the last four weeks before death. At the beginning he had induration of one apex only. The treatment was suspended because of persistent fever and infiltration of lower lobe).

Catarrhal pneumonia was found, but it differed from ordinary catarrhal pneumonia (in which the alveoli when squeezed out have a gelatinous appearance) in that the contents of the alveoli were very watery and turbid—a turbid infiltration; it resembles a phlegmonous condition.

Soft hepatization, which differs from ordinary catarrhal hepatization, in that in the midst of the patches foci of softening become developed, leading to rapid breaking down and excavation.

Development of fresh tubercles; small tubercles giving rise to new ulcers have suddenly appeared, especially in pleura, pericardium, and peritoneum.

Metastasis bacilli mobilized.

Abscesses in the lungs.

Perforating abscesses in respiratory organs.

Burning sensation in both lungs, better in the open air.

Severe burning sensation in apex of right lung, under second rib.

Dry, hacking cough and expectoration of yellow, bloody, streaked mucus.

Chest sore, first in one place then in another.

Early morning cough, sputa streaked with blood.

Hard, dry cough for several days, resulting in the expectoration of yellow mucus mixed with white lumps or a quantity of white, stringy substance looking like thick milk, with soreness of one or both lungs when coughing or taking a deep inspiration.

Sensation of intense anxiety in the region of the heart, especially worse on waking.

Pulsation synchronous with the heart-beat felt in all parts of the body.

|| Slight hacking cough, continuing all day, < at bedtime and on rising; emaciation; dulness on percussion at apex of right lung.—*Burnett.*

|| Girl, aged 15, tall for her age; tonsils enlarged; chronic discharge from nose, < early morning on rising; speech thick; thorax of pigeon-breast type; perspires much across nose; very bad perspiration of chest, armpits, palms, nose, and feet; feels very chilly; spleen swollen; distinct dulness on percussion at

apex of right lung; suffered badly from vaccination; gets chilblains.—*Burnett.*

| | Hectic flush of cheeks; shortness of breath; slight hacking cough; several strumous scars on neck; dusky skin; large, moist rales in both lungs; increased vocal resonance of right lung; amphoric sounds in right lung; large, soft-feeling gland in left side of neck; very pronounced endocardial bruit, best heard at apex beat. Iodoformum 3x in four grain doses for two months, with improvement, followed by Tuberculinum c. in very infrequent doses.—*Burnett.*

| | Incipient phthisis in a boy aged 7; loss of flesh; great prostration; morbid timidity; glands of groins and on both sides of neck very much enlarged and indurated, particularly glands over apex of right lung; as he had suffered much from vaccination, Thuja 30 and Sabina 30 were first given, then Tuberculinum.—*Burnett.*

| | Nocturnal perspirations; notched incisors; indurated glands everywhere, very large and numerous; drumbellied; grinding of teeth at night; great susceptibility to taking cold; perspiration < at back of lungs and on head; big head, with bulging forehead; subject to attacks of fever and diarrhea.—*Burnett.*

| | Incipient tubercular disease; restless at nights; sleepless; grinds teeth; tendency to diarrhea; want of appetite; foul breath; notched teeth; pain after food; vomiting of food; indurated glands; strawberry tongue; naughty; very irritable temper; puny growth; very thin; girl, aged 6.—*Burnett.*

| | A nasty little cough, for seven weeks; much expectoration; pains in right lung; evening fever; liver and spleen enlarged; cough morning after breakfast; neck slightly goitrous; eats hardly any breakfast.—*Burnett.*

| | Cough, < 6 A.M.; notched incisors; thin and puny; cervical and inguinal glands much enlarged and indurated; strawberry tongue; girl, aged 7.—*Burnett.*

| | No respiratory sounds at top of right lung, and vocal

resonance slightly increased; pain in left side; profuse perspiration; girl, aged 18.—*Burnett.*

|| Much fever, < evenings; restless and terribly irritable; much depressed and in almost constant agitation; tongue very red; chronic diarrhea; has lost fourteen pounds during last six weeks; has no appetite; evacuations discharged from bowels as from a pop-gun.—*Burnett.*

|| Bad cough of about twelve months' duration; expectoration of blood; one of apices was audibly diseased; has had pneumonia; chest flat; respiration accelerated; tanned unduly in sun.—*Burnett.*

|| Anemic, sickly, pale; profound debility; dyspnea, cannot mount or hurry; menses irregularight—*Burnett.*

|| Lady, aged 26, in first stage of consumption; dyspnea and rapid breathing; loss of flesh; greasy, dingy skin.—*Burnett.*

|| Stout man, bright, florid complexion, mother died of phthisis, with which disease her sister is suffering; gets pneumonia very often in cold weather; hence travels from place to place to avoid colds; coughs much, brings up much phlegm; perspired profusely and drank great quantities of fluids; wretched sleepless nights, with almost constant fever; glands of neck much enlarged.—*Burnett.*

|| Complains that she has been in consumption for many years; is very thin and consumed with fever; lungs very flat; respiration almost imperceptible; fever; poor appetite; languid.—*Burnett.*

|| Ringworm on scalp; lymphatic glands everywhere palpable; ribs very flat; strawberry tongue, bad cough, < at night; although 11 years old she had practically no teeth, they were rudimentary, and not above level of gums.—*Burnett.*

|| Pronounced phthisical habit; severe piles; constipation; brown cutaneous affection on abdomen.—*Burnett.*

In September, 1905, I was called to see a little Irish girl, named Mary Gilbert, ten years of age, who was suffering with what I thought was an attack of pneumonia, temperature 104, a dry cough with severe pain in chest. I treated her with the usual remedies, Belladonna, Bryonia, etc., with only an apparent amelioration of symptoms. But the child lost flesh and seemed to develop an empyema. About the third week there was a profuse discharge of foul smelling pus-like matter, greenish in colour, from mouth.

The family had been named by the 'household angel' that the child would die—three successive raps on the door at midnight had given the warning. They administered holy water and asked for a consulting physician. Dr. Pugh, who had attended the mother a year previously, in pneumonia, of which she died, was called, made a careful examination and left the following note:

"I think you are completely right. She has I think some empyema on right side (not much), but she has pulmonary tuberculosis of both lungs. I doubt that the hospital would do any good."—(Sgd.) Dr. Chas. E. Pugh.

I had thought of sending her to the hospital as she had the poorest of care at home; but the doctor said it was of no use, nothing could save heright I quite agreed with him, but bethought myself of Tuberculinum. Here was a chance to try it, surely it could do her no harm. She was given a number of doses of the 200, and later higher potencies till I reached the cm., and with continual improvement. The cough diminished, the hectic spots left her cheeks after a number of weeks, but before the real spring came she was a plump and rosy child. All this, too, in a cold, bad winter and with the most unsanitary surroundings.

The child had previously had what I thought at the time were tubercular abscesses, from enlarged cervical glands at the base of the neck.

The family openly said her recovery was a miracle due to prayers to St. Anne, and it was a miracle, only the saint was Tuberculinum. I heard from little Mary this week and she is well, and I mean cured, restored to robust health, not in the least a puny child.

I always hesitate to use the remedy first hand, but have a number of times used it after other remedies failed, and with success, especially where there was a tubercular tendency.—*Scholes*.

Heart—

Palpitation early in morning.

Sensation of heaviness and pressure over heart.

Palpitation with cough and sticking pain in lungs.

By deep inspirations severe palpitation.

Aching in heart.

Palpitation in night < when raising himself up.

Palpitation with pain in the back.

Death from paralysis of heart.—*Libhertz*.

Neck and Back—

Glands in neck and scars swollen and very tender, various lupus points about them showing yellow fluid under epidermis.

Scars in neck softer and flatter; no lupus nodules now perceptible.

Glands cannot now be felt, except the largest, which is now reduced to size of a pea.

Cervical glands much smaller.

Aching like needle-pricks in the back.

Prickly feeling in skin of back.

Weakness in lumbo-sacral region.

Sticking pain over both scapulae; pain in region of spleen; vague pains in back and on chest, with sensation of pressure.

Sticking in back.

Pain in back with palpitation.

(Sensation on his back as if the clothing were moist. —Bac.)

Three red patches on left side of back became much deeper.

Violent reaction, during which pains in loins < by pressure; (case of Addison's disease; two injections given.—*Pick*.

Tuberculosis of sacrum greatly improved.—*Kurz.*

Large boil on back of neck, intensely painful, discharge of green pus and did not heal for two months.

Beating, throbbing pain under inferior angle of right scapula.

Severe pain in left trapezius muscle, from nape of neck to occiput.

When waking after first sleep at 3 A.M. neck and back stiff and painful, wears off during the day.

Unable to turn the head to the left, and when turning to the right, the left side is painful.

Wakened at midnight with twitching at angle of left scapula; passed to right scapula and down the right arm like a convulsive tremor shaking the arm.

|| Indurated cervical glands.

Lump, size of a walnut on cord of neck, is movable and occasionally itches.—*Rose.*

Upper Limbs—

Aching in forearms; vague, stitching pain.

Diminution of inflammation above elbow-joint; disappearance of abscess over olecranon; sinus connected with radius discharging freely a thick yellow pus.

Sensation of luxation with severe pains in right carpal joint; < by effort to move it; ceasing by rest.

Trembling of hands.

Hands and arms so weak am unable to write; must support right wrist with left hand in raising a cup or glass to my mouth; and passing dishes at table.

Unable to dress myself from weakness of the arms.

Lower Limbs—

During night pain referred to right knee; right leg rotated in and flexed slighted at hip and knee; movement of right hip-joint free; 1 P.M., left hip. much more painful and tender, more flexed, abducted and rotated out (disease of left hip in girl of five).

Aching in the hip-joints.

Pain right knee without swelling (Heron, a non-tubercular case).

The knee became easily movable and could be bent to a right angle (tuberculous affection of right knee).

Swelling and tenderness of both knee-joints.—*Heron.*

Sensation of formication in arms and legs.

Great weakness in limbs after dinner.

Sensation of fatigue and faintness in all limbs.

Pains in limbs, fatigue (3 to 4 h. after injection).

Pains in limbs (2nd d.).

Pains in ulnar nerve and calves of legs and knees, left great toe much affected, and became very red and turgid.

Trembling of limbs (in an alcoholic).

Twitching in the limbs.

Dull pain in bones, aggravated from walking and much worse every afternoon and evening.

Left leg painful on walking, must keep weight off it as much as possible; worse sitting than when walking, but pain always worse after exercise.

Severe pain across sacrum, as if parts were massaged with a fist.

Lame feet for three weeks, would walk or stand on sides of feet to rest them.

Cramps in calves.

|| Tubercular swelling of knee; intermittent attacks of pain in it; has expectorated clots of blood and suffered from exhausting sweats; family history of phthisis.—*Burnett.*

|| Tuberculous disease of left knee; for eleven months had been limping; knee much enlarged and very tender; teeth dirty and carious; strawberry tongue.—*Burnett.*

Skin—

Erythematous eruption like measles or scarlatina.

Erythema with subcutaneous indurated nodules.

Great bronze patches on the forehead and temples.

Bronze finger-points.

Finger-points as if touched by *Argentum nitricum.*

Itching all over the body in the evening in bed; changing place after rubbing.

"Rash on chest and abdomen similar, patient says, to what came out when disease first appeared."

Rash on abdomen and back, commencing very red; speedily becoming brownish, resembling ordinary skin eruption of secondary syphilis.

Edematous condition of upper lip.

Edematous condition of eyelids.

Nose swollen, tense, erysipelatous-looking epidermis in lupus patch raised by yellow fluid.

In two cases, at least during the febrile action, old chilblains became again inflamed.

Slight attack of jaundice (several cases).

Site of injection slightly painful and red (2nd d.).

Erythematous blush confined to lupus parts, which were the seat of throbbing pain.

It has repeatedly caused general erythematous eruptions on the skin, and in some, nodular effusions into the cellular tissue.

Boil on right hand near base of little finger; whole hand intensely swollen. Boil opened in about a week, discharging large quantities of green pus.

Eczema: itching, burning, smarting; in patches two or three inches in diameter on lower legs from knees to ankle. < by heat, touch > by cold water; patches elevated, oozing, watery fluid which forms dry scabs; red, so sensitive cannot be rubbed or scratched; < by thinking of it.

Eruption eczematous; itching radiating from patch to patch; burning, stinging, creeping; red, hot, swollen, with nerve shocks all over body; severe stinging sensation over whole body where there is no irritation; > by cold bath or ice bags.

The itching irritation runs over the limbs and through the body, terminating in involuntary shudders that creep over the body continuously; at times limbs burn and throb; there are intervals of a few hours, sometimes a day or two, when hostilities cease only to be renewed with increased vigor without intervals.

At night about 10 o'clock or later, after drinking cold water, there is an acid sensation in stomach like heartburn; limbs are swollen from knees down; look as if the skin had dried; severe reflex irritation over whole body; cannot bear the least heat, this sensitiveness to heat seems to be increasing. Since the skin symptoms became so intensely irritating the normal secretions of the vagina have been greatly lessened.

A fine, red, scaly eruption in patches about an inch in diameter over the entire body, itching intensely when skin was exposed to the air. Rubbing or stratching gave relief, but was followed by soreness.

A rash-like eruption on neck, both sides, for several days.

A fine, red eruption on right wrist extending up the arm in spots, with great itching.

|| Very bad tempered; very much pigmented where sun's rays impinged upon him; teeth dirty, greenish.—*Burnett*.

Eruption of itching blotches all over body, with exception of face and hands.

| Ringworm.

Sleep—

Great desire for sleep; drowsiness during day; after dinner.

Inclination to sleep in mornings.

Shivering when beginning to sleep.

Cold feet in bed.

Troubled sleep; sleeplessness.

Sleep disturbed from 3 A.M.

Sleeplessness on account of constant coughing.

Many dreams: disturbed sleep, interrupted by fearful dreams; gloomy dreams; dreams of shame; cries out in dreams.

Intense restlessness, worse from 3 A.M. until morning.

Great restlessness every night, with distressing frightful dreams, worse towards morning.

Sleepy in the day-time; can sleep all day, but it is unrefreshing.

Waken from 3 to 4 A.M. with terrible dreams; of snakes crawling upon my sister from the back; of dark-green snakes three and four feet long, two inches in circumference, they seem like the snakes in my own country, Colombia.

Awake weeping with fear.

Restless and wakeful after 3 A.M.

Awake with sensation of fear that some evil is impending to my family.

Disturbed distressful sleep.—*Burnett.*

Fever—

Shivering, when beginning to sleep; cold feet in bed.

Freezing and heat alternately; cold and heat for months.

|| Fever.

Violent attack of ague, lasting almost an hour.

Freezing on the back in evening.

Freezing during whole day.

Sensation of heat in evening in bed.

Flush of heat from back to head.

Feverish, nausea, thirsty, with headache, no vomiting (Heron).

Flushes of heat after eating.

High temperature, abating in twelve hours.

Lowering of temperature after each injection (Heron).

Lowering of temperature after a rise (Heron).

Temperature seven hours after injection, 103.80 accompanied by thirst, rigor, increased cough, headache, and pains in joints (Heron).

Sweat in the night.

Much sweat, especially on head in night.

Profuse sweat after light exertion.

A little walk and slight efforts produce sweats.

Short sweats in morning, while walking.

Profuse sweats during slight exertion.

Chilly all day, most severe up and down the spine, followed in afternoon and evening by fever; pulse 104, temperature 102, with thirst and intense restlessness.

Great coldness of hands and feet with general chilliness; compelled to retire in haste.

Wanted much covering with hot applications to feet; hands are cold to waist, as if plunged into ice water; cold sweat on palms of hands.

Fever all afternoon and evening; temperature, 99 4-10; pulse, 86.

Nerves—

Suddenly became unconscious while sewing or talking, began screaming, tearing her hair, beating her head with her fists, or trying to dash it against the wall or floor; attacks daily for a month, then spasms set in, with rolling of head from side to side and moaning; continuing five weeks, followed by a recurrence of fainting fits, at least twice a week; a few hours before an attack of fainting, a shuddering like a chill seemed to go from brain down spine; when questioned about an attack, she said head would suddenly seem to swell over eyes and pain became 'horrid ' and she knew no more; between attacks she was free from all complaints except fatigue and an ever-present frontal headache.—*Swan*.

Generalities—

Feeling of fatigue.

Malaise, depression, headache, somnolence, oppression of breathing, tightness of chest, nausea.

General fatigue in morning; sensation of faintness; great weakness in lower extremities, especially from knees down to feet.

Terribly tired, so that she can scarcely walk.

General excessive fatigue after a short walk, so that he must lean on his companion.

Emaciation (lost six pounds in fourteen days, twenty pounds in five weeks).

In parts affected throbbing pain.

Leucocytosis; diminution of oxyhemoglobin.

Oxyhemoglobin first diminished then increased (Henoque).

Feeling well, but decidedly losing flesh.

Acts principally by very acute irritation of internal organs affected (in the same way as in external organs), causing intense redness and great swelling.

Actual inflammatory processes (not mere hyperemias), and especially active proliferations, occur to an intense degree, in (1) edges of existing ulcers; in (2) neighbouring lymphatic glands, especially bronchial and mesenteric.

Lymphatic glands present a quite unusual degree of enlargement, and notably that form of medullary swelling, characteristic of acute irritations, which is caused by rapid proliferation of the cells in the interior of the glands.

Leucocytosis: various infiltrations of white blood corpuscles over affected parts, especially around the tubercles themselves.

Enormous dangerous swellings in parts near ulcers (even where the surface of the ulcer becomes clean), causing dangerous constriction.

Phlegmonous swelling resembling erysipelatous edema of glottis and retropharyngeal abscess.

Where tubercle is associated with any other specific disease, reaction is so slight as to be scarcely discernible (Heron).

Syphilitic cases are refractory to reaction (Heron).

Children bear the treatment well (Wendt).

Tuberculinum, a typical case: Howard L., 28 years of

age, a resident of Attleboro, Mass., was indisposed in the fall of 1898, troubled with hoarseness and gastric ailments. A neighbouring physician was called who had attended the young man's family for many years. This physician commenced in September, 1898, to inject Tuberculin (Koch's), and up to December had injected his toxin twice a week for several weeks, and then once in two weeks the remainder of the time.

The result ? At the time of the commencement of this treatment Mr. L., could work and eat comfortably; soon his stomach rebelled against food and the bowels became constipated, his hoarseness increased and distressing, suffocative spells set in every forenoon, lasting an hour or so; he would then be able to breathe well the rest of the day.

In January, 1899, I was summoned hastily in the night and found him laboring for breath, the noise of his breathing audible from the street. His first words were: "My God, help me; relieve me, Doctor, or I shall die." Expectoration was scanty, dark green, lumpy, tubercular matteright Examination of the throat revealed a larynx full of tubercular nodes. I saw that his end was near, and told his parents with whom he lived I would rather they would call their family physician. But as they insisted on my keeping the case, I prepared some medicine which relieved him, but the next morning he was again worse, and from that time on was in agony from efforts to get breath. To relieve him intubation (through the mouth) was resorted to, but he could not keep the tube in. He died that afternoon, his great agony being > only by resort to chloroform applied locally. This man had been wild in his youth, had had gonorrhea several times, and of diathesis tubercularight I asked him if he had told his former physician these things and he said he had. This case is typical as far as the use of Tuberculin by injection is concerned, of a score I could mention who have died under the hypodermic use of Tuberculin in this vicinity the past two years.

USTILAGO

Mind—

Depression of spirits in afternoon.

|| Very sad, cries frequently; exceedingly prostrated from sexual abuse and loss of semen; sleep restless.

Could not bear to see or talk to any one.

Irritability, being asked a question or to repeat anything.

The day seemed like a dream.

Melancholia; depression of spirits; oppression and faintness in a warm room. An aversion to or < from warmth in general.

Partial or completeloss of control over the functions of vision and deglutition.

Great irritability, mental weakness and depression.

Head—

Vertigo in attacks, sometimes with double vision, sometimes white specks blot out everything else, later attacks of vertigo with internal heat.

Vertigo at climaxis with too frequent and profuse menstruation.

Headache: all the morning; at 7 A.M.; in evening, < forehead; < walking.

| Nervous headache from menstrual irregularities in nervous women.

Frontal pain: in morning; in forenoon, with smarting in eyes; all day, with aching distress in eyeballs and with fulness of head in morning; with distress in epigastrium.

Scalp dry, head congested, with loss of hair.

Scale-head, watery serum, oozing from scalp.

Prickling in left temple.

Loss of hair.

Bursting congestive sensation to the head; and various parts of the body.

Upward surging of blood with bursting in the head.

Vertigo from such causes, especially at climacteric.

Feeling of fulness with dull pressive headache < by walking.

The headache and vertigo appear to be reflex from ovarian or uterine condition.

Frontal headache, < by walking.

Violent frontal headache as if forehead would burst open.

Sharp flying pains in forehead, congestion of the brain.

Pain on top and side of head; climaxis.

Falling of the hair and nails; complete alopecia, not a hair on the head.

Headache in temples.

Eyes—

Attacks of twitching in eyes, they appear to look (revolve) in circles and dart from one object to another.

Continual watery flow from eyes and nose with occasional chills.

Spasms, with vanishing of vision and head seems to whirl.

Aching in eyes and lachrymation.

Aching and smarting in eyeballs, with profuse secretion of tears.

Hot feeling on closing lids.

Weakness of eyes.

Lachrymation in open air.

Lids agglutinated in morning.

Vision of spots dancing to and fro.

Things whirl before the eyes, appear double; white specks come into view and blot all else.

Dull aching pain in right eyeball.

Ears and Hearing—

Constant dull pain in left ear, caused by extension from inflamed tonsil.

Nose—

Boil in right nostril.

Dryness of nostrils in forenoon, with dry feeling in skin.

Bright epistaxis, > pressure.

Rhinitis, bitter taste, offensive odor noticeable to patient himself.

Dryness of nostrils as if he had taken cold.

Pains at root of nose, extending in toward canthi, and up and out at each eyebrow.

Face—

Sudden pallor in face when sitting, and in evening.

Burning of face and scalp from congestion.

Flushes of heat; the face becomes red and hot.

Teeth—

Sometimes looseness of teeth.

Aching all day in decayed upper first and second molars, which have ached before.

Shedding of teeth (in animals).

Mouth—

Tongue coated in morning.

Prickling in tongue, with feeling as if something were pressing the roots upward, with dryness of nostrils.

Salivation: thin, bitter; profuse.

Taste: coppery; in morning; slimy coppery.

Slimy: slimy, with burning distress in stomach.

Throat—

Tonsils congested, inflamed.

E. tonsil enlarged, congested, dark reddish, right painful on swallowing at 2 P.M.; left painful at 9 P.M.; next morning congestion of left extending along Eustachian tube and causing pain in ear.

Lancinations in right tonsil (fauces were somewhat inflamed when the medicine was taken), next day fauces more hot and sensitive to motion.

Roughness of fauces.

Dryness of fauces, with burning dryness in stomach; difficult deglutition.

Dryness of fauces with difficulty in swallowing, feeling of a lump behind larynx, later frequent efforts to swallow, with feeling as if something had lodged in fauces, afterwards irritation of fauces, and on swallowing feeling of a lump in larynx.

Burning in esophagus at cardiac orifice.

Appetite—

Appetite: craving; poor.

Thirst at night.

Loss of appetite followed by canine hunger.

Stomach—

Eructations: of sour fluid; of sour food.

Cutting in stomach.

Pain in stomach; frequently in afternoon; on full inspiration.

Pain in epigastrium with drawing pain in joints of fingers.

Burning in sternum and cardia.

Distress in stomach in forenoon; in afternoon, < by supper.

Hematemesis: passive, venous, accomuanied by nausea, which is > by vomiting.

Weak, empty, all-gone sensation in the stomach.

Burning in esophagus and stomach; extends to ovaries, heart, face and scalp.

Faint feeling in epigastrium, with pain in region of liver and bowels.

Repeated fine sharp cutting pains in epigastrium.

Constant distress in region of stomach.

Burning distress in sternum and stomach, accompanied by fine neuralgic pains in same region, lasting about three minutes at a time; come on every ten or fifteen minutes for several hours; sharp cutting pain in stomach.

Abdomen—

Periodical cutting in umbilical and hypogastric regions at 6 P.M., < at 8 P.M. by a constipated stool, afterwards grumbling pain in whole abdomen.

(Pain as if intestines were tied in knots.)

Pain: in right lobe of liver; in umbilicus; in umbilicus before natural stool; in left groin when walking.

Drawing pain in right hypochondrium all day.

Distress in umbilicus and right hypochondrium.

Grumbling pains in abdomen all afternoon, followed by dry, hard stool, fine cutting colicky pains every few minutes all day, > by hard constipated stool, followed by dull distress in bowels.

Stool—

Natural stool at 4 A.M.

Loose stool at 4 A.M., with pain and rumbling in abdomen.

Light-coloured diarrhea.

Soft stool, next day dry, lumpy, two days later black, dry, lumpy.

Constipated: black, dry, lumpy stools.

Urinary Organs—

Tenesmus of bladder and incontinence of urine.

Urging, urine light-coloured, increased.

No desire, but uneasiness.

Urine: increased; scanty, red; acid, high-coloured; scanty and dark.

Frequent urination, with pain at meatus as the last drops were passing.

Male Sexual Organs—

| | Spermatorrhea after onanism; emissions every night, talking about women causes an emission; very sad; cries frequently; says he cannot break off habit, has no control of himself when passion is aroused; knows it is fast killing him; cannot work, is so prostrated.

Genitals relaxed.

Erections: when reading at 4 o'clock; frequently during day and night.

Scrotum relaxed and cold sweat on it.

Pain in testes, < right

Pain in testes, sometimes neuralgic; in paroxysms, sometimes causing faintish feeling.

Desire depressed.

Chronic orchitis, irritable testicle.

| Erotic fancies.

Seminal emissions and irresistible tendency to masturbation.

Irresistible tendency to onanism; frequent emissions; is prostrated, dull, with lumbar backache. Despondent; irritable.

Irritable weakness and relaxation of the male sexual organs, with erotic fancies and seminal emissions.

Female Sexual Organs—

Yellow and offensive leucorrhea.

Tenderness of left ovary, with pain and swelling.

Burning distress in ovaries.

| | Intermittent neuralgia of left ovary; enlarged, very tender to touch.

| Uterus: hypertrophied; prolapsed; cervix sensitive, spongy.

Menses: too scanty with ovarian irritation; too profuse

and too early; blood clotted; as if everything would come through.

Between periods constant suffering under left breast at margin of ribs.

Vascular system of ovaries is most powerfully affected, producing congestion, enlargement, and great irritation, with ovaralgia, dysmenorrhea and especially menorrhagia.

|| Oozing of dark blood, highly coagulated, forming occasionally long, black, stringy clots.

|| Extreme pain during period; flow very profuse and did not cease entirely until next period; most of time confined to bed.

Suppression of menses.

|| Vicarious menstruation from lungs and bowels.

| Constant aching distress at mouth of womb.

Menses that had just ceased returned, bright coloured, soreness and bearing down in left side preceding the flow and partially ceasing with it.

Menses copious, bright red, not coagulating easily (in a woman who thought she had passed the climacteric, as there had been no discharge for over a year), it stopped as suddenly as it began, no path, only faintness and confused feeling in head.

| Menorrhagia at climaxis; active and constant flowing with frequent clots.

Bland leucorrhea.

Abortion.

| Deficient labor pains; os soft, pliable, dilatable. Constant flooding.

Puerperal peritonitis.

|| Lochia too profuse, partly fluid, partly clotted; prolonged bearing-down pains; uterus feels drawn into a knot.

| Hypertrophy and subinvolution of uterus with great atony.

Hemorrhage: mixed character, partly liquid, partly coagulated. The flow is passive, slow, protracted. A tonic condition of pelvic organs; deficient labor pains, with dilatable os.

Metrorrhagia, with vertigo during climacteric.

| Menorrhagia, with displaced uterus.

The ligaments of the uterus are relaxed; prolapsus, with bearing down sensation, as if all the pelvic organs would be expelled.

Flabby, relaxed condition of pelvic organs, a tonic condition of uterus; a state of weakness, relaxation and atony.

Flushes of heat, and disturbances of circulation similar to those occuring at the climaxis, or from premature suppression of the menses; ovaries inflamed, irritable, sensitive, and swollen; burning distress in both ovaries.

Sharp pains commence in ovaries and run down the legs. Aching distress referred to the uterus.

| Metrorrhagia after miscarriage, confinement or at the climaxis.

Discharge of blood on the slightest provocation; after digital or mechanical examination; cervix swollen, bleeding easily when touched.

Uterus remains large after miscarriage or confinement; sub-involution delayed.

Hemorrhage bright red, but more frequently dark, clotted and stringy; post-parturn oozing from flabby atonic uterus.

Uterus hypertrophied, heavy, feels soft, spongy or boggy.

Complaints of the lying-in woman; profuse debilitating lochia.

Milk deficient or superabundant; nursing increases the lochial discharge.

Acute pain < in left ovary, with swelling; pains intermittent; shoot rapidly down legs.

Ovaritis, constant pains in ovary, sharp pains passing down legs rapidly; ovary much swollen and tender, with scanty menstruation.

|| Ovaritis; took cold after menstruation; constant dull

pain in right groin and back, three or four times an hour; sharp neuralgic pains in ovary; walking painful; bowels torpid, very languid.

|| Ovarian irritation, constant pain in left ovary passing down hip, has to limp when walking; pains sharp and at times pass down leg with great rapidity; every few clays has quite a swelling in left groin; cannot bear pressure over ovary.

|| Every day from 12 M. to about 4 P.M., constant pain from left ovary to uterus; every few minutes, pain in ovary is intensely severe, cutting like a knife; pain in right ovary and hypo-gastric region, but all starting from left ovary; ovary can be distinctly felt in groin about as large as a hen's egg and very hard; when pressed upon gives intense pain; every day thinks she has fever with paroxysm of pain, but no chill; slight leucorrhea; loss of appetite; constipated.

Displaced uterus with menorrhagia; cervix tumefied; bleeds when touched.

|| Uterus hypertrophied, sensitive, blood bright, fresh, without coagula.

||Subserous or interstitial fibroid of uterus (two cases), fibroid much diminished.

| Cervix tumefied, bleeds when touched.

|| For days oozing of dark blood with small coagula; uterus enlarged, cervix tumefied or dilated.

Chronic uterine hemorrhage, and passive congestion.

| Blood dark, but so thin as to scarcely colour fingers.

|| Profuse menstruation, flow lasting from ten days to two weeks, at first very abundant, gradually wearing off; always < from motion; discharge dark and quite painless.

|| Menses every three weeks, with dark coagulum; profuse, with gushes of bright-red blood when rising from a seat, or after having been startled or frightened; two days before menses, a heavy backache with sharp pain across abdomen from hip to hip, followed by expulsive pains; pains diminish after flow commences and stop with it; between menstrual

periods heavy dragging backache on exertion; pain shooting up back from hips to shoulder; abdomen tender to touch; excessive bearing down; pressure in head; sensation of contraction in vertex, and feeling as if head were lifting off; vertigo; excoriating, albuminous leucorrhea, < before menses; ravenous appetite; excessive tired feeling; pulse 80 and weak; mental depression.

|| Subject to profuse menstruation; childless; large, fleshy, flabby, bloated-looking, with a very sallow complexion, inclined to be (and formerly had been) dropsical from excessive loss of blood; profuse menstruation, which seems to her to be principally water and clots', says there is no outward flow when she lies still, but clots and water pass out of uterus when she gets up; feels so full in uterus that she must rise to get rid of clots; flowed fearfully during night; very low, scarcely able to speak aloud.

|| Severe menorrhagia for past twelve years at every menstrual period, lasting a week or ten days, sometimes longer; pale, thin, weak, very nervous.

|| Profuse discharge of dark, clotted blood of fetid odor, with pain and tenderness in one or both ovaries.

| Dysmenorrhea of a congestive character, with much ova, rian irritation; severe pain in ovaries; uterus and back every few minutes; scanty, pale flow accompanied by false membranes; poor appetite, thickly-coated tongue.

|| Subject to headaches ever since menstruation appeared at age of fifteen; headache mostly on top of head; appetite poor; pain in left chest with some cough; total suppression of menses for last eight months; severe pain in back, is unable to ride in carriage; pain in uterine region, especially over ovarian region, < left side; vomiting of mucus and blood daily; no sleep; some leucorrhea; hysterical; no uterine displacement, but great congestion in pelvic region.

| Suppression of menses without apparent cause; troublesome cough; considerable expectoration; sometimes also dry cough; stitching pains in chest, especially left side; night sweats; loss of appetite; pain in ovaries, especially left;

general debility, headache; leucorrhea; chlorotic; anemic, as if in first stage of consumption.

|| Menses suppressed for last fourteen months; very irritable and depressed; uneasiness in region of stomach; pain in ovarian region, especially left; skin hot and dry; constipation, stools dry and hard; no appetite; stitching pains in chest, < worse in left side; constant hacking cough; considerable expectoration; night sweats; general prostration; great uneasiness in lower extremities.

|| Mild leucorrhea.

| Climaxis: vertigo; frequent flushing; metrorrhagia.

Pregnancy. Parturition. Lactation—

Abortion: bearing-down pains, as if everything would come from her; in flabby constitutions; from general atony of uterus: with or without hemorrhage.

|| Has aborted a number of times at third month; is now about three months pregnant; for last ten days has had more or less hemorrhage every day, some days quite bad; not so much at night; blood passes a number of times through day, in dark-coloured clots.

| Post-partum hemorrhages from a flabby, atonic condition of uterus.

| Constant flooding; every few minutes, expulsion of a large clot of bright red blood, with bearing-down pains.

Persistent hemorrhage of brownish blood, with want of uterine contraction.

|| One and a half hours after delivery commenced to flow violently.

| Passive hemorrhage after miscarriage, blood in lumps, flooding for days and weeks.

|| Severe flooding two weeks after labor; large bright-red clots; no pain; very weak.

Very profuse lochial discharge, very dark in colour, almost black.

|| Agalactia; chronic inflammation, and induration of mamma.

Galactorrhea.

| | Promotes expulsion of foreign bodies from the uterus.

| Puerperal peritonitis, with constant flooding; high fever; secretion putrid; abdomen excessively tender and tympanitic.

| | Puerperal peritonitis; aborted about two days since, at about three months: constant fever; pulse 120; cannot bear least pressure on any portion of bowels; about six times today has had sharp, cutting pains in left ovary; has flowed constantly for two days; blood dark, not copious, nor attended with bearing-down pains; cannot move in bed; is compelled to lie upon her back; constant, dull, frontal headache; loss of appetite, tongue furred.

| | For last year vertigo every day, some days so bad she has to go to bed; menses every three weeks for last year; last about ten days and profuse; flows as much again as she did when in health; constant aching distress under left mamma; rheumatic pains in shoulders and back; very weak, not able to work.

| Fibroids and induration of os.

| | Discharge of blood from uterus, bright-red, partly fluid, partly clotted; passive congestion of uterus, so that there is a slight oozing of blood after each examination; tissues of uterus feel soft and spongy; os patulous.

Gave Mrs. —— Ustilago 1m., four doses, for aching distress and extreme soreness of os -uteri. After twenty-four hours she was cured, but had the following symptoms, never before felt by her: Headache in temples. Pains at root of nose, extending in toward canthi, and up and out at each eyebrow. Pain in back of neck. Great pains in bones all over body, and especially in calves, which are somewhat cramped. Pain in both shoulders, especially in raising arms. Stiffness in shoulder-joints on bringing down the arms on waking—the arms are extended over head when sleeping. Thirst for cold drinks. Felt chilly externally, but not internally. Frequent urination, with pain at meatus as the last drops were passing.

Chest—

Spasmodic tearing at top of left side and passing to sixth or seventh rib, at 3 P.M. when standing or reading, < breathing.

Pain in left infraclavicular region in morning.

Drawing pain in left inframammary region, waking me at 3 A.M., > turning on back from right side.

Aching, burning distress in sternum and under it in stomach, with neuralgic pains.

Oppression along median line.

Constriction with pain.

Heat and pressure.

Heart—

Sudden flying pain from heart to stomach, arresting breathing.

Burning pain in cardiac region.

Respiratory Organs—

Feeling as if there were a lump behind larynx, which produces constant inclination to swallow.

Back—

Pain in back extending to extreme end of spine.

Severe rheumatic pain in lumbar region, < by walking; aching distress in small of back.

Pain in back of neck.

Pain in region of right kidney, < sitting still; next day in region of left kidney, > moving about, with heat, fulness, soreness on deep pressure (but it relieved the pain), with uneasiness in left thigh, frequent desire to urinate, stream very small, the following day it requires considerable effort of will to empty the bladder, which is done slowly, pain and soreness in left loin continue; heavy in lumbar region, in bed with uneasiness about bladder (had had no desire to urinate on going to bed), woke early in morning With distended feeling in bladder, micturition slow and difficult, urine scarcely coloured, pain in back < next night, < lying on face, > lying on right side.

Bearing down in sacral region as in dysrnenorrhea, changing to left ovarian region and gradually extending through hip.

Upper Limbs—

Pain in both shoulders, especially in raising arms.

Pain in shoulder joints; rheumatic, in muscles of right shoulder, all night.

Intermittent, numb tingling sensation in right arm and hand every day.

Stiffness in shoulder-joints on bringing down the arms on waking—arms extended over head when sleeping.

Pain in right elbow, < by motion.

Stitching along metacarpal bone of right index.

Rheumatic drawing pain in finger-joints, < second joint of right index, all afternoon.

Hypertrophy or loss of nails.

Rheumatic pains in arms, hands and fingers.

Dull rheumatic pains in right elbow joint on motion.

Severe drawing pains in joints of all fingers.

Fine, sticking pains along metacarpal bone of right forefinger, every few seconds.

Sharp, cutting pains along metacarpal bones of right hand.

Lower Limbs—

Pain in left knee when walking, increasing to cramp, obliging me to lean upon the arm of a friend; the pain, with occasional cramps, lasted all the evening, < raising foot so as to press upon toes.

Cramp-like stiffness in left leg, < raising foot so as to press upon toes.

Feet swollen in morning.

Cutting in bones of right hand and foot.

Frequent rheumatic symptoms in arms, fingers and legs.

Rheumatic pains in legs.

Flying rheumatic pains in metatarsal bones of right foot.

Great pains in bones all over body, and especially in calves which are somewhat cramped.

Skin—

The scalp became one filthy mass of inflammation, two-thirds of the hair came out, the rest matted together, with oozing of watery semen from scalp, eruption like rubeola on neck and chest, gradually extending to feet, thickest on chest and joints, itching < night, rubbing any part brought out the eruption, on face and neck it was in patches like ringworm, but not vesicular.

Tendency to small boils.

Boils on nape.

Congested feeling in skin.

Skin dry and hot; congested.

Painful, destructive disease of nails.

Paresthesia of the skin; pricking, burning, itching, a marked erythema of the skin of the uncovered parts of the body, followed by a parchment-like, dark brown skin with rhagades < by warmth.

Roullin observed loss of hair and sometimes the teeth occurred both in animals and men; that mules fed on it often cast their hoofs, and that fowls laid eggs without shells; it has caused loss of hair on animals, and cured complete alopecia.

Pustular ulceration of the skin, scald-head and various forms of eczema.

Copper-coloured spots on skin; secondary syphilis; macula.

Negro, urticaria of six years' standing, troubled more or less all the time; every night itching, scratching parts produces large pale welts on body, arms and legs.

Sleep—

Difficult falling asleep and then unpleasant dreams.

Restless night; with fever; with troubled dreams.

Sexual dreams; without emission; and disgusting, waking him, arose and urinated with difficulty and tenesmus.

Fever—

Chills running up and down back.

Heat at night, during sleep.

Internal heat; with vertigo; < eyes, which are inflamed and sensitive to light, eyeball sore to touch; intermittent; pulse normal.

Burning in face and scalp.

Skin dry; at night; and hot.

Relapsing agues; very profuse sweat; slight nausea; oppression of chest; cerebral disturbance, and great irritability.

Thirst for cold drinks.

Chilly externally, but not internally.

Generalities—

Neuralgic pains in forehead, hands and feet.

Rheumatic pains all up and down left side, with cutting in left knee and calf if I pressed any weight upon toes or flexed knee with any weight upon it.

Rheumatic pains in muscles of arms, hands, fingers, and small of back, those in back < walking.

Symptoms of a cold.

Malaise as if I had taken cold; felt sick with a cold, continual watery flow from nose and eyes, with occasional chills.

Languor: during the day, with headache, < noon, and with burning frontal headache at 9 P.M.; in morning on rising; at 2 P.M.

Faint feeling at 11 A.M. in a warm lecture-room.

Faint spells beginning in epigastrium, with small pains in hypochondrium and bowels.

COMPARE:

SECALE	USTILAGO
Burning; in all parts of the body, as if sparks of fire were falling on patient.	Burning; in esophagus, stomach, overies, heart, face, scalp; less on the skin.
< warmth, covering affected parts; < from heat, all diseases.	Faintnessand oppression in a warm room; < from warmth less marked.
Adapted to thin, scrawny, feeble, cachectic women; irritable, neverous, pale, sunken countenance.	Adapted to weak, relaxed, atonic patients; irritable, despondent, weak mentally.
Hemorrhage; copious, thin, black, watery, decomposed, bloody; hemorrhagic diathesis; the slightest wound may bleed for weeks; defibrinated.	Hemorrhage; passige, oozing, dark, clotted, bloody, forming long, black, string clots; partly dark, partly clotted and stringy, or thin and watery.

RELATIONS.—Compare: Mel., Med., Mez., Psor., Vine, m., in crusta lactea and other scalp affections of childhood; Bry., Ham., Mill., Phos., in vicarious menstruation; Agar., Mur., Sep., in bearing down and uterine collapse; Helon., Lys., Natr. h., Sec., delayed subinvolution; Malan., Sec., affections of the hair and nails; Act., Caul., Thuj., Sul., Vib. o., in left ovarian pain; Bov., Elaps, Graph., Ham., in intermittent flow; Sang., Urt. ur., pain and rheumatic affections of right shoulder; Sang., left inframammary pain extending to scapula; Lac c., Kali bi., Puls., erratic rheumatic pains; Sul., faint all-gone sensation at 11 A.M.; Cob., backache and seminal emissions; Bov., flow midway between the periods; Canth., Pyright, Sec., in expelling foreign bodies from the uterus.

VARIOLINUM

Dr. Fellger gave Variolinum reports, giving Variolinum to hundreds of people, and none of them were ever attacked with small-pox. In one family where the father had confluent small-pox, he gave Variolinum as a prophylactic, and of the others, although not one had been vaccinated, not one of them took the disease.

He reports case of a broker in Philadelphia who was well pitted from small-pox; when a child he was vaccinated, and he became idiotic in consequence. When sixteen years old he had a violent attack of small-pox, after which he recovered his reason.

Variolinum is indicated in small-pox where there is not much pain; the patient can even eat fairly well; the skin looks natural between the pustules; the appearance of the eyeball is white and natural; the mild uncomplicated cases of small-pox are the ones calling for Variolinum.

Mind—

Delirium with initial fever.

Fear of death; wild excitement and begging to know if he was to die, and before the sentence was complete drops into a heavy sleep with loud breathing.

Head—

Vertigo.

Syncope in attempting to rise.

Forehead very hot, face red and bloated, carotids pulsating violently.

Headache: with or after a chill; all over head; particularly in forehead; severe in vertex; as if a band tightly encircled head; severe lancinating, throbbing; < with every pulsation.

Intolerable pain in occiput.

Crazy feeling through brain, hard to describe.

Eyes—

Keratitis, with small-pox and after vaccination.

|| Chronic ophthalmia with loss of sight.

|| Pupils contracted.

Ears—

Deafness.

Face—

Skin of face and neck deep dark-purple hue.

Jaw falling when asleep, with trembling when aroused.

I once made a beautiful cure of a most intractable case of acne with Variolinum, which I was led to prescribe because the man's face was so disfigured by cicatricial marks so as to resemble one who had been afflicted with small-pox.— *W. J. Guernsey.*

Teeth—

Teeth covered with thick brown slime.

Mouth—

|| Thick, dirty yellow coating on tongue.

|| When asleep tongue protruded, black coating, when raised it is with difficulty drawn back; looks like a mass of putrid flesh.

| Tongue coated white, as with a piece of white velvet, in variola with headache, backache and high fever.

Throat—

Throat very sore, redness of fauces.

|| Pharynx and fauces deep purplish crimson, with gangrenous appearance; breath horribly offensive.

Painful deglutition.

Sensation as if throat were closed.

Sensation as of a lump in right side of throat.

Diphtheria with horrible fetor oris.

Appetite—

Food, especially water, tastes sickish sweet.

Stomach—

Soreness in pit of stomach and across epigastric region.

Severe pain in precordial region, frequent nausea and vomiting of bilious and bloody matter.

|| Frequent bilious vomiting.

As soon as he drinks milk he vomits it up.

Stool—

Thin, bloody stools.

Several brown, green, at last grass-green stools, painless, loose, of intolerable fetid odor; no thirst; last stool slimy, with small quantity of blood.

|| Dysentery.

Constipation.

Urinary Organs—

Urine: high-coloured, like brandy; turbid, and offensive; stains a rose tea-colour, difficult to remove.

Male Sexual Organs—

Enlargement of testicle.

Hard swelling of left testicle in consequence of a contusion.

Respiratory Organs—Oppressed respiration.

|| Asthma.

Troublesome cough, with serous and sometimes bloody sputa.

Hawking up thick, viscid slime, smelling bad.

Neck and Back—

Stiffness of neck, with tense drawing in muscles, < on motion.

Pain in base of brain and neck.

Chills like streams of ice-water running down from between scapulae to sacral region.

Intolerable aching in lumbar and sacral region.

Pain in muscles of back like rheumatism; < on motion.

Upper Limbs–

Hands icy cold during invasion.

Swelling of arm which had been half-paralyzed.

Lower Limbs–

Muscular rheumatism; < on motion.

Petechial eruptions, erythematous, on lower abdominal region, apex of triangular form being at pubis, and the base crossing the abdomen transversely, in neighbourhood of umbilicus; also on lateral surface of trunk to axilla, invading folds of axilla, corresponding portion of arm and pectoralis major.

|| Terrible pains in back on right side of spine, and over and below shoulder blade; muscles sore to touch, nausea, pains all over especially in legs; tongue clean; pulse 120; Variolin. cm.; body completely covered with large pustules, face one mass of confluent pustules, pulse still high, constant expectoration of viscid mucus, mouth and fauces lined with pustules, even tongue covered with them; bowels constipated, mild delirium at times; eight days later temperature 104½; pulse 120, very weak and stopping at intervals; great fear of death; begging to know if he must die, and before sentence was completed would drop into a heavy sleep with stertorous breathing, jaw dropped on breast, pupils contracted, teeth covered with thick brown slime, centre of tongue perfectly black, mucous membrane of mouth and pharynx of a deep purplish-crimson, with gangrenous appearance and breath horribly offensive; skin of face and neck of a deep dark purple; odor from body like a fetid stream; little control over tongue or jaw, latter hanging down, and tongue protruding like a mass of decayed liver when asleep; an effort to speak when roused

up caused violent trembling of jaw and tongue, which was drawn back into mouth with difficulty, was stiff, but looked like a mass of putrid flesh; urine dark coloured, passing freely through whole attack; had continued the cm. till now, gave one dose cmm. dry on tongue; next day almost convalescent; made a good recovery with but few marks.

|| Severe chill followed by high fever; severe pain, in back as if broken; pain all over head, very severe and constant in occiput; frequent bilious vomiting; thick, dirty, yellowish coating on tongue; wild delirium and spasms; night before eruption appeared obstinate constipation; on third day very thick eruption of small-pox pustules, soon assuming confluent form, Variolin. cmm.

|| Small-pox; peculiar smell causes intense sickness of stomach; congestion toward head, palpitation of heart; two hours after took a dose Variolin. 30; an hour later crawling in back and feeling of coldness in lower extremities; cold feet; lame, heavy feeling in left arm; no appetite; sleep disturbed by heat; toward morning some perspiration over body; next day continuous pressing headache, especially in occiput; pulse somewhat irritated; disinclined to mental work; when reading heat in head and forehead; weak when walking; pain in joints of upper and lower extremities, as if lame; toward evening again feverish; pressing pain in small of back down to sacrum (Glonoin. 3 relieved headache); in bed, drawing in upper jaw and teeth; sleep full of dreams; toward morning again perspiration; urine smells ammoniacal; on fourth day red pimples on back of left hand, staying for several days without filling with pus; mental work still causes heat in forehead and pressure in head; escaped smallpox.

|| On third day of eruption, when pustules had filled, and were confluent on face, intense itching; Variolinum 1m. in water, every two hours; on second day itching nearly gone, pustules shrinking; third day drying; fifth day crusts fell from face; seventh day other crusts fell off, and tongue clean.

Have used and seen it used in many and severe cases,

and when treated with Variolin. 200 disease is shortened nearly or quite one-half, sufferings of patients much mitigated, secondary fever either absent or very much lighter, pustules do not burst, but wither or wilt and- fall off, suppurative stage immeasurably hastened and shortened, and patients are not marked.

Mrs. —— and Miss —— took Variolinum m. (Fincke), one dose, Nov. 22 and another dose Nov. 23. On the 24 a vesicle appeared on left side of neck, which became sore and itched severely where top was broken. It was red and angry, with a sharply defined areola about an inch in diameter; from the inflamed base were light-yellow, ray-like scales, like psoriasis. It ran its course in about two weeks. Several similar spots appeared on different parts of the body, with intense itching at times, but without systemic symptoms. On both, the eruption was similar in character and ran the course. Both had been vaccinated years before, but neither had any eruption of any kind.

Skin—

Exanthema of sharp, pointed pimples, usually small; seldom large and suppurating, dry, resting on small red areola, frequently interspersed with spots of red colour, sometimes severe itching.

Petechial eruptions.

Varight 30 warded off an attack of small-pox after intense sickness of stomach had been caused by the smell of a case.

Var 1m in water every two hours, given on third day of eruption of a confluent case, cut short the attack.

Shingles.

Fever—

Very severe chill, followed by hot fever.

Intense fever, commencing with chills running down back like streams of cold water, causing shivering and chattering of teeth.

Fever with intense radiating heat, burning hot to touch.

Hot fever, no thirst.

Very profuse, bad-smelling sweat.

VACCININUM

Mind—

Crying.

Ill-humor, with restless sleep.

Nervous depression, impatient, irritable; disposition to be troubled by things.

Morbid fear of taking small-pox.

Confusion, she does not remember things at the time she wants them.

Head—

Frontal headache.

Forehead felt as if it would split in two in median line from root of nose to top of head.

Stitches in right temple.

Eruption like crusta lactea.

Aching and heat in whole head, especially forehead.

Stinging in both temples.

Aching in forehead the whole forenoon.

In middle of night, waked up by pain in forehead and eyes like split, and stinging in both temples.

Severe headache all over head.

Prickling in left temple, as if going to sleep.

Eyes—

Tinea tarsi and conjunctivitis in a woman, aet. 28, remaining as result of variola in infancy, conjunctiva painfully sensitive.

Weak eyes; falling out in forehead as if it were split.

Inflamed eyelids.

Redness of eyes and face, with small pimples on face and hands.

Keratitis after vaccination.

Pain in forehead and eyes as if split.

Gausy sensation before eyes in morning, cannot see well.

Puffed red face and red eyes, with small pimples on face and hands.

Soreness in inner corner of left eye.

Peculiar dull sensation at left lower lid.

Nose—

Full feeling of head, with running of nose.

Bleeding at nose preceded by a feeling of contraction above and between eye-brows, soon after eating meat; menses rather profuse and too frequent; cured by revaccination.

Neck—

Swelling of the neck under right ear (parotid gland), with sensation like being cut.

Coolness at throat, anteriorly down the breastbone, in and outwardly.

Face—

Redness and distension of face, chill running down back, till afternoon.

Puffed red face and red eyes, with small pimples on face and hands.

Mouth—

Tongue coated, dryish yellow, with papilla showing through coat.

Dry mouth and tongue.

Appetite—

Appetite gone, disgust to taste, smell, and appearance of food.

Coffee tastes sour.

Good appetite.

Stomach—

Aching in pit of stomach, with short breath.

Bellyache.

Abdomen—

A stitch in hepatic region, at margin of last lower rib, axillary line.

Stitch in splenic region.

Blown up with flatulence.

Urinary Organs—

Nephritis with albuminuria, hematuria, and dropsy, developed eleven days after vaccination; child recovered.

Respiratory Organs—Short breath with aching in pit of stomach, and pressure in region of heart.

Whooping-cough.

Chest—Stitch in left side of chest, anteriorly, under short ribs.

Stitches in right side under short ribs in front from right to l., then at corresponding place in left side, but from left to right, lasting five minutes, felt in liver and spleen.

Drawing down left side of chest and back.

Heart—

Febrile action of heart and arteries.

Aching at heart.

Back—

Backache.

Aching pain in back, < in lumbar region, extending around waist.

Twisting pains in lower back.

Weakness in small of back coming on suddenly > by lying down.

Upper Limbs—

Severe pains in left upper arm at vaccination mark, could not raise it in the morning.

Rheumatic pains in wrists and hands.

Sensation of heat passing from dorsum of hand, as of steam.

Cheloids on re-vaccination marks.

Left upper arm feels stiff, somewhat tremulous.

Redness on left upper arm.

Slight tearing from left wrist into forepart of radius anteriorly.

Prickling in left fourth finger, as if going to sleep; also in left middle finger.

Aching of left fourth finger.

Drawing at left elbow up arm.

Left hand feels hot.

Left fourth finger burns; a warmth streams through left arm.

Lower Limbs—

Tearing in left thigh downward.

Soreness of lower extremities, as if heated or over-exerted.

Legs ached immoderately, hardly able to get about, a break-bone sensation, and a feeling as if bones were undergoing process of comminution.

Twisting pains in both knees.

Skin—

Skin hot and dry.

A general eruption similar to cow-pox.

Small pimples develop at point of vaccination with fourth dilution.

Red pimples or blotches in various parts, most evident when warm.

Eruption of pustules with a dark-red base and a roundish or oblong elevation, filled with pus of a greenish-yellow colour, at left side of trunk, between shoulders, on left shoulder, behind right ear, resembling varioloid, some as large as a pea, some less, without depression in the centre, coming with a round, hard feel in the skin (like a shot), very itchy.

Tingling burning in skin over whole body, most intense in skin of forehead and in lower and anterior portion of hairy scalp, which parts are tinged with a scarlet blush, or efflorescence, similar to the immediate precursor of variolous eruption.

Vaccininum 6, in water, for one day with strict diet, repeated for eight days, acted as preventive in six hundred cases.

Treated a great many cases of variola and varioloid during last eighteen years, some of them of the most desperate character, and yet never lost a case when employing vaccine virus as a remedy; moreover, none of the cases so treated were ever troubled with hemorrhage, or with delirium, or secondary fevers, or were ever disfigured with pitting.

Vaccininum 200th quickly > severer symptoms of variola occurring in a child, aet. six months; two days before appearance of eruption had been re-vaccinated (after an interval of eight days) on a navus near right nipple; deglutition difficult through implication of tongue and fauces; pustules, many of large size, scattered over scalp, face, body, and limbs.

Eruption of small, red vesicles on left upper arm and chest, dying off after a few days.

Pustule filled with matter, with a depression in centre and red halo on left shoulder.

Pustules suddenly much depressed.

Eruption all over body of small pustules, some with a central depression, some brown.

Sleep—

Waked in middle of night by pain in forehead and eyes as if split, and stinging in temples.

Restless sleep.

Fever—

Fever, with heat, thirst, tossing about, crying, aversion to food.

Chill with shaking. The following night she could hardly get warm.

After lying down profuse perspiration broke out, after which chill, redness, and pimples disappeared.

Generalities—

Restlessness.

General malaise.

Languor, lassitude.

Tired all over, with stretching, gaping feeling; unnatural fatigue.

Child wants to be carried.

Many persons faint when being vaccinated.

Weakness.

PROVINGS OF THE X-RAY

If Constantine Hering had never given the homeopathic profession anything but his admirable pathogenesis of Lachesis he would have been remembered in gratitude for all time by the homeopathic world.

If Bernhardt Fincke had never given the homeopathic profession anything but his proving of the X-ray, his name, too, would be held in grateful remembrance by posterity, for its possibilities in the cure of many of the most obstinate of chronic diseases appear almost limitless.

We are indebted to Dr. John B. Campbell, one of the original provers, for the discovery of the great value of this dynamic agent in rousing the reactive vitality of the system, both mentally and physically, and thus bringing to the surface suppressed symptoms of persons laboring under a combination of dyscrasia, the miasms of Hahnemann. This is especially true of the deep-seated constitutional ailments, sycotic in character, which so often terminate in malignant disease, especially cancer.

When the sycotic or syphilitic virus is grafted on a psoric or tubercular diathesis; when from the paucity of presenting symptoms it is almost impossible to be certain of the predominant diathesis, in consequence of which the best selected an-tipsoric, Calcarea, Medorrhinum, Psorinum, Sepia, Sulphur, Syphilinum, or Tuberculinum, fails to relieve or to rouse the overpowered vitality to a sufficient degree to throw off or bring to the surface the predominant toxine, the X-ray bids fair to be our curative remedy.

Every physician who has had even a limited experience

in the treatment of the toxic effect of the X-rays on either a bone or soft tissue will not need any proof of its deep-seated character and the extreme difficulty under any form of treatment of arousing the overpowered vitality and effecting a cure. An Xray burn, so-called, whether of the bone or skin, is almost impossible to heal, and despite the best efforts of the ablest practitioner, the best treatment known to medical science of the present day, is often fatal.

Here is a field of action in which the potentized dynamic remedy bids fair to be unrivaled, for there is no known homeopathic gent, either crude or potentized, that in its primary action is so deep-seated or long-acting in results. Neither is there any known agent that will more surely suppress and render incurable many chronic diseases as this, or none which better illustrares what Shakespeare said so long ago, that, "Fools rush in where angels fear to tread," or where

"A little learning is a dangerous thing,
Drink deep or touch not the Pyerion spring."

There is no therapeutic agent that so often cures, and so often fails where we think it ought to cure, in its empirical use, as this. If when its empirical use has roused latent vitality and restored suppressed symptoms we could correctly observe and interpret them, and for them find the similimum, what possibilities lie in the future?

As maintained by Hahnemann, Hering and Fincke and demonstrated by the work of the Austrian Provers' Union, the dynamic potentized drug is the chief factor in both proving and healing. Like Magnetis Polus Australis and other imponderabilia, electricity and the X-ray are both capable of potentization, and the potentized dynamic remedy is just as superior to the crude drug as Aurum, Lycopodium, Silicea or Sulphur.

A very able description of the discovery of the X-ray by Professor Roentgen was given in the *Homeopathic Physician* (March, 1896), by Dr. Walter M. James, and concluded with the words:

"Why should not the homeopathist seek to procure a proving of the effects of the X-ray upon the animal economy of the human being? An inviting field is there opened up to the experimenters of our school. May it soon be cultivated !"

March 27, 1897. A drachm vial filled with absolute alcohol was exposed to a Crook's tube in operation for half an hour, and then brought up to the sixth centesimal potency. With this smallest globules were moistened and the vials containing them presented to the members of the Brooklyn Hahnemannian Union, which met the same evening in regular session.

Of course everyone was curious of trying the new remedy and took a small number of globules on the tongue at once, and lo! it began to reveal its existence immediately, and during the two hours of our being together a number of symptoms were observed, which were at once announced and taken down by our diligent Secretary. Some of the members from that time have been seriously affected, that they would not for any consideration try any more of that mysterious power.

The following is a narrative of its action upon the several provers, being perfectly healthy up to that time, which lasted from the beginning to two months. The action reveals not only new symptoms, but also hunted up many old ones.

If it is assumed that glass is opaque to the X-ray, it was not so in our case, for the alcohol in the vial was certainly affected by it, as the result of the provings show. If the X-ray penetrates certain tissues of the body in order to make the condition of the opaque organs, such as the bones and foreign bodies contained in the body, visible, it also shows its penetration into that invisible interior of the human being, which is under the dominion of the life-force.

Dr. Alice B. Campbell, one of the provers, said:

"Dr. Fincke presented each of us with a bottle of the X-rays, and said: ' It is a sample, you can take a dose.' Each of us took a dose. I thought it was such a low potency that it would not have any effect, and that was the reason I took it. We did not know what it was going to do. I took just the one dose."

I was in the best of health and spirits when I began to use the X-ray; was a healthy girl, never had a doctor until pregnancy.

Nov. 24, 1906. A lady, aged 56, hereditary cancer in her family; mother died of it at 52. For an injury of right breast, which resulted in a tumor, which would probably develop into cancer, the X-ray was used for months, reduced its size and entirely relieved the pain. Some time after a stiffening of neck on left side appeared, to which little attention was paid. Suddenly one morning it went to right side, with intense pain, from which I have never been free for a moment since. Pain severe every night, and occurs in paroxysms during the day. Sudden 'cricks' attack first one side, then the other < on getting cold, and turning the head nearly produces convulsions. The pain is more severe behind the ears, the mastoid process. A sickening grating is heard between the bones of the cervical spine on turning the head. Skin behind the ears red and sore to touch.

The grating is heard and felt in nearly all the joints, especially the shoulders; toe pains are steady, but at times will appear in sharp 'cricks,' then in streaks down the course of the nerves < by moving head or neck; moving the head on pillow at night is agony. Sometimes the pain is relieved on keeping perfectly quiet, again gentle motion relieves.

Have read all the stiff neck symptoms in Lippe, Hering, Raue, T. F. Alien and other works; the indicated remedy has failed to give me slightest relief.

Dec. 1, 1906. Last three days left side of head and neck pain intensely and constantly, at times paroxysms of cramping pain in cord, from left shoulder to head, and sharp shooting pain in head, back and above left earight Cords feel too short. Only relief I have is in walking the floor. Skin is so sore, cannot bear the slightest touch, though hard pressure relieves for an instant. I am nearly mad with pain. (Dr. G—— has said frequently in the last month that he was afraid that I was getting too much X-ray; I though not, although I thought it very queer he could not relieve my pain.)

Jan. 9, 1907. Have taken no X-ray treatment since Nov. 23. Have not been out of the house for six weeks. Suffered torture for four weeks at every motion of head, neck or shoulders. The neuralgic pains were torturing, and the best selected remedies had little or no effect. Spigelia partially relieved severity of pains, but they appeared on the right side of head and neck, yet never left the left side for an instant. Atropin relieved the right sided pain for 24 hours, but neck and shoulder are still lame. I now have no severe pain, if I lie still on left side of face and body, but am unable to lift head from pillow without taking my hands, and then only by a slow circular motion.

I can sit up or stand for 15 or 30 minutes, and then clutching, shooting, aching pains begin behind left ear, and in muscles of left side of neck, and I must lie down on left side, and in a few minutes am free from pain. The stinging, contracting of the muscles relieved, but the pain in back of head is still persistent. Massage, at times, has given slight relief, at other times the slightest touch is so painful that it cannot be borne. Heat relieves the pains at times, but Arsenic does not.

Jan. 14. Improving some; yesterday could lie with a much higher pillow, first time in six weeks. Should be able to bear the pains could the darting, aching, clutching pain in the bone behind the left ear, which makes its appearance every time I sit up over twenty minutes, be relieved. The stinging, contracting pain is better, and notwithstanding all the suffering from the last few weeks, I do not look as if I had been ill; colour good and gaining weight.

The tumor in breast is softening some, and decreasing in size.

The X-ray treatment was always the very lightest possible, and never once coloured the skin red, although tanning it very brown. . Took it at first but once a week; the effect being so good, applied it every third or fourth day. The first pain I had was a slight stiffness of neck on left side. In March it was only felt on turning in bed at night; increased slightly and gradually until Nov. 1st; though I had one severe paroxysm of pain in right side of neck in May, relieved by hot applications, which still give some relief at times. Sitting in the hot sun shining on my neck gives some relief. Have suffered intensely of late from flushes of heat, similar to those I had during climacteric; better afternoons and evenings. The back of head at times seems perfectly well—next moment cannot bear slightest touch or lift my head from the pillow without great pain on both sides in muscles of neck.

1. *Dr. B. L. B. B.,* after one dose of X-ray 6 cent.

A magnetic thrill in right hand extending up forearm, immediately.

No particular symptoms the next day.

Next morning awaked earlier than usual by dull aching in the left side of occiput, and immediately in left sacro-iliac region, then on posterior aspect of left thigh and calf, a dull ache. These pains extend from above downward, not severe, lasting fifteen minutes.

In afternoon suddenly a sharp ache in left side of occiput on a small area. This occurred two or three times at intervals of some hours without regularity.

After that in the course of two or three days a trouble which he had once before, a catarrhal condition of inflammation of rectum with discharge of mucus, slightly bloody, after action of bowels.

Corns on soles of feet more sensitive than formerly, consisting of thickening of cuticle, and sometimes a little pin-head depression which does not scale off.

2. *Dr. Miss Alice B. C.,* after one dose X-ray 6 cent.

A feeling on the external orbital margin as if it might be an ache, immediately.

Buzzing in right ear with pressure extending to temples.

Bearing down of eyelids.

Woke with headache next morning, continuing at intervals during whole day.

A pressing across forehead, with a miserable feeling generally as though going to be sick.

Sleepy with headache.

Bloody mucus from nose.

No appetite for anything, only sweet pudding or cake most tolerable.

Aversion to meat.

Heaviness and fullness in lower abdomen after eating small quantity.

Uneasy feeling in lower abdomen at intervals like fomentation, as though diarrhea would follow.

Most distress after midday and evening meal.

Abdomen distended with full feeling.

(Pulsatilla, which a year ago helped for months a train of symptoms, had only very slight effect.)

Drawing gnawing in the region of appendix as though inflammation were beginning.

Sensation in right lower abdomen as though bubbles were forming and wanting to burst (relieved by Taraxacum for twenty-four hours).

Flatulence with ineffectual desire for stool.

Seven days after taking the medicine was roused out of bed at 4 A.M. with desire for stool, and complete evacuation of immense quantity followed by nausea and vomiting, profuse sweat.

Colicky pain in right lower abdomen, sometimes extending behind hip, and retained urine.

Tenestnus vesicae continuing for twelve hours to 4 P.M., when the urine came freer.

Vomiting ceased though colic-pains remained for twelve days.

Moving aggravated pains especially on right side of abdomen, which seemed to adhere to the walls, feeling as if being torn off. Had to keep a large towel-pad between abdomen and thigh to support abdomen and prevent the excruciating pain.

Ate nothing for three days.

Thirst for cold drinks, though nothing tastes good.

Tongue thickly coated.

Breath foul.

Only snatches of sleep during these twelve days, always followed by terrible mental depression, did not want to answer questions, did not want to see anybody nor speak to anybody, misanthropy.

Chills as soon as beginning to sleep running up back, preventing sleep.

Dreams of distressing nature. Recurrence of a dream that used to trouble her many years ago. This dream was repeated at wide intervals over twenty years ago. Now it came every night for five times.

Seven days from beginning of the attack had a return of renal colic with vomiting, continuous nausea, cold sweat and retention of urine on left side. A clutching pain from kidney to bladder that never relaxed for four hours, causing the wildest demonstration of agony, ghastly face, blue rings around sunken eyes, violent trembling, frightful restlessness, cold sweat, urine retained in ureter, giving a perfect picture of Tabacum which also relieved the symptoms. As soon as the pains in the ureter relaxed, the urine seemed to fill up the bladder and then passed without pain. Some spasm remained and was relieved by Cantharis in five minutes. (He had something like this before, about a year ago, by all means not so severe, a mere strangury.)

Varicose veins inside of knees and legs, with swelling and soreness (after years returned).

The palms of the hands, which were rough and scaly and bleeding at times, became entirely smooth during proving. Healing action. After that the hands went back to former condition while general health improved.

Prostration for a long time.

During the continued action of the X-ray she suffered so much that for some time she had to take medicine to counteract it. All these symptoms have been thrown out.

3. *Dr. John B. C.*, March 28th, 1897, took X-ray 6 cent., three doses in globules ten minutes apart.

Five minutes after second dose.

Sensation of fullness of head with slight full feeling in both ears, worse in right ear.

Feeling in head and nose as if coryza were about to commence, with some slight desire to sneeze.

Sense of pressive fullness starting from posterior prominence of vertex in a straight line to bridge of nose, followed by fullness in entire vertex extending to bridge of nose.

Tingling in both arms as of an electric current, or as if asleep.

Intermittent, slightly burning rheumatic-like pain in right carpo-metacarpal articulation extending from index-finger up outside of forearm.

Aggravation of fulness over vertex worse along centre to nose, worse stooping.

Dull pain in right sciatic nerve, worse on walking.

Wandering pains in chest, sticking in character, worse on right side.

Sticking pains in different parts of head and face.

Rheumatic pains in different parts of head and face.

Rheumatic pains in front of right thigh.

March 29th. Bad taste in forenoon.

Disagreeable fulness of head all morning, with bland coryza and stoppage of nostrils.

General tired and sick feeling.

Symptoms gradually increasing in severity after noon.

Headache gradually extending to frontal region, worse in centre of forehead.

Sense of pressure in centre of forehead.

Dull headache in morning, worse stooping and after rising.

Symptoms all intermittent in character, they have all returned.

Sensation of sulphur-vapor in nose, with much sneezing.

Aching pain across top of head, coronal suture, on blowing nose and after it.

Pain in dorsal region.

Sulphur-vapor sensation in throat and nose.

Intermittent noise as of deep steam whistle in left ear, and ringing in head.

Mental processes not clear; writes wrong words in letters.

Stitching pain in right upper chest, going through to upper part of scapula.

Rheumatic pain in left wrist and forearm.

Lame and stiff in back.

Aching whole length of spine.

Chilly while undressing in warm room.

March 30. Constant ache in vertex, worse on waking, also worse coughing, sneezing, motion or head low.

Rheumatic twinge in last two phalangeal articulations of index and middle finger for a short time in forenoon.

Appetite diminished.

Nose stopped, worse on left side.

Throat painful on swallowing.

Sense of painful lump about left tonsil, worse swallowing.

Very vivid lewd dreams repeated night after night.

Dreams of strife, busy dreams.

Sleep not unrefreshing, though apparently dreaming all night.

Remark of the Prover. This medicine resurrects old troubles that have been long dormant, and remedies that formerly helped have little, if any, effect against the renewed difficulty, In five provers old symptoms were brought to light. In some cases the symptoms had been absent one year, some six, twelve or even thirty years.

May 24. No appetite for breakfast (an old symptom absent for years).

Re-appearance of an old slight pimply eruption on left side of forehead.

Persistent exhaustion and languor; this last was marked and not attributable to spring.

Return of a slight eruption on outside of lower legs, burning when scratched, worse after scratching (absent for months).

Observation of the Prover. It seems this medicine might be used in three ways: 1 To develop old troubles or those which might become latent from any cause including suppression. 2. To develop acute symptoms already present as against its own pathogenetic phenomena. 3. As an antipsoric somewhat like Sulphur.

4. *Dr. Miss C.,* March 27, 9 P.M., one dose X-ray 6 cent.

An indescribable sensation in esophagus, immediately.

Pain in right side of head above temple.

Palpitation during evening, causing cough.

Pulsations greatly diffused and violent, provoking an exclamation which was repressed, accompanied with a desire to walk in open air, and entirely relieved by lying down.

Before going to sleep, dull pain in upper jaw on right side.

Scraping pain in lateral incisor, aggravated by noises and jarring of cars.

March 28. After waking at daybreak next morning sensation in dorsal region of spine, as if its convexity were anterior and drawn far forward, lasting but a minute, and followed by a very uncomfortable feeling in that region, lasting a much longer time.

In morning after rising and before eating, a cough caused by an irritation in larynx, accompanied by a pain in right side just above crest of ilium; eating relieved cough, but side felt bruised when bending, or jarring, or pressing it.

Red, smooth eruption on right side of face.

Sore pain in cartilage of left ear, felt when pressing it, later in right ear.

March 29. Pain darting upward in region of left ovary, when sitting, walking or standing.

March 3left After eating at noon, a sensation of a long and narrow foreign body lodged in pharynx, unmoved by swallowing, aggravated by swallowing. After this passed away, pharynx felt hollow and sore on deglutition.

Sharp pain at apex of heart, better by lying on left side.

Had always heat and swelling of feet in spring which is betternow. Healing action.

5. *Dr. St. C.*, after one dose X-ray 6 cent. Threatening headache, pressure through temples, immediately.

Aching of extensor muscle of forearm, going up to shoulderight

6. *Mrs. E. C.*, after one dose of X-ray 6 cent.

Drawing, aching discomfort in right thigh through hip and knee down through toes, immediately.

Sciatic pain in right hip.

Palpitation of heart.

In less than a week began to cough, with tearing sensation in bronchi, hoarseness, palpitation.

Chilliness on moving or from draft.

Eyeballs sore.

Lame and sore all over.

Wave-like sensation as if would break out in perspiration.

Stools green though normal in consistency.

Teeth-covered with a gray-green deposit.

Menses dark green one day.

Second day of menses violent sick headache, pulsating pressure outward in forehead as if bursting, vomiting, pain relieved by hot water application.

Phlegm of greenish hue causing cough in crawling up.

7. *Dr. L. M. L.*, after one dose of X-ray 6 cent.

Drawing in and heaviness across brow approaching nose and resting there.

Ears more clear from ringing and from dullness of hearing than for many years. Healing action.

Rheumatic pains in right wrist and arm.

Headache across brow and a different pain in temples.

Eyelids feel sleepy and heavy.

Tingling like pins and needles in left hand.

Improvement of hearing continues.

8. *Dr. F. H. L.,* after one dose of X-ray 6 cent.

Tingling in right hand, immediately.

Pain across brow over bridge of nose.

9. *Dr. Miss R.* After one dose X-ray 7 cent.

Lower part of both legs asleep, tingling feeling as if from electric battery increased in right, immediately.

A feeling as if some one were drawing icy hands over the thigh downward aggravatingly slow. (Return of an old symptom twelve years ago after a nervous shock which did not return for five years.)

Three years ago proved Uranium nitrate. Up to that time had never missed a regular menstruation, but it has been irregular ever since. Had not menstruated for six months till after taking X-ray, when it was almost prostrating.

Three or four days previously felt from waist down as if bursting and wanting to hold herself up, with distention and weight in abdomen, relieved by flow, violent, profuse, without pain. Flow lasting seven days.

Mental condition upset, felt as if she would like to kill somebody.

Heavy pressure on vertex as from a hand (old symptom absent a year).

10. *Mr. Davis S.* took one dose X-ray 6 cent. 1897, March 28. Next day mental irritability.

Trembling all over.

Body tired and exhausted.

Pain on right side of head passing around base of brain to left ear, followed by paralytic numbness.

Nervous.

Powerlessness of limbs.

Slightly sick of stomach.

A sensation of hyperesthesia or nervous concentration in bridge of nose.

Sore feeling across loins as after a heavy cold.

Fullness in ears, worse in right ear, worse by inserting finger.

Pressing outward in ears.

Sensation as of a cool drop of sweat going down left side of spine.

Sense of contraction across middle chest.

Chills going down back, followed by paralytic feeling in right cheek.

Muscles feel soft subjectively.

Tongue felt dry, rough, sore, scraped.

Soreness in small of back.

Sleepy and unable to sleep for some hours after retiring.

On rising in morning expectoration of considerable mucus.

Generally worse in open air.

Nasal discharge thin.

Mentally irritable.

Headache and soreness worse toward afternoon.

Mental and physical aggravation markedly pronounced toward evening.

Bitter taste.

Pain in left temple, worse at 8 P.M.

Contraction of chest at night, relieved by belching.

Slight electric current sensation in left side of tongue and face, passing over and disappearing on right side of face at 8.25 P.M.

Much expectoration of tough lumps as large as fingers ends, whitish like gelatine, raised easily.

At first had desire for sweets.

The sleeplessness, which was getting constant and troublesome, seemed to be relieved permanently by a bottle of Pabst Malt Extract.

May 1st. Drowsy at night when sitting up.

Drowsiness leaves the instant he lies down, so he cannot sleep.

Reappearance of many symptoms which occurred during an attack of inflammatory rheumatism, twenty-five years ago.

Painful bulging of left chest over the cardiac region.

Sensation in right eye as though bulging.

Right eye sore to touch.

On closing eye in dark sees old women's and old men's ugly faces.

A paralytic sensation extending from spine down left leg.

Twitching internally in various parts of body.

All symptoms worse towards evening and at night.

On inside of left knee sensation in different spots, painful as if hairs were being pulled out, worse on walking, better on rubbing and scratching.

Sexual desire lost.

Raising of jelly-like mucus, worse in forenoon, tenacious and tough.

Grayish expectoration.

While lying on left side, heart-sounds keep him awake.

Goes to sleep on right but wakes on left side.

Symptoms better after Bell, or Acon, for a short time, better from ale, which puts him to sleep.

Sleepy during day.

Waking frequently at night from no apparent cause.

Spells of feverishness, perspiration and weakness.

On straining at stool, a sore sensation in nates.

Rheumatic-like fever in trunk, pain steady and dull going steadily from trunk to legs and finally to heels, worse left knee, worse stepping on heel, on underside.

Head feels empty as though scraped out, worse at night in bed.

Can't hold things in left hand, being powerless or clumsy.

All symptoms worse in bed.

Third day after taking.

Slight nose-bleed on left side at 4:30 P.M.

Sensation of swooning at times during day and night, feeling like dying.

Rheumatic pains in limbs (an old symptom of rheumatism resurrected even to an old soreness in heels).

Soreness worse in legs and arms and around heart, dull and constant.

No hunger, goes till he feels faint, can eat plenty but does not enjoy it.

Frequent urination, worse after getting into bed.

Testes relaxed, impotent feeling.

Pressure in small of back as from congestion about kidneys.

Sharp stabbing pain in left temple, which staggered him, followed by clearing up of mental functions—the heart immediately felt this impulse.

Left chest bulged out (like enlargement of heart in old rheumatism twenty-five years ago).

A sensation in left side as if fingers pressed the cartilages in, followed by sensation as though something broke inside, with temporary relief.

Sensation of drops of water trickling down on inside of chest.

Wind around heart, flatus and flatulence as though diarrhea would commence.

Unnatural lewd or disgusting dreams, occurring on several nights, or several times in one night.

Mind and Disposition—

Mental irritability.

Clearing up of mental function after sharp stabbing pain in left temple staggering him, the heart feeling the impulse immediately.

Mental depression after snatches of sleep for twelve days.

Mental processes not clear, writes wrong words in letters.

Mental condition upset during profuse menstruation, would like to kill somebody.

Misanthropy during renal colic, did not want to answer questions, did not want to see anybody or to talk to anybody, being completely prostrated.

Head—

A feeling at right external orbital margin as if it might be an ache, immediately (the first symptom observed).

A pressing across forehead with a miserable feeling generally as though going to be sick.

Awoke with headache next morning, continuing at intervals through whole day.

Sleepy with headache.

Headache gradually extending to frontal region, worse in centre of forehead.

Sense of pressure in centre of forehead.

Dull headache in morning, worse when stooping and after rising.

Headache and soreness, worse toward afternoon.

Head feels empty as though scraped, worse at night in bed.

Sensation of fullness of head with slight full feeling in ears, worse in right ear.

Pain in right side of head above temple.

Threatening headache, pressure through temples.

Headache across brow, and a different pain in temples.

Pain in right side of head, passing around base of brain to right ear, followed by paralytic numbness.

Pain in left temple, worse 8 P.M.

Sharp stabbing in left temple, followed by clearing up mental function, the heart immediately feeling the impulse.

Feeling in head and nose as if coryza would set in, with slight desire to sneeze.

Sense of pressive fulness starting from posterior prominence of vertex in a central straight line to bridge of nose, followed by fulness in entire vertex extending to bridge of nose.

Aggravation of fullness over vertex, worse along the centre to nose and when stooping over.

Disagreeable fulness of head all morning, with bland coryza and stoppage of nostrils.

Aching on top of head across along coronal suture on blowing nose and after it.

Constant ache in vertex, worse on awaking, also on coughing, sneezing, or head low.

Drawing in and across the brow approaching nose and resting there, immediately.

Pain across brow over bridge of nose.

Heavy pressure on vertex as from a hand (old symptom, absent a year).

'Sticking pains in different parts of head and face.

Sickening grating between the bones of the cervical spine on turning the head.

Pains steady, but at times appear in sharp 'cricks,' then in streaks down the course of the nerves < by turning the head or neck; moving the head on pillow at night is agony; > keeping-perfectly quiet; again by gentle motion.

Pain in left side of head and neck, intensely and constantly, at times paroxysms of cramping pain in cord, from left shoulder to head, back and above left ear. Cords feel too short.

Cannot bear slightest touch, though hard pressure relieves for an instant; > by walking the floor.

Pain > by lying on left side of face and body.

Unable to lift head from pillow without taking hands, and then by a slow circular motion.

Pain in back of head > at times by massage slightly, also by heat.

Back of head at times seems perfectly well, next moment cannot bear slightest touch or lift my head from the pillow without great pain on both sides and in muscles of neck.

Morning awaking earlier than usual with dull aching in left occiput, and immediately in left sacro-iliac region, lasting fifteen minutes.

Suddenly sharp ache in left occiput on small area, recurring two or three times at intervals of some hours, without regularity.

Violent sick-headache second day of menses, pulsating pressure outward in forehead as if bursting, vomiting, pain relieved by hot water applications.

Neuralgic pains.

Neck—

Stiffness on left side of neck, turning in bed.

Stiffness on right side of neck, with intense pain at night; occurs in paroxysms during the day > somewhat by hot applications.

Sudden 'cricks' attack first one side of neck, then the other, < on getting cold; turning the head nearly produces convulsions. Pains more severe behind the ears—the mastoid process.

Aching pains in left side of neck.

Clutching, shooting, aching pains begin behind left ear and in muscles of left side of neck on sitting up over twenty minutes; > by lying on left side.

Pain on both sides and in muscles of neck when lifting head from pillow.

Pain relieved on keeping perfectly quiet; sometimes by gentle motion.

Stinging contracting pain.

Eyes—

Bearing down of eyelids.

Eyeballs sore.

Sensation in right eye as if bulging.

Right eye sore to touch.

Congestion of eyes in forenoon, worse on rising.

On closing eyes in dark sees old men's and women's ugly faces.

Eyelids heavy and sleepy.

Ears—

Sore pain in cartilage of left ear when pressing it, later in right ear.

Pressing outward in ears.

Buzzing in right ear with pressure extending to temples.

Fullness in ears, worse in right ear, worse by inserting finger.

Fullness in ears, more right, and fullness in head.

Intermittent noise as of deep steam-whistle in left ear, and ringing in head.

Ears more clear from ringing and dullness of hearing than for many years, an improvement lasting up to this day. Healing action.

Nose—

Bloody mucus from the nose.

Sensation of sulphur-vapor in nose with much sneezing.

Sulphur-vapor sensation in throat and nose.

Congested sensation in head and nose as before coryza.

Nose stopped on left side.

On blowing nose and after it aching across top of head along coronal suture.

Sensation of hyperesthesia or nervous concentration in bridge of nose.

Nasal discharge thin.

Flowing coryza with stoppage of nostrils and fullness in head, forenoon.

Face—

Dull pain in right upper jaw.

Paralytic feeling in right cheek, preceded by chills going down back.

Slight electric current sensation in left side of tongue and face, passing over and disappearing in right side of face.

Red, smooth eruption on right side of face.

Stinging pains in different parts of head and face.

Mouth—

Tongue dry, rough, sore and scraped.

Scraping pain in lateral incisor, aggravated by noises and jarring of cars.

Teeth covered with a gray-green deposit.

Tongue slightly coated.

Throat—

Sulphur-vapor sensation in nose and throat.

Throat painful on swallowing.

Sense of painful lump about left tonsil, worse swallowing.

Indescribable sensation in esophagus, immediately.

Foul breath.

After eating at noon, sensation of a long and narrow foreign body lodged in pharynx, removed by swallowing, aggravated by swallowing. After this passed away, pharynx felt hollow and sore on deglutition.

Appetite—

No appetite for anything except sweet pudding or cake.

Aversion to meat.

Ate nothing for three days.

No appetite for breakfast (old symptom absent for two years).

Appetite diminished.

Desire for sweets.

Most distress after midday and evening meal.

No hunger, goes till he feels faint.

Can eat plenty but does not enjoy it.

More thirst than usual.

Thirst for cold drinks, though nothing tastes good.

Bad taste in forenoon.

Bitter taste.

Nausea, Vomiting—

Nausea and vomiting with profuse sweat after immense stool at 4 A.M., seven days after taking.

Slightly sick at stomach.

Vomiting ceased, though colic pain remained in lower abdomen for twelve days.

Abdomen—

Abdomen distended with full feeling. (Pulsatilla, which a year ago helped for months a train of symptoms, had only very slight effect.)

Flatulence with ineffectual desire for stool.

Heaviness and fullness in lower abdomen after eating small quantity.

Uneasy feeling in lower abdomen at intervals like fomentation, as though diarrhea would follow.

Wind around heart, flatus and flatulence as though diarrhea would commence.

Drawing gnawing in region of appendix, as though inflammation were beginning.

Sensation in right lower abdomen, as though bubbles were forming and wanting to burst (relieved by Taraxacum for twenty-four hours).

Flatulence with ineffectual desire for stool.

Colicky pains in right lower abdomen, sometimes extending behind the hip, and retained urine.

Moving aggravates the colic pains, especially on right of abdomen, which seemed adhered to walls, feeling as if torn off. Had to keep a large towel pad between abdomen and thigh to support abdomen and prevent the excruciating pain.

Pain in right side just above crest of ilinm, with an irritation in larynx causing cough in morning after rising, and before eating; eating relieved cough, but the side felt bruised when bending, or jarring, or pressing it.

Stool–

Catarrhal inflammation of rectum, with discharge of mucus slightly bloody after action of bowels, in course of two or three days (a trouble he had once before).

Seven days after taking medicine roused out of bed at 4 A.M. with desire for stool and complete evacuation of immense quantity, followed by nausea and vomiting, profuse sweat, pain in right lower abdomen, retained urine, vesical tenesmus continuing for twelve hours, till 4 P.M., after which urine became freer, vomiting ceased; colic pains remained for twelve days.

Stools green, though normal in consistency.

On straining at stool a sore sensation in nates.

Ineffectual urging to stool, with flatulence.

Urine–

Retained urine, vesical tenesmus after enormous evacuation, vomiting for twelve hours to 4 P.M.

Seven days from beginning of attack return of renal colic with vomiting, continuous nausea and retention of urine on left side. A clutching pain from left kidney to bladder that never relaxed for two hours, causing the wildest demonstration of agony, ghastly face, blue rings around sunken eyes, cold sweat with trembling, frightful restlessness, urine retained in ureter (giving a perfect picture of Tabacum which relieved at once). As soon as the pain in ureter relaxed after it, urine was filling up the bladder and then passed without pain. Some spasm remained and was relieved by Cantharis in five minutes. (She had something of a like trouble a year ago, but not so severe as this, only a strangury.)

Great prostration followed this attack.

Frequent urination, worse after getting into bed.

Pressure as from congestion about kidneys.

Male Sexual Organs–

Sexual desire lost in man.

Testes relaxed, impotent feeling.

Unnatural or disgusting, lewd dreams on several nights, or several times in one night.

Female Sexual Organs–

Menses dark green one day.

Pain darting upward in region of left ovary when sitting, walking or standing.

Second day of menses a violent sick headache, pulsating pressure outward in forehead as if bursting, vomiting (pain relieved by hot water application).

After cessation of menstruation for six months it reappeared again, violent, profuse, without pain but prostrating, the flow lasting several days.

Three or four days before menstruation, felt from waist down as if bursting with distention and weight in abdomen, and wanted to hold herself up, relieved by the flow. Mental condition upset, she would like to kill somebody (three years ago she proved Uranium nitrate. Up to that time had never missed a regular menstruation, but irregular ever since).

Flushes of heat; better afternoons and evenings.

Air Passages–

Cough caused by palpitation during evening.

In morning after rising and before eating, a cough caused by irritation in larynx, accompanied a pain in right side just above the crest of ilium, eating relieved cough, but side felt bruised when bending, jarring or pressing it.

In less than a week a cough with tearing sensation in bronchi, hoarseness, palpitation.

Phlegm of greenish hue causing cough in crawling up.

On rising in morning expectoration of considerable white mucus.

Much expectoration of tough mucus as large as fingers' ends, whitish like gelatine, raised easily.

Raising of jelly-like mucus, worse in forenoon, tenacious and tough.

Grayish expectoration.

In two cases of gonorrhea, obstinate in character, deficient in symptoms, on which to make an accurate prescription, due, probably, to the deep sycotic diathesis, the X-ray not only developed all the acute symptoms of original attack but revealed the remedy (Merc. cor.) which promptly and permanently cured the disease and an old catarrhal deafness as well.

In two other cases, which had resisted the best of treatment for months, the remedy developed numerous sycotic excrescences on glans and the symptoms calling for the similimum were sharply indicated, and it cured permanently. The physical and mental incubus, which for months had made one patient's life a burden, was immediately removed on the reappearance of the condylomata, which had followed suppression by injections and were subsequently disbursed by cauterization.

Chest—Wandering sticking pains in chest, worse on right side.

Stitching pain in right upper chest going through to upper part of scapula.

Sense of contraction across middle chest.

Contraction of chest at night relieved by belching.

Left chest bulged out like enlargement of heart (old symptom of inflammatory rheumatism twenty-five years ago).

Sensation of drops of water trickling down on inside of chest.

Sensation in left side as if fingers pressed costal cartilages in, followed by sensation as if something broke inside, with temporary relief.

HEART.—Palpitation during evening causing cough.

Pulsations greatly diffused and violent, provoking an exclamation, which was suppressed, accompanied with a desire to walk in open air, and entirely relieved by lying down.

Sharp pain at apex of heart, better by lying on left side.

Palpitation with a cough with tearing sensation in bronchi and hoarseness.

Painful bulging of left chest over cardiac region (old symptom of inflammatory rheumatism twenty-five years ago).

Heart's sounds keep him awake while lying on left side.

Dull and constant soreness around heart, and worse in legs and arms.

Wind around heart; flatus and flatulence as though diarrhea would begin.

Back—

Awakened earlier than usual by dull aching in left occiput, and immediately in left sacro-iliac region, then posterior thigh and calf for fifteen minutes.

Pain in dorsal region.

Lame and stiff in back.

Aching whole length of spine.

After waking at daybreak next morning, sensations in dorsal region of spine as if its convexity were interior and drawn far forward, lasting but a minute, and followed by a very uncomfortable feeling in that region, lasting a much longer time.

Sore feeling across loins as after a heavy cold.

Sensation as if a cool drop of sweat going down left side of spine.

Soreness in small of back.

A paralytic sensation extending from spine down left leg.

Rheumatic-like fever in trunk, steady dull pain going

steadily from trunk to legs, and finally to heels, worse in left knee, worse stepping on heel, on underside of heel (old symptom of inflammatory rheumatism twenty-five years ago).

Pressure in small of back as from congestion about kidney.

Upper Extremities—

Magnetic thrill in right hand, extending up forearm.

Tingling in both arms as of electric current, or as if asleep.

Intermittent, slightly burning, rheumatic-like pain in right carpo-metacarpal articulation, extending from index finger up outside of right forearm.

Rheumatic pain in left wrist and forearm.

Rheumatic twinge in last two phalangeal articulations of index and middle fingers for a short time in forenoon.

Grating heard in shoulder joints, as well as nearly all other joints of the body.

Aching extensor muscles of right forearm going up to shoulder.

Rheumatic pain in right wrist and arm.

Tingling like pins and needles in left hand.

Tingling in right hand.

Can't hold things in left hand, powerless or clumsy.

Palms of hands, which were rough and scaly and bleeding at times, became smooth and natural during the proving. Healing action. (Afterward they went back to former state when general health improved.)

Lower Extremities—

Lower part of both legs asleep, tingling, as if from electric battery more in right, immediately.

Sciatic pain in right hip.

Rheumatic pains in limbs.

Dull aching posterior aspect of thigh and calf in morning, from above downward.

Pain in right sciatic nerve on walking.

Rheumatic pains in front of right thigh.

Drawing aching discomfort in right thigh through hip and knees down through toes, immediately.

Feeling as if somebody were drawing icy hands over thigh downward, aggravatingly slow. (This occurred first twelve years ago after a nervous shock and did not return for five years.)

Varicose veins inside of knees and legs, with swelling and soreness (returned after years).

Had always heat and swelling of feet in spring, which is better now, although it is spring. Healing action.

On inside of left knee sensation in different spots painful as if hairs were being pulled, worse walking, better rubbing or scratching.

Rheumatic-like fever in trunk, steady dull pain going steadily down to legs and finally to heels, worse in left knee, worse stepping on heel, on underside of heel (old symptoms of inflammatory rheumatism twenty-five years ago).

Fever—

Chills as soon as beginning to sleep, running up back, preventing sleep.

Chilly whilst undressing in warm room.

Chilliness on moving or from draft.

Chill going down back, followed by paralytic feeling in right cheek.

Wave-like sensation as if it would break out in perspiration.

Profuse perspiration on getting into bed, keeping him awake.

Spells of feverishness, perspiration and weakness.

Sleep—

Kept awake by heart's sound while lying on left side.

Sleepy with headache.

Only snatches of sleep during these twelve days, always followed by mental depression, during suffering from nephralgia.

As soon as she begins to sleep, chills running up back preventing sleep.

Sleepy, but unable to sleep for some hours after retiring.

Sleeplessness constant and troublesome (relieved permanently by a bottle of Pabst Malt Extract).

Drowsy all night while sitting up.

Drowsiness leaves the instant when lying down, so cannot sleep.

Goes to sleep on right side, but wakes on left side.

Symptoms worse when getting into bed, worse after sunset.

Profuse perspiration on getting into bed, keeping him awake.

Sleepy during day.

Waking frequently at night from no apparent cause.

All symptoms worse in bed.

Frequent urination, worse after getting in bed.

(Symptoms better after Bell, or Aeon, for a short time; better from ale, which puts him to sleep.)

Dreams of distressing nature.

Sleep not unrefreshing, though apparently dreaming all night.

Awaking with a headache lasting all day.

Recurrence of a dream which used to trouble her many years ago. (This dream was repeated at wide intervals over twenty years ago; now it came every night for five times.)

Dreams of strife, busy dreams.

Very vivid lewd dreams, repeated night after night.

Unnatural lewd and disgusting dreams, occurring on several nights and several times in one night.

General Symptoms—

General tired and sick feeling.

Persistent exhaustion and languor, not attributable to spring.

Lame and sore all over.

Trembling all over.

SKIN.—Reappearance of an old, slight, pimply eruption on left side of forehead.

Return of a slight eruption on outside of lower legs, burning when scratched, worse after scratching.

August 28, I took a dose of a few globules of X-ray 45m. for some urinary trouble, which ameliorated without being removed. September 13 I felt a stinging and smarting on a place behind the left hip joint while sitting at the dinner table. In the course of the afternoon this symptom disappeared and reappeared on the right side, precisely corresponding to the place on the left side. Toward evening it burned like fire, and, on examination, a place as large as a silver dollar on the right buttock was red and tough as if the skin were abraded. On going to bed a blister as large as a hickory nut, not unlike a fish bladder, was present, from which smaller blisters extended down in a curve. The redness and roughness was enlarged to about three inches in diameter. On being quiet there was no pain, but on the least motion or friction, the part burned like fire, or a severe burn. In the night the blister opened, and another had come opposite to the first, as large as a chestnut. The pains on motion, touch, or friction, continued like a real burn. The skin was red, rough and inflamed, like raw meat, for four inches down, with small blisters of different size extending downward. The large blister discharged gradually, and a scab formed, which, under cessation of pain, fell off, so that by the end of September the skin was as sound as before.

This reminds me of a similar experience observed from repeated action of the X-rays upon the skin, resulting in a denudation of the tibia for the space of about six inches, as far as the leg was exposed to the rays, because it would not heal from an ulcer consequent upon an injury.

"On the red erythematous surface elevations begin to appear, of different sizes and which may be acuminate or papular. In the early stage they are barely visible, and resemble ordinary congestion papules. If, however, their surface is scratched with a needle, a yellow serous slightly opaque fluid exudes and the papule disappears. These elevations, though of small size, are in reality vesicles. They occur in groups or disseminated over the surface, and ultimately develop into vesico-bulle, or vesico-pustules which have the appearance of an ordinary eruption."

"In a weeping eczema the exudation disappears after one to four exposures, and does not return."

"In pruriginous eczema the itching often ceases after a single application."

"On dry eczema the effect of the rays is most marked." A single application is frequently sufficient. "It is in the more obstinate, chronic, and recurring types that they are the most useful."

To quote now from Dright Hall-Edwards:

"The disease generally makes its first appearance in the form of a mild erythema around the roots of the nails. The nails begin to thicken and their substance to degenerate, until they become shapeless masses. The skin becomes uniformly red, and later small warty growths appearight These gradually increase in size and number, whilst the skin generally becomes dry and wrinkled. At this stage, apart from the disfigurement, the patient suffers no inconvenience. The warty growths continue to increase in size, and the skin loses its elasticity to such an extent that it cracks with the slightest exertion. These cracks are very painful and difficult to heal. Pain of an almost indescribable character, which appears to come from the bones, and which is aggravated by holding thehands downwards, is felt. Loss of power in the arm muscles is also experienced. At this stage the skin between the warty growths exhibits marked telangiectasis, is considerably thickened, and is tied down to the subjacent tissues. There is an ever-present sensation of burning and extreme itching, so that it requires no small amount of self-control to keep from scratching. The bases of some of the larger warts become inflamed, and the thickened mass may come away, leaving an ulcer which takes months to heal. These ulcers are so tender and painful that words fail to convey any idea of the suffering of the patient. They occasionally refuse to heal, become gradually larger, and may assume malignant characteristics, which demand operative interference."

Dr. J. T. Pitkin, in a paper read before the "American Roentgen Ray Society," in 1903, thus graphically describes the sufferings of this terrible disease:

"For a description of the pain and suffering, hyperesthesia and paresthesia, no language, sacred or profane, is adequate. The sting of the honey bee or the passage of a renal calculus is painful enough, but they are comparative pleasure; being paroxysmal, they have a time limitation. Extreme tenderness to the slightest touch, hot and cold waves and flashes, warmth, tingling, pricking, throbbing, stinging, crawling, boring, and horning sensations, as if the parts were on fire and contained bugs and other living things; feelings as if the anatomical structures were being removed from one position to another; all of these sensations are proportionate to the depth of the inflammatory process."

GENERAL SYMPTOMS.—General tired and sick feeling.

Persistent exhaustion and languor, not attributable to spring.

Lame and sore all over.

Trembling all over.

Body tired and exhausted.

Nervous powerlessness in limbs.

Sensation of swooning at times during day and night, feeling like dying.

Prostrated for a long time.

All symptoms worse in bed.

All symptoms worse toward evening and at night.

Mental and physical aggravation markedly pronounced toward evening.

Symptoms intermittent in character, the first observed symptoms have all returned at irregular intervals.

Muscles feel soft objectively.

Generally worse in open air.

Twitching internally in various parts.

Symptoms gradually increasing in severity after noon.

For many years have removed the sensitiveness of nervous persons in electric storms with electricity cm.

Case of Dr. John B. Campbell. A patient for three years has gout, which is the summing up of a history of suppressed chills. He got X-ray 30th cent., which seems to have helped him somewhat. Swelling of legs and knees disappeared, after being present for weeks. Some of the pains were better. 1897, March 29, 2:30 P.M., took X-ray 30 cent., one powder; at 5 P.M., the second—no symptom—at 1 P.M. the third, which produced little itching. At 10 P.M. took a hot bath with some improvement, and 11 P.M. the fourth powder, all of the 30 cent.

After that decided glow of heat all over body with some itching.

Little rash on both legs, with decided pricking on both legs from knees to toes.

Pain in region of spleen for one hour which passed away in bed, during which time no twitching or jerking of muscles, could stretch out both legs comfortably.

Very good night's sleep.

March 30th, 7 A.M., slight perspiration on legs from knees to toes.

March 31st, took the remaining powder of same potency.

Some itching on left shoulder blade and arm from shoulder to elbow, with considerable increase of pain in elbows and hands, and sensation of heat all over body, but no fever.

Stiffness of back and neck, necessitating moving of whole body to turn his head.

Slight rash on left leg above knee.

Some itching of arms and chest in bed, especially when beginning to get warm.

Could walk a little better the first two days after taking medicine.

More thirst than usual.

Had no chill since 21st, until today, when he had a slight chill from 2 to 4 P.M.; no fever thirst or sweat.

Appetite and bowels extremely good.

Some itching or prickling pains above knees.

The swelling from legs and feet has gone down immensely, though pain does not abate.

Relations—

Compare: the Calcareas, Caust., Hepar, Med., Nat. mur., Psor., Puls., Sili., Sulph., Thuja, Tub., for its power to reproduce old or suppressed symptoms and conditions; Act., Lil., Lac can., Plat., Sep., Pyr., for nervous reflexes and neuralgic conditions from ovarian or uterine irritation; Agaright, Curight, Tar., Zinc., for irritation of the cord, spinal reflexes, neurasthenia; electric storms, thunder storms, Agar., Med., Nat. c., Phos., Psoright, Rhod., Sep., Sil., Syph., Thuja.

Antidotes—

Nux, Sulph. and the dynamic potencies of the remedy.

Aggravation—

In bed; towards evening and at night (both mental and physical); in the open air; in the afternoon.

"Six years ago I received a severe X-ray burn on my left hand and fingeright Eighteen months afterwards warts appeared—one seedy old chap, near knuckle of left index finger, second joint, gave me much concern. Various remedies were tried. Five months ago it became exceedingly annoying to me, and then I looked up the Materia Medica carefully, and there, sure enough, was the remedy. I took Causticum 200, and one dose, after awhile, of the cm. I am usually a high potency man. The result was a cure. Then I recalled the article of Dr. W. P. Wesselhoeft, in October issue, 1906, *Medical Advance,* under 'Reminiscences,' and had I remembered it I could have been cured of the unsightly warts long before. Some day I may write up the case for the *Medical Advance.* It may help out some one suffering from these X-ray warts, so common from X rays." Sgd. *J. W. King, M. D.*

Kienbock lays down this axiom: "The stronger the dose given at a seance, the shorter the period of latency, the sharper the reaction, and the longer its duration."

" The first degree of intensity is characterized by hyperemia and infiltration of the skin, accompanied by exfoliation of minute scales and a considerable amount of itching. Atrophy of the appendages of the skin—glands, hair and nails—may follow.

"The second degree of dermatitis is characterized by the occurrence of vesiculation and phlyctenule. Inflammatory signs are severe, the tension considerable and the pain intense. Under the phlyctenule the bares chorion appears red and discharging.

"The third degree is characterized by total destruction and sloughing of the irradiated tissues. These show the usual signs of dry gangrene; the sloughs separate slowly, leaving behind an ulcer of a very torpid nature, which sometimes remains unhealed for years.

"In radiotherapy one should endeavor to irradiate the tissue with the exact quantity necessary to produce a definite result. In the use of other therapeutic agents we are often obliged to vary the dose. A given drug may have a tonic action in a small dose, an emetic action in a moderate dose, and a poisonous action in a large dose. The same may be said of X-rays. Take, for example, their action on the scalp. In mall fractional doses they have a stimulating effect on the hair, whereas in large doses they cause epilation, and in still larger doses vesiculation, ulceration, and sloughing."

Scalp—

"At first sight it may seem contradictionary that the same agent will, in one case, cause the hair to fall out, and in another case favour its growth. The contradiction, however, is only apparent, as the results depend on the amount of rays absorbed by the hair papilla and the consequent inflammatory reaction. It is evident that if this factor is varied the results will be altered.